Handbook of Radiosurgery in CNS Disease

Handbook of Radiosurgery in CNS Disease

EDITORS

Michael Lim, MD
Wesley Hsu, MD
Daniele Rigamonti, MD
Lawrence R. Kleinberg, MD

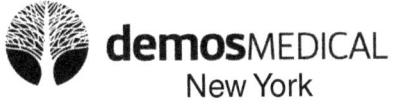

New York

Visit our website at www.demosmedpub.com
ISBN: 9781936287444
e-book ISBN: 9781617050893

Acquisitions Editor: Rich Winters
Compositor: Newgen Imaging

© 2013 Demos Medical Publishing, LLC. All rights reserved. This book is protected by copyright. No part of it may be reproduced, stored in a retrieval system, or transmitted in any form or by any means, electronic, mechanical, photocopying, recording, or otherwise, without the prior written permission of the publisher.

Medicine is an ever-changing science. Research and clinical experience are continually expanding our knowledge, in particular our understanding of proper treatment and drug therapy. The authors, editors, and publisher have made every effort to ensure that all information in this book is in accordance with the state of knowledge at the time of production of the book. Nevertheless, the authors, editors, and publisher are not responsible for errors or omissions or for any consequences from application of the information in this book and make no warranty, express or implied, with respect to the contents of the publication. Every reader should examine carefully the package inserts accompanying each drug and should carefully check whether the dosage schedules mentioned therein or the contraindications stated by the manufacturer differ from the statements made in this book. Such examination is particularly important with drugs that are either rarely used or have been newly released on the market.

Library of Congress Cataloging-in-Publication Data
Handbook of radiosurgery in CNS disease / Michael Lim ... [et al.], editors.
   p. ; cm.
 Includes bibliographical references and index.
 ISBN 978-1-936287-44-4—ISBN 978-1-61705-089-3 (e-ISBN)
 I. Lim, Michael
 [DNLM: 1. Central Nervous System Diseases—surgery. 2. Radiosurgery—methods. WL 301]

  617.4′8—dc23

                                                  2013001000

Special discounts on bulk quantities of Demos Medical Publishing books are available to corporations, professional associations, pharmaceutical companies, health care organizations, and other qualifying groups. For details, please contact:

Special Sales Department
Demos Medical Publishing, LLC
11 West 42nd Street, 15th Floor
New York, NY 10036
Phone: 800–532-8663 or 212–683-0072
Fax: 212–941-7842
E-mail: specialsales@demosmedpub.com

Printed in the United States of America by Courier Digital Solutions.

13 14 15 16 17 / 5 4 3 2 1

Contents

Preface   ix
Contributors   xi

SECTION I: RADIOBIOLOGY   1
(Section Editor—Lawrence R. Kleinberg)

1. **The Fundamentals of Radiosurgical Radiobiology**   3
   Chun Po Yen, David Schlesinger, and Jason Sheehan

SECTION II: TECHNOLOGY AND TECHNIQUES OF RADIOSURGERY   11
(Section Editor—Lawrence R. Kleinberg)

2. **Technology and Techniques of Cranial Radiosurgery**   13
   Jacob Ruzevick and Michael Lim

3. **Technology and Techniques for Spinal Radiosurgery**   27
   Maziyar A. Kalani and Stephen Ryu

SECTION III: RADIOSURGERY FOR BRAIN TUMORS   33
(Section Editors—Jacob Ruzevick and Michael Lim)

4. **Intraparenchymal Tumors**   35
   A. **Radiosurgery for Primary Brain Tumors**   35
      Andy Trang, Marko Spasic, Winward Choy, and Isaac Yang

   B. **Radiosurgery for Brain Metastases**   45
      Lawrence R. Kleinberg

5. **Skull-Base Tumors**   59
   A. **Radiosurgery for Skull-Base Meningioma**   59
      Mario Moreno, Timothy Bui, and Gordon Li

B. Role of Radiosurgery for Hemangiopericytomas   67
   Bowen Jiang, Anand Veeravagu, and Steven D. Chang

   C. Stereotactic Radiosurgery for Glomus Jugulare Tumors   77
   Zachary D. Guss, Anubhav G. Amin, and Michael Lim

   D. Radiosurgery for Vestibular Schwannomas   83
   Jacob Ruzevick, Michael Lim, and Daniele Rigamonti

   E. Stereotactic Fractionated Radiation Therapy for Optic Nerve Sheath Meningiomas   93
   Neil R. Miller

   F. Role of Radiosurgery for Sellar Lesions   103
   Bowen Jiang, Wendy Hara, and Gordon Li

6. Imaging Changes Following Radiosurgery for Metastatic Intracranial Tumors: A Review of Differentiating Radiation Effects From Tumor Recurrence   111
   Jacob Ruzevick and Lawrence R. Kleinberg

SECTION IV: RADIOSURGERY FOR INTRACRANIAL VASCULAR LESIONS   121
(Section Editor—Daniele Rigamonti)

7. Radiosurgery for Arteriovenous Malformations   123
   Jacob Ruzevick, Sachin Batra, Michael Lim, and Daniele Rigamonti

8. Role of Radiosurgery for Dural Arteriovenous Fistula   137
   Omar Choudhri and Raphael Guzman

9. The Role of Radiosurgery for the Treatment of Cerebral Cavernous Malformations   147
   Peter A. Gooderham and Gary K. Steinberg

SECTION V: RADIOSURGERY FOR FUNCTIONAL DISEASES   153
(Section Editor—Lawrence R. Kleinberg)

10. Role of Radiosurgery for Trigeminal Neuralgia   155
    Alessandra Gorgulho and Antonio A. F. De Salles

11. Radiosurgery for Drug-Resistant Epilepsies:
    State of the Art, Results, and Perspectives   161
    *Jean Régis, Romain Caron, Fabrice Bartolomei,
    and Patrick Chauvel*

SECTION VI: RADIOSURGERY FOR SPINE LESIONS   181
(Section Editor—Wesley Hsu)

12. Tumors of the Osseous Spine   183
    A. Stereotactic Radiosurgery for Primary Osseous
    Spinal Tumors   183
    Joseph A. Lin, Mohamad Bydon, Mohamed Macki, and Ali Bydon

    B. Stereotactic Radiosurgery for Metastatic Spine Tumors   195
    Wesley Hsu

13. Radiotherapy and Radiosurgery in the Management of
    Intramedullary Spinal Cord Tumors   203
    Mari Groves and George Jallo

14. Radiotherapy and Radiosurgery in the Management of Sacral
    Tumors   213
    Mari Groves, Patricia Zadnik, and Daniel Sciubba

15. Radiosurgery of Vascular Disorders   221
    Samuel Ryu

16. Complications and Dose Selection of Radiosurgery for Spine
    Lesions   225
    Edward A. Monaco III and Peter C. Gerszten

Index   237

Preface

In recent years, there has been increasing appreciation of the value of radiosurgery for many central nervous system indications, improving outcome and reducing risks. This has been possible because the technology for imaging and delivering treatment has improved greatly. It is now routinely possible to image small abnormalities with high resolution and precision, robust noninvasive immobilization techniques have been validated, and image guided treatment technologies can now be used in the treatment of spinal disease with great precision. In addition, the increasingly rapid diffusion of these technologies, beyond the few specialty centers that pioneered radiosurgery, has enabled the accumulation of supporting data.

When Lars Leksell first developed the Gamma Knife stereotactic treatment system, invasive immobilization was ingeniously utilized to solve the problem of precisely relating imaging to treatment targeting. Reference points created by the frame system, visualized on imaging and well localized on the treatment machine allowed correlation between imaging abnormalities and treatment targeting. Initially, the indications were limited as modern three-dimensional imaging was not yet available and primarily included vascular abnormalities such as AVM visualized by angiography. Later, CT scanning and MRI scanning, which could be performed in the frame, expanded the indications to many other diseases such as meningioma and brain metastasis.

The frame-based Gamma Knife system provided highly accurate treatment, but also had the limitation that all imaging and treatment must be performed with the same frame placement. Frame based systems were also developed using standard radiotherapy linear accelerators modified to provide high precision and stability in aim. These systems were confined to indications where all needed imaging could reasonably be obtained, treatment planned, and radiation delivered, all in a single-frame placement. This was, in addition, not suited to treatment given over more than one day or outside the brain.

While frame-based systems remain quite useful, systems using non-invasive custom immobilization head masks have allowed stereotactic precision treatment to be administered with more comfort and with easy use of fractionation. Fractionation can increase safety to normal tissues. This approach has allowed this technology to be applied to lesions larger than those generally considered safe to treat with single dose therapy (> 3 cm) or in close proximity to critical sensitive structures, including the optic nerve and brainstem. Research continues into optimizing dose selection using fractionation, and it is still not clear if this is appropriate for certain benign or vascular abnormalities such as arteriovenous malformation.

The need for invasive frame immobilization had confined this treatment approach to intracranial lesions. With noninvasive body immobilization and image-guided targeting, treatment of spinal cord and vertebral column lesions is now possible. These image-guided technologies may include linear accelerators with built in CT scanners to verify positioning, placement of fiducials that may be detected using x-ray imaging on the linear accelerator, or robotic image-guided therapy which has the potential advantage of repeated imaging to adjust for any motion. Breath hold or respiratory cycle gating of therapy may be utilized under some circumstances. Spinal indications include primary intramedullary lesions such as AVM or metastasis, epidural disease, meningioma, and vertebral metastasis. This approach is routinely utilized to intensify treatment, and ongoing trials will provide information to further guide patient selection and the treatment parameters.

In this textbook, the current data related to the expanding uses of CNS radiosurgery is reviewed. The major recent developments have been: (1) the use of radiosurgery without whole brain radiotherapy to improve outcome and reduce toxicity for patients with multiple brain metastasis; (2) greater data demonstrating that radiosurgery is an appropriate choice for benign lesions such as vestibular scwhannoma, and meningioma, balancing risks of surgery against limitations of radiosurgery treatment; (3) radiosurgery for spinal metastasis, with or without epidural disease; (4) approaches to therapy of larger lesions, especially arteriovenous malformation; and (5) an increased understanding that the effects of radiosurgery on MRI imaging can mimic progression. In addition, techniques for treatment for other indications have continued to evolve with accumulation of more relevant data and improvements in technology.

Michael Lim
Wesley Hsu
Daniele Rigamonti
Lawrence R. Kleinberg

Contributors

Anubhav G. Amin, MD
Department of Neurosurgery, Johns Hopkins Hospital, Baltimore, Maryland

Fabrice Bartolomei, MD, PhD
Service de Neurophysiologie Clinique, Universite de la Mediterranee, Marseille, France

Sachin Batra, MD, MPH
Department of Neurological Surgery, Johns Hopkins University School of Medicine, Baltimore, Maryland

Timothy Bui, BA
Department of Neurosurgery, Stanford University School of Medicine, Stanford, California

Ali Bydon, MD
Department of Neurosurgery, Johns Hopkins University School of Medicine, Baltimore, Maryland

Mohamad Bydon, MD
Department of Neurosurgery, Johns Hopkins Hospital, Baltimore, Maryland

Romain Caron, MD
Department of Stereotactic and Functional Neurosurgery, Timone University Hospital, A.P.M., Marseille, France

Steven D. Chang, MD
Department of Neurosurgery, Stanford University School of Medicine, Stanford, California

Patrick Chauvel, MD
Department of Stereotactic and Functional Neurosurgery, Timone University Hospital, A.P.M., Marseille, France

Omar Choudhri, MD
Stanford University School of Medicine, Stanford, California

Winward Choy, BA
Department of Neurological Surgery, University of California, Los Angeles, California

Antonio A. F. De Salles, MD, PhD
Departments of Neurosurgery and Radiation Oncology, Head of Stereotactic Surgery Section, University of California at Los Angeles, Los Angeles, California

Peter C. Gerszten, MD, MPH, FACS
Neurological Surgery and Radiation Oncology, University of Pittsburgh Medical Center, Pittsburgh, Pennsylvania

Peter A. Gooderham, MD
Division of Neurosurgery, Department of Surgery, University of British Columbia, Vancouver, British Columbia, Canada

Alessandra Gorgulho, MD, MSc
Stereotactic Section, University of California at Los Angeles, Los Angeles, California

Mari Groves, MD
Department of Neurosurgery, Johns Hopkins Hospital, Baltimore, Maryland

Zachary D. Guss, BA
Johns Hopkins University School of Medicine, Baltimore, Maryland

Raphael Guzman, MD
Division of Pediatric Neurosurgery, Lucile Packard Children's Hospital, Stanford University School of Medicine, Stanford, California

Wendy Hara, MD
Department of Radiation Oncology, Stanford University Medical Center, Stanford, California

Wesley Hsu, MD
Department of Neurosurgery, Wake Forest Baptist Medical Center, Winston-Salem, North Carolina

George Jallo, MD
Division of Pediatric Neurosurgery, The Johns Hopkins Hospital, Baltimore, Maryland

Bowen Jiang, BS
Department of Neurosurgery, Stanford School of Medicine, Stanford, California

Maziyar A. Kalani, MD
Department of Neurosurgery, Stanford Hospital and Clinics, Stanford, California

Lawrence R. Kleinberg, MD
Department of Radiation Oncology, Johns Hopkins University School of Medicine, Baltimore, Maryland

Gordon Li, MD
Department of Neurosurgery, Stanford University School of Medicine, Stanford, California

Michael Lim, MD
Department of Neurosurgery, Johns Hopkins University School of Medicine, Baltimore, Maryland

Joseph A. Lin, BA
Department of Neuroscience, Spinal Outcomes Laboratory, The Johns Hopkins Hospital, Baltimore, Maryland

Mohamed Macki, BA
Department of Neurosurgery, Johns Hopkins University School of Medicine, Baltimore, Maryland

Neil R. Miller, MD, FACS
Department of Ophthalmology, Johns Hopkins Hospital, Baltimore, Maryland

Edward A. Monaco III, MD, PhD
Department of Neurological Surgery, University of Pittsburgh Medical Center, Pittsburgh, Pennsylvania

Mario Moreno, BA
Department of Neurosurgery, Stanford University School of Medicine, Stanford, California

Jean Régis, MD
Department of Stereotactic and Functional Neurosurgery, Timone University Hospital, A.P.M., Marseille, France

Daniele Rigamonti, MD
Department of Neurosurgery, Johns Hopkins University School of Medicine, Baltimore, Maryland

Jacob Ruzevick, BS
Department of Neurological Surgery, Johns Hopkins University School of Medicine, Baltimore, Maryland

Samuel Ryu, MD
Department of Radiation Oncology and Neurosurgery, Henry Ford Health System, Detroit, Michigan

Stephen Ryu, MD
Department of Neurosurgery, Palo Alto Medical Foundation, Palo Alto, and Department of Electrical Engineering, Stanford University, Stanford, California

David Schlesinger, PhD
Department of Neurological Surgery, University of Virginia, Charlottesville, Virginia

Daniel Sciubba, MD
Department of Neurosurgery, Johns Hopkins Hospital, Baltimore, Maryland

Jason Sheehan, MD, PhD
Department of Neurological Surgery, University of Virginia, Charlottesville, Virginia

Marko Spasic, BA
Department of Neurosurgery, David Geffen School of Medicine at UCLA, University of California at Los Angeles, Los Angeles, California

Gary K. Steinberg, MD, PhD
Department of Neurosurgery, Stanford University School of Medicine, Stanford, California

Andy Trang, BS
University of California at Los Angeles, Department of Neurosurgery, Los Angeles, California

Anand Veeravagu, MD
Department of Neurosurgery, Stanford University School of Medicine, Stanford, California

Isaac Yang, MD
Department of Neurosurgery, David Geffen School of Medicine at UCLA, UCLA Jonsson Comprehensive Cancer Center, University of California at Los Angeles, Los Angeles, California

Chun Po Yen, MD
Department of Neurological Surgery, University of Virginia, Charlottesville, Virginia

Patricia Zadnik, BA
Department of Neurosurgery, Johns Hopkins University School of Medicine, Baltimore, Maryland

Section I

Radiobiology

Section Editor

Lawrence R. Kleinberg

Chapter 1

The Fundamentals of Radiosurgical Radiobiology

Chun Po Yen, David Schlesinger, & Jason Sheehan

Radiosurgery originally denoted the destruction of intracranial targets or induction of desired biological effects in target tissue through the use of a single, high dose of focused ionizing beams through the intact skull. The concept of radiosurgery has, however, been expanded to include one to five fraction treatments and now involves targeting of the spine as well. The radiobiology of radiosurgery appears distinctly different from that of fractionated radiation therapy, and the clinical effectiveness of radiosurgery is not fully explained by traditional radiobiology. This chapter covers basic concepts of medical physics and radiobiology for stereotactic radiosurgery.

TYPES OF IONIZING RADIATION

Ionizing radiation refers to radiation that has sufficiently high energy to dislodge electrons from the atoms or disrupt the bonds between the atoms or molecules. Two radiation sources are used in radiation treatment—artificially produced radiation from machines and spontaneously generated radiation from radionuclides. Two basic forms of radiation are produced from the aforementioned sources, including electromagnetic radiation and particle radiation.

Electromagnetic Radiation

Electromagnetic radiation carries energy via oscillating electric and magnetic fields. The electromagnetic spectrum spans a range from infrared waves, through the visible light spectrum, to high-energy x-rays and gamma rays. It is the high-energy x-rays and gamma rays that are commonly used in radiation therapy and radiosurgery. Such high-energy waves exhibit a dual nature; they can be described as waves, and they can also be described in terms of small packets of energy called photons.

X-rays are produced either as a result of the interaction between a high-speed electron and a nucleus (*bremsstrahlung x-rays*) or when electrons in the outer shell of an ionized atom fall from a high to a low energy level to fill a vacancy created by an electron that has been ejected (*characteristic x-rays*). X-rays may be the product of radioactive decay or created by human intervention. For example, linear accelerators generate x-rays by accelerating electrons and directing them to strike a target comprising a substance with a high atomic number (1). Gamma rays are photons from the nucleus of a radioactive atom when it decays from an excited to a more stable state. An example is Cobalt-60 (^{60}Co), a common gamma-ray source used in stereotactic radiosurgery.

High-energy photons are indirectly ionizing. When interacting with tissue, photons cause the liberation of charged particles (electrons), which then go on to cause the majority of the ionization and, thus, the biological effects. High-energy photons exhibit a property called the "buildup region" when they enter tissue. This occurs because the electrons near the skin surface are scattered in a mostly forward direction and deposit their energy deeper in the tissue. This gives photons an advantage known as the "skin-sparing" effect (Figure 1.1).

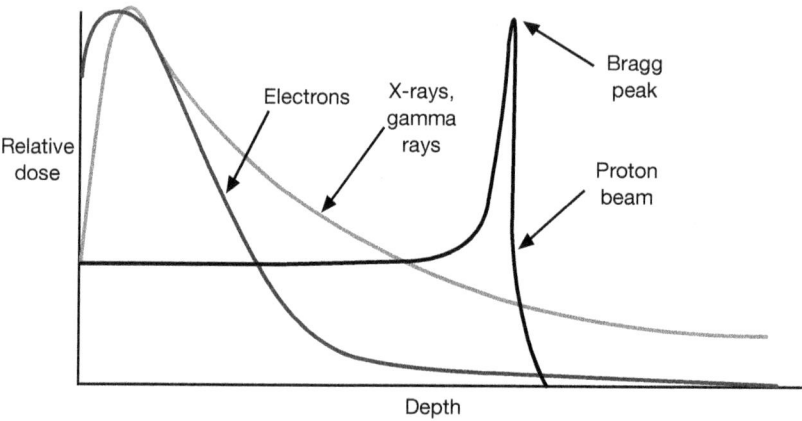

FIGURE 1.1 A relative comparison of the radiation deposition using photon beams, electron beams, and proton beams. Notice that photon beams have a "buildup region" that provides a measure of skin sparing at the surface of the patient. Electron beams exhibit less skin sparing and a sharper dose falloff. Proton beams deposit most of their dose at the end of their range, a phenomena known as a "Bragg peak." Photons also have a maximum dose range in tissue.

Particle Radiation

Particle radiation differs from photon radiation in that the energy of the radiation propagates as the kinetic energy of the particle itself. High-energy, charged particles such as electrons and protons are directly ionizing forms of radiation. They have sufficient kinetic energy to ionize atoms as they interact with tissue. Unlike high-energy photons, which tend to sparsely interact with matter and can travel long distances before being absorbed, high-energy particles tend to have predictable ranges of penetration in tissue. The particles used most frequently for therapeutic purposes are electrons and protons. There are a few centers that employ heavy ions and attempts have also been made to use neutrons.

High-energy electrons are usually produced in linear accelerators by replacing the target used for x-ray production. Electrons begin depositing an appreciable dose near the surface of tissue, have a predictable range where they deposit the majority of their energy, and exhibit a rapid dose falloff. This gives electron therapy a particular advantage in the treatment of cutaneous or subcutaneous lesions (Figure 1.1).

Proton particles are produced in particle accelerators such as cyclotrons. Protons are much heavier particles than electrons. Therefore, at a particular velocity, protons have much greater kinetic energy and do not scatter as easily. Hence, protons can potentially cause less damage to surrounding tissues. Also, most of the energy absorption from protons occurs at the distal end of the track. The precisely defined area of intense ionization at the end of the track following the passage of protons is called a Bragg peak (Figure 1.1). Protons have a defined range in which they are deposited into tissue, so there is little to no exit dose. The beam may be altered to spread the Bragg peak to conform to the thickness and depth of the volume to be treated. Taking advantage of the Bragg peak effect as well as crossfiring of a number of proton beams, a localized volume of high radiation delivery can be produced and has been applied in a radiosurgical setting (2,3).

RADIOCHEMISTRY

Radiation damage at a subcellular level occurs in one of two ways: (a) *direct action* whereby the ionization breakage of the DNA strand is the primary effect; (b) *indirect action* in which the DNA damage is produced by free radicals, which are products of the radiation effect on other molecules, especially water molecules.

Free Radicals

When cells are irradiated with ionizing radiation, photons can interact with water molecules by stripping an electron from a hydrogen atom, resulting in a fast electron and an ionized water molecule. The resulting fast electrons further interact with water molecules through additional ionizing events. The positively charged water molecule exhibits a short half-life before dissociating into an H^+ ion and an OH^- free hydroxyl radical. The hydroxyl radical is reactive and has sufficient energy to break chemical bonds in nearby molecules. This indirect effect of radiation through a free radical intermediary is traditionally believed to be responsible for the majority of radiation-induced damage. The chemical reactions are enhanced by the presence of oxygen. Tissue hypoxia (partial oxygen pressure lower than 30 mmHg) will lessen the production of free radicals and, thereby, lower the damaging effects of radiation.

Radiation Injuries to DNA

Evidence suggests that DNA is the most important target for cellular damage by ionizing radiation. The reactive water derivative may interact with DNA and creates permanent cell injury or death. Radiation can also interact directly with DNA.

Damage to DNA can take the form of single-strand breaks, in which one of the two intertwined helixes is broken or double-strand breaks in which both are broken. Single-strand breaks (the more common form of damage) are potentially fixable by DNA repair enzymes that use the undamaged strand as a template for repair. Double-strand breaks are more difficult if not impossible to repair; these cause the most serious biological damage. Double-strand breaks may be a result of a single particle or the interaction of two single-strand breaks caused by separate particles occurring at close temporal and spatial distances. Studies on synchronously dividing cell cultures have demonstrated that cells in the G2 and M phase of the cell cycle are most susceptible to double-strand DNA breaks.

RADIOBIOLOGY

Radiobiology of Conventional Radiotherapy

Radiation damages the DNA of tumor cells as well as the DNA of normal cells in its path. Normal tissue, however, is generally more capable of DNA repair than tumors. This is in part due to an aberrant cell cycle control mechanism in tumors. Abnormal metabolic patterns may also make tumors more susceptible to increased oxidative stress compared to normal cells.

Cells require time to repair DNA damage, and the normal cell response to irradiation is to delay the cell cycle. Cells are most sensitive to the effects of ionizing radiation when in the M and G2/M interphase. They are least sensitive in the late S phase and demonstrate intermediate sensitivity in the G1 and early S phase. Therefore, the radiobiology of differential cell repair is of paramount importance for conventional radiotherapy. Repair plays a less critical role as the number of fractions decreases.

Cell survival after single doses of radiation is a probability function of absorbed dose, measured in the gray unit (Gy). Typical mammalian cell survival curves obtained after single-dose irradiation in culture have a characteristic shape, including a low-dose shoulder region followed by a steeply sloped portion at higher doses (4,5). The shoulder region is interpreted as accumulation of sublethal damage at low doses with lethality resulting from the interaction of two or more such sublethal events. As previously noted, single-strand breaks in DNA may be repaired and therefore represent sublethal damage to the cell. However, double-strand breaks may result in severe cellular changes and cell death. Such a model can be described by the following probabilistic equation in which probability (cure or complication) = $\exp[-K \times \exp(-\alpha D - \beta D^2)]$ ("exp" represents exponential, K equals the number of clonogens, "α" and "β" are constants that are related to single-event cell killing and cell killing through interaction of sublethal events, respectively, and D represents dose). The α/β ratio is the single dose at which overall cell killing is equally attributable to both components of cell killings ($\alpha D = \beta D^2$ or $D = \alpha/\beta$) (6). The validity of the linear-quadratic formula for single-dose radiosurgery has been questioned (7). Nevertheless, it still is used to provide a meaningful way of relating radiosurgery to fractionated radiation schemes.

The α/β ratio varies depending upon the tumor and normal tissue type (Figure 1.2). Late-responding tissues such as the brain or benign brain tumors have an α/β ratio of approximately 2, whereas many malignant tumors have an α/β ratio of nearly 10. α/β ratios for skin or mucosa are approximately 5 to 8. Tumors with low α/β ratio (i.e., a small alpha or single-hit component for radiation kinetics) will have less of a desired effect when a low radiation dose per fraction scheme is used than when comparable tissues with a high α/β ratio are treated.

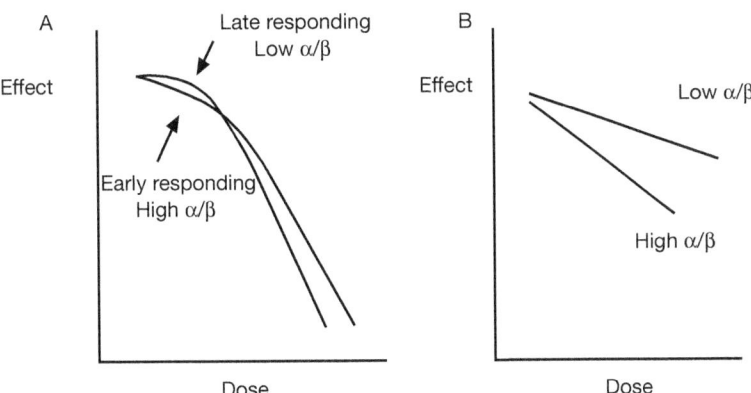

FIGURE 1.2 Comparison of single-dose effect curves *(A)* and fractionated dose effect curves *(B)* for low and high α/β tissue. The small advantage seen in the low-dose region sparing low α/β tissue is amplified through dose fractionation.

Conventional fractionated radiation therapy relies on the four Rs of radiobiology, namely, repair of nonlethal injury, reoxygenation of hypoxic tumor cells, repopulation of tumor cells, and reassortment of tumor cells into more susceptible phases of the cell cycle. Depending upon the clinical scenario, one may prove superior to the other.

The standard approach to radiotherapy includes daily treatments preceded by the dose-delivery simulation, which means approximately positioning the patient in reference to the treatment machine from appropriate beam entrance and exit. The most commonly prescribed fraction of absorbed dose is 1.8 to 2 Gy, which has proved to be well tolerated in most areas of the body and can be repeated a specific number of times, depending on the region involved and the therapeutic target. For practical purposes, the tolerance of the whole brain is considered to be 45 to 50 Gy in 20 to 25 fractions, although it is recognized that this dose may yield substantial side effects manifested by leukoencephalopathy on MRI and seen clinically with dementia and memory loss with time (8,9).

Radiobiology of Radiosurgery

A therapeutic advantage may also be achieved by depositing a much higher radiation dose in the tumor than in the surrounding normal tissue. Radiosurgery achieves this through the use of stereotactic fixation and crossfiring of numerous radiation beams.

A single, low-dose radiation beam entering a patient is directed to the target. The dose progressively increases at the target, where multiple radiation beams are crossfired. In contrast to the radiation buildup region, the surrounding normal nervous tissue is spared from the high doses of radiation. This rapid falloff of radiation dose is the basic principle employed to spare normal tissue in radiosurgery. This approach is in distinct contrast to the addition of margins to a tumor volume in conventional radiotherapy (i.e., an expansion of the gross tumor volume to a larger planned treatment volume). This concept of stereotactic radiosurgery was first described by Lars Leksell in 1951. He believed that radiation could replace the scalpel or an electrode for performing functional neurosurgery. In so doing, the biology of differential repair was discarded, and the main biologic advantage became the ability to destroy focally identified areas and avoid the normal brain by physical means.

Leksell's initial radiosurgery concept was intended for the treatment of functional neurological disorders (10), but it has expanded to become a standard treatment option for benign and malignant central nervous system pathologies. In radiosurgery, the surgeon does not attempt to spare some tissues and treat others but to achieve inactivation or destruction within the targeted volume. Obliteration of vascular supply with accompanying endothelial damage of vessels to the tumors also plays a much more significant role in radiosurgery than radiation therapy. This is illustrated by histopathologic studies of resected tumors and the similar tumor control rates between radiosensitive and radioresistant tumor pathologies after radiosurgery (11–13).

CONCLUSION

Although similar in some ways to fractionated radiation therapy, the principles of radiosurgery and its underlying mechanisms differ substantially. The clinical effectiveness of radiosurgery is not fully explained by the linear-quadratic model. Through refinements in our understanding of the radiobiology of radiosurgery and advances in medical physics, the application of radiosurgery for central nervous system pathologies has expanded, and the safety profile has improved.

REFERENCES

1. Khan FM. *The Physics of Radiation Therapy*. Baltimore, MD: Lippincott, Williams and Wilkins; 2003.
2. Kjellberg RN, Koehler AM, Preston WM, Sweet WH. Stereotaxic instrument for use with the Bragg peak of a proton beam. *Confin Neurol*. 1962;22:183–189.
3. Kjellberg RN, Sweet WH, Preston WM, Koehler AM. The Bragg peak of a proton beam in intracranial therapy of tumors. *Trans Am Neurol Assoc*. 1962;87:216–218.
4. Dale RG. The application of the linear-quadratic dose-effect equation to fractionated and protracted radiotherapy. *Br J Radiol*. 1985;58(690):515–528.
5. Fowler JF. The linear-quadratic formula and progress in fractionated radiotherapy. *Br J Radiol*. 1989;62(740):679–694.
6. Hall EJ, Giaccia A. *Radiobiology for the Radiologist*. Baltimore, MD: Lippincott Williams & Wilkins; 2006.
7. Hall EJ, Brenner DJ. The radiobiology of radiosurgery: rationale for different treatment regimes for AVMs and malignancies. *Int J Radiat Oncol Biol Phys*. 1993;25(2):381–385.
8. Chang EL, Wefel JS, Maor MH, et al. A pilot study of neurocognitive function in patients with one to three new brain metastases initially treated with stereotactic radiosurgery alone. *Neurosurgery*. 2007;60(2):277–83; discussion 283.
9. Lawrence YR, Li XA, el Naqa I, et al. Radiation dose-volume effects in the brain. *Int J Radiat Oncol Biol Phys*. 2010;76(3 suppl):S20–S27.
10. Leksell L. The stereotaxic method and radiosurgery of the brain. *Acta Chir Scand*. 1951;102(4):316–319.
11. Mathieu D, Kondziolka D, Cooper PB, et al. Gamma knife radiosurgery in the management of malignant melanoma brain metastases. *Neurosurgery*. 2007;60(3):471–81; discussion 481.
12. Sheehan JP, Sun MH, Kondziolka D, Flickinger J, Lunsford LD. Radiosurgery in patients with renal cell carcinoma metastasis to the brain: long-term outcomes and prognostic factors influencing survival and local tumor control. *J Neurosurg*. 2003;98(2):342–349.
13. Szeifert GT, Kondziolka D, Atteberry DS, et al. Radiosurgical pathology of brain tumors: metastases, schwannomas, meningiomas, astrocytomas, hemangioblastomas. *Prog Neurol Surg*. 2007;20:91–105.

Section II

Technology and Techniques of Radiosurgery

Section Editor

Lawrence R. Kleinberg

Chapter 2

Technology and Techniques of Cranial Radiosurgery

Jacob Ruzevick & Michael Lim

Fractionated radiation therapy (RT) and stereotactic radiosurgery (SRS) form the mainstay of treatment for primary, recurrent, and metastatic brain tumors and have been used with increasing frequency in patients with vascular and functional disorders, especially when surgery cannot be pursued. Fractionated RT (also known as fractionated SRS) refers to delivering a uniform dose of radiation, albeit to both normal brain tissue as well as the tumor. In contrast, SRS refers to the delivery of multiple beams of radiation, which converge at the site of the intracranial lesion to deliver a high dose of conformal radiation to the lesion while sparing normal brain tissue (Figure 2.1). There are three basic forms of SRS: particle beam (proton), Cobalt-60 (photon), and linear accelerator based (LINAC, photon). Although many differences exist between radiotherapy and SRS, the general strategy of both modalities is similar and is summarized in Table 2.1. In this chapter, we review the technologies used to deliver radiation to intracranial pathologies and include discussions on immobilization, targeting, dosage considerations, complications, and guidelines to consider in preventing complications.

FRACTIONATED RADIATION THERAPY

RT is a common adjuvant treatment for primary, recurrent, and metastatic brain tumors. In fractionated RT, the dose delivered to the tumor bulk usually includes normal brain tissue or critical structures. The efficacy of this treatment relies on the following general principles. These include (a) normal parenchyma's ability to repair DNA damage relative to tumor cells' defective DNA repair machinery; (b) reoxygenation of normally hypoxic, radiation-resistant tumor cells; and

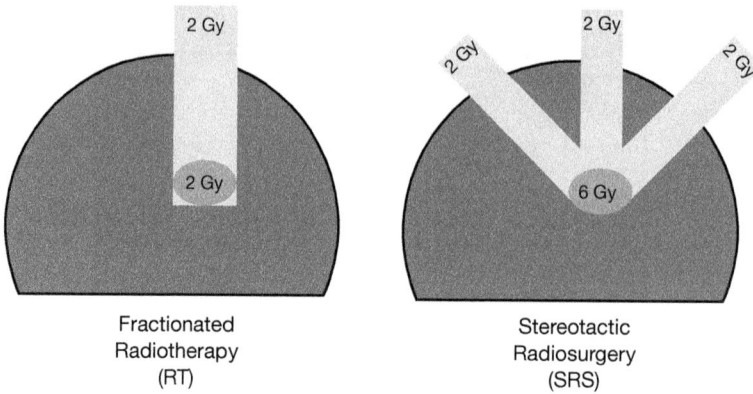

FIGURE 2.1 Schematic of fractionated radiotherapy and stereotactic radiosurgery. In conventional RT, the same dose of radiation that is delivered to the intracranial pathology is also delivered to the normal brain tissue in which the radiation beam travels. It is important to note that fractionated RT can be delivered at different angles. In SRS, multiple beams of radiation converge on the intracranial pathology. Unlike conventional RT, the dose of radiation delivered to the pathology is greater than that delivered to the normal brain that the radiation beams pass through. In this schematic, the same intracranial pathologies would receive 2 Gy via RT and 6 Gy via SRS limiting exposure of any normal range to 2 Gy.

TABLE 2.1 General Principles of Radiosurgery for Intracranial Lesions

Establishment of a fiducial system
Stereotactic imaging and planning
Dosing
Treatment

(c) tumor cells' tendency to proceed through the radioresistant "S" phase of the cell cycle following delivery of an initial radiation dose. Treatment using low doses of radiation is spread over several days or weeks to optimize treatment effect against tumor cells, allowing normal brain parenchyma to repair itself.

The decision to pursue RT depends on multiple factors, including the nature of the primary pathology, volume, and proximity to critical structures (such as cranial nerves) and eloquent brain structures. Fractionated RT is recommended for pathologies greater than 4 cm because the required therapeutic dose for SRS would also subject the surrounding normal tissue to higher doses of radiation, thereby negating the benefits of SRS. Similar logic applies to pathologies near cranial nerves, especially near the optic or vestibulocochlear nerves, or eloquent brain locations if the dose exceeds 10 Gy (1,2). Finally, the location of the pathology is a critical variable in the decision to pursue fractionated RT as lesions located in the thalamus, basal ganglia, midbrain, or pons were associated with significant toxicity in patients treated for arteriovenous malformations with SRS

(3). Fractionated RT uses high-energy photons that are generated by LINACs and delivered using up to 10 beams to conform to the tumor volume for conventional treatments.

Treatment usually requires patients to be immobilized using either a biteblock or a customized thermoplastic mask system with fiducial markers (which provide the axial, coronal, and sagittal lasers that intersect at the isocenter). This setup allows fractionated RT to have an accuracy of less than 5 mm (4,5) and have precise localization that can be reliably replicated over weeks of therapy. Following immobilization, different imaging modalities and protocols are used to reconstruct the tumor volume. Axial computed tomography (CT) imaging, often with contrast to enhance the tumor margin, is the most basic modality used. T1 and T2 MRI can be combined with CT imaging with many computer simulation programs (6). Metabolic imaging protocols using positron emission tomography (PET) and single photon emission tomography (SPECT) can also be fused with CT imaging to enhance identification of the tumor margin and eloquent brain regions (7). Once the tumor volume is determined from a single or combination of imaging techniques, the final volume is expanded by 1 to 5 mm (planning target volume) with conventional LINACs to account for uncertainty, subtle differences in patient position over multiple sessions, and expansion of tumor cells beyond the visible tumor margin.

Planning and dosing of radiation is based on delivering maximum radiation to the tumor bulk while sparing normal parenchyma. This is accomplished using three-dimensional conformal radiotherapy (3DCRT) or intensity-modulated radiation therapy (IMRT). 3DCRT is performed manually by optimizing beam arrangements and uses multiple converging beams shaped to the tumor volume. Dose volume histograms are then used to optimize the dose and conformality of radiation delivered to the tumor bulk. A representative conventional RT unit is shown in Figure 2.2.

INTENSITY-MODULATED RADIATION THERAPY

Intensity-modulated radiation therapy is a fractionated radiation schema for delivering nonhomogenous doses of radiation to a treatment volume. The goal of IMRT is delivering radiation that conforms to the patient's pathology, such that a maximum dose of radiation is delivered to the pathology while sparing normal brain parenchyma. The ability of IMRT to use 3D reconstruction and back planning allows this delivery method to be particularly useful in concave lesions and those in eloquent brain regions (8,9).

IMRT allows for specifying the dose and distribution of radiation to be delivered and then backcalculating the appropriate beam delivery parameters. Having the ability to focus different doses of radiation at different points within the pathology allows for a simultaneous boost that can be delivered to the tumor bed. However, a resulting consequence of the ability to conform to many different shapes is increased inhomogeneity of radiation delivered to the lesion. This

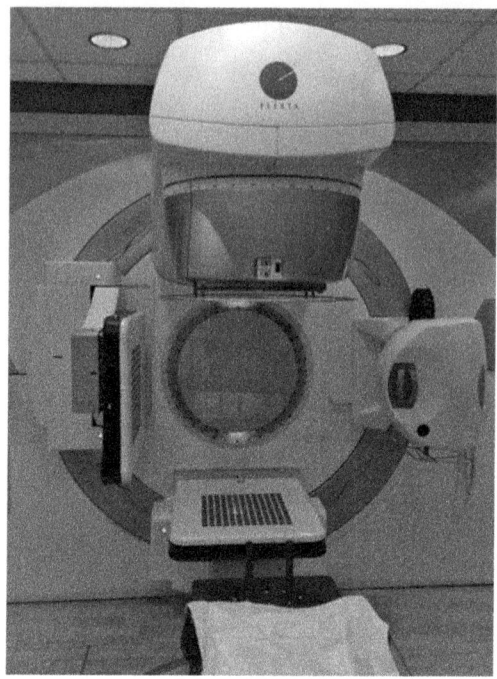

FIGURE 2.2 Representative image of an Elekta XRT unit with integrated CT scanner used to verify patient positioning.

inhomogeneity, resulting in both "cold-" and "hot-spots," can effect treatment outcomes due to incomplete tumor control in the case of "cold-spots" or damage to critical structures when "hot-spots" are present.

The delivery of IMRT as well as the radiation intensity in each beam can be completed using a variety of normal radiation delivery techniques. Radiation delivery platforms include compensator based IMRT, robotic LINAC IMRT (CyberKnife), and the use of multileaf collimator systems. Notably, IMRT is designed for highly fractionated plans and the margins are often in centimeters rather than the millimeter margins that are required for stereotactic treatments.

STEREOTACTIC RADIOSURGERY

SRS is a radiation delivery modality typically used to treat smaller (less than 3.5 cm) intracranial pathologies. Unlike conventional RT, SRS can deliver a target dose of radiation in a single session with steep radiation falloff outside of the targeted volume. SRS is usually delivered in a single fraction although it can be given in up to five fractions. There are multiple approaches/devices to delivering SRS and a brief comparison of the various devices and approaches is listed in Table 2.2.

TABLE 2.2 Comparisons of Dose Characteristics of SRS

	Gamma Knife	Proton Beam	LINAC
Dose falloff	90% to 20% zone	80% to 20% zone	90% to 20% zone
	7 to 8 mm	7 to 8 mm	7 to 8 mm
	(10)	(11)	(12)
Dose distribution	Spherical with equal falloff in all dimensions	—	Nonspherical with unequal falloff in all dimensions
Percentage of normal tissue receiving greater than 80% of target dose	Small target size: +	Small target size: +	Small target size: +
	Large target size: ++++	Large target size: ++	Large target size: ++++

Leksell Gamma Unit (Gamma Knife)

The Leksell Gamma Unit uses an array of 201 ^{60}Co sources that are rigidly arranged on a half-hemisphere shell with each ^{60}C-derived beam (1-mm wide, 20-mm long) aimed at a single isocenter (Figure 2.3). Each beam is collimated by the primary collimator as well as a second collimator shell to which the patient is attached at the time of treatment. The multiple collimators allow for homogenous spherical distributions at the isocenter with diameters of 4, 8, 14, or 18 mm. At the time of treatment, the patient is positioned so that the isocenter overlays the pathology. In the case of large or irregularly shaped lesions, multiple treatments using different isocenters with overlapping spheres can be used.

Treatment planning for patients receiving Gamma Knife surgery begins with MRI, CT, or angiography at the time of treatment using a stereotactic frame that is attached to the skull under local anesthesia. Once the pathology is confirmed, treatment computers can determine the best array of isocenters and radiation characteristics to optimize treatment. Irregular pathologies can be treated by forming multiple isocenters with different collimator sizes and weightings (13).

Overlapping spheres of radiation created by the intersection of 201 collimated beams are created to deliver a therapeutic conformal dose of radiation. The plans have a steep dose falloff to protect normal tissue. Because both the Gamma Knife unit and patient are rigidly immobilized during treatment, treatment with multiple isocenters in a short period of time is possible. Furthermore, up to 100 of the collimator holes can be plugged to further customize the beam arrangements. When mobilization of the patient is needed to align a new isocenter, mechanical motors are able to move the stereotactic frame, decreasing the time normally needed to manually change the location of the new isocenter.

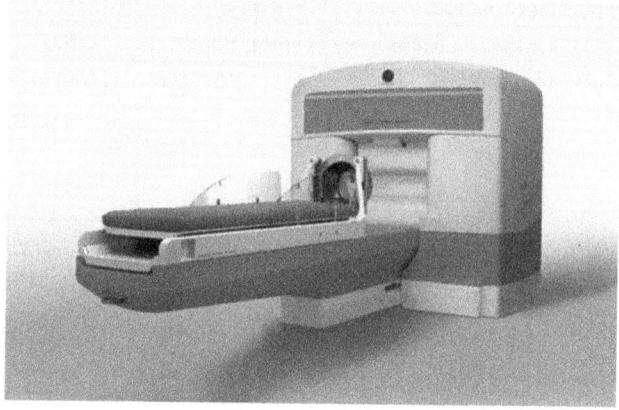

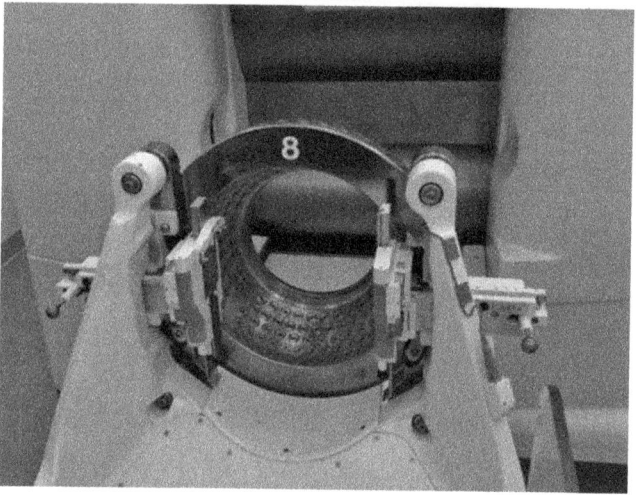

FIGURE 2.3 Representative image of a Leksell Gamma Knife Unit 4C (*above*, courtesy of Elekta) and stereotactic frame *(below)*.

Proton Beam

The properties of proton beam in tissues make proton beam delivery systems an attractive method of delivering radiation to intracranial pathologies, especially for those pathologies that are large and/or near eloquent brain locations. As compared to electrons, protons travel in relatively straight lines and deliver an increased amount of energy to tissue as they slow down. These properties give rise to a Bragg peak, which is only several millimeters thick. As such, the proton beam must be altered to create a spread-out Bragg peak to cover the entire pathology. Furthermore, the dose of radiation falls off to nearly zero, 1 cm deep to the target. The 80% to 20% falloff distance has been reported as 8 mm (11).

Proton beams can be delivered using gantry or horizontal systems. Using a gantry the patient remains immobilized with the gantry delivering beams of radiation from any angle. In a horizontal delivery system, the radiation beam remains fixed and the patient rotates around the radiation beam to achieve different beam angles. Comparing the two systems, a greater range of angles, as well as greater patient comfort, can be achieved through a gantry system.

Following planning, patients may be immobilized using a Gill–Thomas–Cosman frame, which is then bolted to the treatment bed. The gantry system can then be aligned with the fiducial system that was used and custom collimators inserted to modify the beam path. Treatment typically lasts 30 to 40 minutes with only minimal posttreatment monitoring needed to assess immediate treatment side effects.

Proton beam delivery generally uses four to five beams to cover the entire intracranial pathology as the dose of radiation in each beam is unlikely to cause adverse effects to normal brain tissue. Custom collimators that manipulate the beam to the shape of the distal side of the tumor, in combination with correct planning, can deliver homogenous doses of radiation to the entire pathologic bulk while minimizing cold-spots in the region being irradiated. Unlike Gamma Knife and LINAC systems, the beam size of proton beams can reach 10 cm, eliminating the need for multiple isocenters. This property makes proton beam therapy a recommended radiation delivery platform treatment of large or irregular targets.

The physical properties of protons make their targeting both accurate and precise. However, meticulous attention to the quality of pretreatment CT images is required as the stopping power of proton beams is calculated from the density of these images. If errors get incorporated into the planning and calibration due to imprecise CT images, a section of tumor will receive subtherapeutic levels of radiation, potentially leading to recurrence. Another potential danger is the issue of alignment as planning for depth could lead to portions of tumor not receiving radiation due to a small error in the entry angle of the proton beam.

Proton therapy differs from Gamma Knife or LINAC treatment in that planning and treatment are completed over multiple days to weeks due to the need to manufacture custom collimators. Similarly, a stereotactic head frame system is not used and multiple options exist for creating a coordinate system to use for treatment planning. Identification of the target is determined using CT with contrast enhancement. If this imaging modality is not optimal for the individual pathology, MRI, PET, or angiograms may be adapted with the CT images to provide optimal tools for planning. Like all other SRS modalities, dosing is determined by a team, including a radiation oncologist, a neurosurgeon, and a medical physicist with the goal of maximizing radiation to the intracranial pathology while limiting radiation exposure to normal tissue.

Linear Accelerator

LINAC systems are another modality that can be used to delivery x-ray beams to intracranial pathologies. The general principle of LINAC-based therapy is to deliver highly conformal doses of radiation with overlapping spherical isocenters that are created by administering radiation with a fixed number of arcs. The x-ray beams are created using a tertiary collimator and arcs of radiation are delivered with the goals of (a) maximizing the angle between arcs in order to decrease the radiation dose to normal tissue and (b) maximize the dose of radiation reaching the target. Many protocols for beam delivery have been used and are summarized elsewhere (12,14–17).

The isocenter produced by LINAC beams are spherical (70%–90% isodose) and can be altered when targeting pathologies near eloquent brain locations by modifying the length and weight of the arcs. To target pathologies with odd or nonspherical shapes, multiple isocenters (i.e. multiple arcs separated by 40°–60° or dynamic radiosurgery, which uses a single arc while rotating the treatment couch as well as the gantry) are generally required and result in nearly overlapping isocenters. However, this can lead to nonhomogenous dosing for nonspherical lesions. To prevent this, LINAC systems are now able to take advantage of miniature multileaf collimators (18). This allows one to create optimum dosing and target protocols to decrease nonhomogenous dosing that arises from using multiple isocenters for nonspherical lesions.

Similar to the other SRS modalities, studies begin with stereotactic CT, MRI, or angiographic imaging on the day of treatment. A stereotactic headframe with fiducial markers is placed on the morning of treatment. The patient's head, now fixed, is bolted to the treatment bed and aligned with the LINAC system. In some cases, headframes are not needed as several delivery systems only require an aquaplast mask due to on-board cone-beam CT imaging capabilities. Once treatment is initiated, each isocenter requires approximately 30 minutes to irradiate. To minimize the number of isocenters used in nonspherical targets, various collimators and arc distribution protocols can be used to precisely target the lesion.

Several challenges exist for LINAC-based therapy. One disadvantage of the LINAC system is the rotational movement of both the patient and the gantry. The LINAC system rotates the patient in the horizontal plane while the gantry rotates around the isocenter. The multitude of moving parts can lead to small inaccuracies in targeting, although this inaccuracy is reported as ±1 mm (19). A second challenge in using LINAC systems is the exponential falloff of dose with increasing depth. This quality causes an increase in radiation delivered to normal tissue as compared to that of the target, especially when only a small number of beams are used. This quality can be overcome by increasing the number of beams, thus decreasing the dose to normal tissue where the beam enters. Finally, the planning required to optimizing isocenters while sparing normal brain can be challenging, especially when more isocenters are required. However with the development of miniature multileaf collimators, inverse planning can produce adequate target conformity while sparing normal brain.

CyberKnife

The CyberKnife system is one of the most common LINAC systems currently in use for treating central nervous system (CNS) pathologies. It is a frameless radiation delivery platform that is composed of a robotic arm with a lightweight LINAC attached that can move with 6 degrees of freedom and is controlled in real time using on-board image-tracking software with real-time correction capabilities (Figure 2.4). Using 6-MV photon beams that are regulated by 12 available collimators, radiation can be delivered up to a rate of 4 Gy/min. There are two diagnostic x-ray sources, one of which can move freely to adjust to the position of the patient. The x-ray detection system is

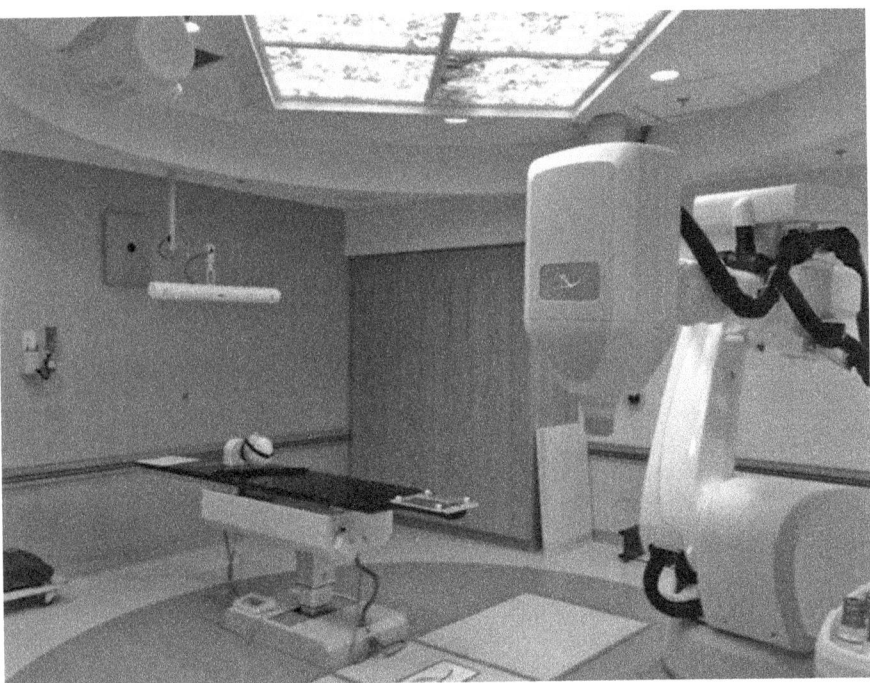

FIGURE 2.4 Representative image of the CyberKnife unit and treatment suite at Johns Hopkins Hospital.

coupled to the robotic delivery system, eliminating the need for a stereotactic frame as radiographic reference points, as opposed to external fiducial markers that are used for localization of the target. Finally, extraordinary treatment flexibility is possible as radiation can be delivered from 101 specific points in space, each with 12 approach angles. The accuracy of the CyberKnife system is less than 1 mm, which is comparable to frame-based systems.

COMPLICATIONS FOLLOWING RADIOTHERAPY AND SRS

The acute, subacute (6 weeks–6 months), and long-term (greater than 6 months) side effects of radiation for intracranial lesions are summarized in Table 2.3. In brief, constitutional symptoms can arise in the acute, subacute, or long-term setting, whereas noticeable neurologic side effects due to radiation damage to normal brain tissue generally require at least 6 weeks to be clinically apparent. The scoring criteria for both early and late morbidities were published by the Radiation Therapy Outcomes Group and are summarized in Table 2.4. In general, the presence of early side effects is not predictive of late side effects.

SRS can also be used as a boost after whole-brain radiotherapy (WBRT). In patients previously treated with WBRT, the prevalence of radionecrosis was 5%, 8%, and 11% at 6, 12, and 24 months, respectively (20). Despite providing an overall survival benefit, boost treatment with SRS was also associated with a higher incidence of grade 3 and 4 toxicities (21).

Finally, although reportedly rare, delivery of radiation to intracranial pathologies is associated with a low rate of radiation-induced neoplasms (22–24). Despite its low incidence, more accurate rates are likely to emerge after longer follow-up periods.

TABLE 2.3 Possible Side Effects of Radiation Treatment for Intracranial Pathologies

Acute	Subacute	Long-term
Alopecia; radiation dermatititis; fatigue; transient neurologic deficits due to edema, nausea, vomiting, otitis externa	Somnolence, fatigue, neurologic deterioration, transient demyelination	Radiation necrosis, diffuse leukoencephalopathy, hearing loss, retinopathy, cataract, visual changes, endocrine abnormalities, vasculopathy, moyamoya syndrome, decreased learning ability, short-term memory loss, decreased problem-solving skills

Adapted from Hansen E, Roach M. *Handbook of Evidence-Based Radiation Oncology.* 2nd ed. New York, NY: Springer Science+Business Media; 2006 (25).

TABLE 2.4 Radiation Therapy Oncology Group Acute and Long-term Morbidity Scoring Criteria

Grade	Acute	Long-term
I	Fully functional, minor neurologic findings, no medication	Mild headache, lethargy
II	Neurologic symptoms requiring some home care, nursing home assistance required, medications required	Moderate headache, more severe lethargy
III	Neurologic symptoms requiring hospitalization for management	Severe headaches, severe CNS dysfunction
IV	Serious neurologic impairment, including coma or seizures that occur more often than three times per week despite medication use; hospitalization required	Seizures, paralysis, coma
V	Any toxicity that causes death	Any toxicity that causes death

Adapted from Hansen E, Roach M. *Handbook of Evidence-Based Radiation Oncology.* 2nd ed. New York, NY: Springer Science+Business Media; 2006 (25).

STRATEGIES TO PREVENT RADIATION TO CRITICAL STRUCTURES

To prevent damage to eloquent brain areas, precautions can be taken and include: (a) using orthogonal beams to avoid overlap in nontarget tissue; (b) avoiding beams that traverse eloquent areas, but if necessary having the beam travel tangential to the structure; (c) decreasing the radiation dose carried in a beam aimed through eloquent brain regions; and (d) aiming beams through homogenous brain regions to avoid changing beam characteristics as the beam travels between different cellular densities. Finally, the dose tolerances of different structures are provided in Table 2.5.

TABLE 2.5 Dose Tolerances of Different Eloquent Brain Regions

Modality	Location	Dose
Conventional radiotherapy 1.8–2 Gy/fraction	Whole brain	50 Gy
	Partial brain	60 Gy
	Brainstem	54 Gy
	Chiasm	50–54 Gy
	Retina	45 Gy
	Lens	10 Gy
	Inner ear	30 Gy
SRS	Brainstem	12 Gy
	Optic nerve and chiasm	8 Gy
	Visual pathway	12 Gy

Adapted from Hansen E, Roach M. *Handbook of Evidence-Based Radiation Oncology.* 2nd ed. New York, NY: Springer Science+Business Media; 2006 (25).

CONCLUSION

Radiotherapy and SRS have emerged as safe and efficacious techniques for the treatment of intracranial pathologies. Although the Gamma Knife unit is the most common SRS modality in use, both proton beam and LINAC units are able to deliver homogenous doses of radiation to irregularly shaped targets. Similarly, advances in patient immobilization allow for more accurate targeting while minimizing radiation delivered to normal brain tissue. Although radiotherapy requires several sessions to deliver the total dose to the target, SRS is able to deliver its treatment dose in a single day and with a more rapid dose falloff. Finally, no matter which modality is used, a coordinated team of neurosurgeons, radiation oncologists, and medical physicists is required to achieve optimum planning, dosing, and long-term outcomes.

REFERENCES

1. Ito K, Kurita H, Sugasawa K, Mizuno M, Sasaki T. Analyses of neuro-otological complications after radiosurgery for acoustic neurinomas. *Int J Radiat Oncol Biol Phys.* 1997;39(5):983–988.
2. Stafford SL, Pollock BE, Leavitt JA, et al. A study on the radiation tolerance of the optic nerves and chiasm after stereotactic radiosurgery. *Int J Radiat Oncol Biol Phys.* 2003;55(5):1177–1181.
3. Flickinger JC, Kondziolka D, Lunsford LD, et al. Development of a model to predict permanent symptomatic postradiosurgery injury for arteriovenous malformation patients. Arteriovenous Malformation Radiosurgery Study Group. *Int J Radiat Oncol Biol Phys.* 2000;46(5):1143–1148.
4. Verhey LJ. Immobilizing and positioning patients for radiotherapy. *Semin Radiat Oncol.* 1995;5(2):100–114.
5. Gilbeau L, Octave-Prignot M, Loncol T, Renard L, Scalliet P, Grégoire V. Comparison of setup accuracy of three different thermoplastic masks for the treatment of brain and head and neck tumors. *Radiother Oncol.* 2001;58(2):155–162.
6. Lattanzi JP, Fein DA, McNeeley SW, Shaer AH, Movsas B, Hanks GE. Computed tomography-magnetic resonance image fusion: a clinical evaluation of an innovative approach for improved tumor localization in primary central nervous system lesions. *Radiat Oncol Investig.* 1997;5(4):195–205.
7. Sweeney RA, Bale RJ, Moncayo R, et al. Multimodality cranial image fusion using external markers applied via a vacuum mouthpiece and a case report. *Strahlenther Onkol.* 2003;179(4):254–260.
8. Woo SY, Grant WH III, Bellezza D, et al. A comparison of intensity modulated conformal therapy with a conventional external beam stereotactic radiosurgery system for the treatment of single and multiple intracranial lesions. *Int J Radiat Oncol Biol Phys.* 1996;35(3):593–597.
9. Kramer BA, Wazer DE, Engler MJ, Tsai JS, Ling MN. Dosimetric comparison of stereotactic radiosurgery to intensity modulated radiotherapy. *Radiat Oncol Investig.* 1998;6(1):18–25.

10. Flickinger JC, Maitz A, Kalend A, Lunsford LD, Wu A. Treatment volume shaping with selective beam blocking using the Leksell gamma unit. *Int J Radiat Oncol Biol Phys.* 1990;19(3):783–789.
11. Urie MM, Sisterson JM, Koehler AM, Goitein M, Zoesman J. Proton beam penumbra: effects of separation between patient and beam modifying devices. *Med Phys.* 1986;13(5):734–741.
12. Lutz W, Winston KR, Maleki N. A system for stereotactic radiosurgery with a linear accelerator. *Int J Radiat Oncol Biol Phys.* 1988;14(2):373–381.
13. Flickinger JC, Lunsford LD, Wu A, Maitz AH, Kalend AM. Treatment planning for gamma knife radiosurgery with multiple isocenters. *Int J Radiat Oncol Biol Phys.* 1990;18(6):1495–1501.
14. Hartmann GH, Schlegel W, Sturm V, Kober B, Pastyr O, Lorenz WJ. Cerebral radiation surgery using moving field irradiation at a linear accelerator facility. *Int J Radiat Oncol Biol Phys.* 1985;11(6):1185–1192.
15. Schell MC, Smith V, Larson DA, Wu A, Flickinger JC. Evaluation of radiosurgery techniques with cumulative dose volume histograms in linac-based stereotactic external beam irradiation. *Int J Radiat Oncol Biol Phys.* 1991;20(6):1325–1330.
16. Houdek PV, Fayos JV, Van Buren JM, Ginsberg MS. Stereotaxic radiotherapy technique for small intracranial lesions. *Med Phys.* 1985;12(4):469–472.
17. Podgorsak EB, Olivier A, Pla M, Lefebvre PY, Hazel J. Dynamic stereotactic radiosurgery. *Int J Radiat Oncol Biol Phys.* 1988;14(1):115–126.
18. St John TJ, Wagner TH, Bova FJ, Friedman WA, Meeks SL. A geometrically based method of step and shoot stereotactic radiosurgery with a miniature multileaf collimator. *Phys Med Biol.* 2005;50(14):3263–3276.
19. Bova F, Spiegelmann R, Friedman WA. A device for experimental radiosurgery. *Stereotact Funct Neurosurg.* 1991;56(4):213–219.
20. Shaw E, Scott C, Souhami L, et al. Single dose radiosurgical treatment of recurrent previously irradiated primary brain tumors and brain metastases: final report of RTOG protocol 90–05. *Int J Radiat Oncol Biol Phys.* 2000;47(2):291–298.
21. Andrews DW, Scott CB, Sperduto PW, et al. Whole brain radiation therapy with or without stereotactic radiosurgery boost for patients with one to three brain metastases: phase III results of the RTOG 9508 randomised trial. *Lancet.* 2004;363(9422):1665–1672.
22. Balasubramaniam A, Shannon P, Hodaie M, Laperriere N, Michaels H, Guha A. Glioblastoma multiforme after stereotactic radiotherapy for acoustic neuroma: case report and review of the literature. *Neuro-oncology.* 2007;9(4):447–453.
23. Sheehan J, Yen CP, Steiner L. Gamma knife surgery-induced meningioma. Report of two cases and review of the literature. *J Neurosurg.* 2006;105(2):325–329.
24. Shin M, Ueki K, Kurita H, Kirino T. Malignant transformation of a vestibular schwannoma after gamma knife radiosurgery. *Lancet.* 2002;360(9329):309–310.
25. Hansen E, Roach M. *Handbook of Evidence-Based Radiation Oncology.* 2nd ed. New York, NY: Springer Science+Business Media; 2006.

Chapter 3

Technology and Techniques for Spinal Radiosurgery

Maziyar A. Kalani & Stephen Ryu

Neoplastic involvement of the vertebral column is very common, accounting for up to 70% of bony metastases in cancer patients (1,2). The standard management recommendation for most patients with spinal tumors consists of some combination of surgery, chemotherapy, and radiation (3). Although surgical advances have rendered most tumors accessible, the majority of spine metastases do not present with significant neurological compromise. Therefore, radiation therapy is often the mainstay of treatment for metastatic spine disease (4,5).

The overarching goals of radiation therapy for spinal tumors are tumor control and preservation of normal surrounding tissue (6). More specifically, we aim for oncological control through progression-free survival, for maintenance of neurological function, for structural preservation, and for the reduction of pain.

Advanced CT and MRI have improved conformational radiotherapeutic planning. Three-dimensional stereotactic planning allows for precise conformal targeting with respect to surrounding structures, factors that affect dose delivery and potential complications. Stereotactic radiosurgery (SRS) takes advantage of such precision targeting of a lesion with respect to a known fixed structure. As such, spinal tumors can be treated by referencing off the spine as a reference structure. But unlike the skull, which can be fixed in a frame, spinal SRS now relies on technologies that obviate the need for a bulky fixed frame.

Modern frameless spinal tumor SRS developed as adjuvant treatment for patients who had undergone prior surgical resection of spinal metastases with or without conventional radiation, allowing for additional precisely defined high-dose radiation to treatment areas while preserving surrounding structures (3). Since then, growing experience has made spine SRS a widely accepted first-line and adjuvant treatment for spinal tumors.

CURRENT TECHNOLOGIES/IMMOBILIZATION

Spinal SRS systems vary generally in the source of the radiation delivery (i.e., fixed source, fixed linear accelerator [LINAC], or portable LINAC) and the immobilization methods. The delivery of the higher dose radiation for stereotactic methods requires very accurate targeting capabilities. This requires precisely determining the location of the target usually with respect to known reference locations in space prior to dose delivery. Early attempts at spinal immobilization required rigid techniques that are now impractical with the exception of the Gamma Knife Perfexion (Elekta, Stockholm, Sweden), which uses the familiar fixed cranial frame to extend treatment down to the upper cervical spine.

Digital radiographic techniques allow for real-time target and surrounding tissue position monitoring, which leads to accurate delivery of the treatment dose without rigid immobilization. Implanted fiducials have been used in the past, but with improved resolution and software, this is now rarely required. Current LINAC-based systems are able to treat the entire spine from occiput to ilium without the need for a fixed frame. Rather than rigid immobilization, these can rely on conformal body cradles such as the BodyFix vacuum body-fixing device (Philips Medical Systems, Cleveland, Ohio), alpha cradle, or other semirigid molds to stabilize the body. This roughly positions the patient and target while some form of image-guided localization device compares anatomic landmarks from the initial planning images for fine-tuning of targeting in space (7).

A fixed LINAC system, such as the Novalis TX (BrainLAB AG, Heimstetten, Germany), has a dimensionally constrained dose-delivery device. As such, this requires the patient to be moved into accurate alignment with the treatment beam. The gantry-mounted LINAC has an integrated multileaf microcollimator. Its ExacTrac alignment system consists of infrared optical tracking of surface makers that are imaged at the time of treatment planning and automated registration of bony structures based on stereoscopic x-ray imaging. This is interfaced with the treatment beam, and adjustments of the patient table are made to account for changes in positioning and to deliver the treatment accurately (7).

A portable LINAC system, such as the CyberKnife (Accuray, Sunnyvale, CA), has a very dimensionally unrestricted dose-delivery device. As such, this system requires the treatment beam to be moved into accurate alignment with the patient. Its Xsight Spine tracking system consists of real-time stereoscopic x-ray imaging that identifies landmarks of the patient and correlates them with the treatment planning imaging. Once so accounted, the system can identify changes in patient movement in real time and adjust the treatment beam paths to adapt to patient movement (7,8).

Other less commonly applied technologies for spinal SRS include ultrasound image-guided radiosurgery (9), CT-based intensity-modulated radiotherapy

(IMRT; CereTom, Accuray, Sunnyvale, CA), and proton beam treatment. Overall, most commonly used spinal SRS systems are found to deliver equivalent target dose coverage, but each has certain differences in dose delivery that are yet to be of noted clinical significance.

TARGETING

In general, MRI is the imaging modality of choice for spine tumors because it provides superior definition of the extent of disease, can help distinguish malignant from benign disease, and is noninvasive. MRI specificity is 97% to 98%, sensitivity of 93% and positive predictive value (PPV) of 98% for spinal malignant disease (10).

After three-dimensional images are acquired and imported into a treatment planning system, the target and critical organ volumes can be delineated based on CT, MRI, and other imaging modalities such as positron emission tomography (PET). Relying on only one modality can be limiting, especially in complex and previously treated cases. Depending on the system used and the pathology, optimal targeting often requires the combination of information from the MRI, CT, and/or other modalities.

Advanced software allows us to fuse different modalities for planning. CT and MRI fusion images are very useful to delineate the location of the bony spine with respect to the soft tissue of the lesion, which can be difficult with bony invasion. Targeting the metabolically active parts of a PET fused to a CT or MRI can be of use. In prior treated cases, overlaying prior radiotherapy and SRS plans can also be helpful.

DOSING CONSIDERATIONS

SRS treatment of spinal tumors continues to become more prevalent; however, treatment has not been standardized, and various institution-specific regimens exist for different pathologies. Though pathology-specific treatment protocols will be discussed in subsequent chapters, some general treatment considerations merit discussion.

Dosing of SRS for spinal tumors depends on the type of pathology, the size of the lesions, the history of prior radiation and/or surgical resection, and the proximity of critical structures—spinal cord and surrounding organs.

More aggressive or radio-resistant pathologies generally require higher treatment doses. Smaller lesions can be safely treated with higher doses than larger ones. Lesions greater than 3 cm in size can be difficult but not impossible to treat (e.g., whole vertebral bodies). Prior radiation decreases the cord tolerance; the prior plan needs to be studied to determine the aggregate dose delivered.

Proximity of critical structures limits the deliverable dose, but of greater concern is the fundamental trade-off that arises in tumors that are very close to the spinal cord and other critical structures. Under treatment of the lesion can limit normal tissue injury, but over treatment of the lesion can improve consequent tumor response. This trade-off requires an understanding of dose physics (e.g., dose drop-off) and the goals of treatment.

Doses are specified as the amount of radiation delivered to an isodose curve in number of fractions (e.g., 21 Gy to the 80% isodose curve in three fractions). Dose is selected from known information or best estimate of the dose–volume relationship. Generally it is best to err on less dosage and to understand and pay close attention to the dose drop-off curve to maximize treatment and minimize injury.

To take advantage of radiobiology, fractionated techniques are easily accomplished with frameless technologies. As such, it is not uncommon to treat spinal lesions in one to three fractions routinely and even up to five to ten fractions in select cases. There is still much debate as to the need or amount of fractionation required (11–14).

Although effective treatment doses can be determined and administered, a major limiting factor has been the tolerance of the spinal cord and cauda equina. The actual cord tolerance to radiation is unknown. From XRT literature, maximum intraparenchymal cord dosing ranges from 4500 to 6000 cGy delivered over 5 weeks, associated with a 5% risk of myelopathy in 5 years (TD5/5) (14,15). Early spinal SRS studies limited dosing to 800 cGy, which is now considered very conservative (16). More detailed discussion of this topic is contained in Chapter 16.

The true cord tolerance to single-dose irradiation is unknown, including situations in which a spinal cord has been previously exposed to radiation. It is unknown if the cervical, thoracic, and lumbar spinal cord have different susceptibilities to radiation (17). No data yet support differences in response to the length of cord treated.

Other structures that are of concern with spinal SRS are the cauda equina and exiting spinal nerve roots, esophagus, and intestines. The TD5/5 of the cauda equina was determined to be 60 Gy (16). Though there is no concrete data, the resistance of terminal nerves is generally felt to be greater than that of the spinal cord. Esophagus and bowel exposure should be considered and limited to around 2000 cGy.

COMPLICATIONS / AVOIDANCE PEARLS

Regular quality assessment and phantom evaluation are critical to maintaining the accuracy of an SRS system. It is important to verify the collimator size routinely as some systems do not provide an interlock for this. Clear planning of the lesion and review with the treatment team are useful. Often, additional shielding structures can be used to "tweak" the plan to make it less toxic to critical structures. Use of these structures and running multiple scenarios is key to good planning technique and avoidance of complications.

Although there is no definite absolute threshold for the onset of myelopathy, standard doses and conventionally fractionated treatments present a risk of myelopathy that varies from 0.2% to 5% at 5 years (18). Fractionation of treatment can be used to mitigate but never eliminate the risk.

Radiation toxicity has been characterized by several early and late reactions. Irreversible, tumor necrosis-associated neurological damage is the toxicity that causes the greatest concern in spinal SRS. A latency of 6 to 20 months can precede the onset of these symptoms (19). L'Hermitte's sign is an uncommon and early manifestation that develops within the first few months of treatment and is rarely progressive (20). A second rare toxicity syndrome is characterized by acute paralysis, presumed to be secondary to ischemia (21). Lower motor neuron disease manifestations have also been reported (22).

The issue of reirradiation to the spinal cord is less studied. Work with animal models has suggested that significant recovery can occur after initial irradiation and, therefore, with allowance for sufficient time, reirradiation can be considered (23). Clinical experience also suggests that the spinal cord can be retreated with meaningful doses leading to functional outcomes (24). It is critical to discuss all these risks, albeit small and delayed, as a part of informed consent.

REFERENCES

1. Fornasier VL, Horne JG. Metastases to the vertebral column. *Cancer*. 1975;36:590–594.
2. Grant R, Papadopoulos SM, Greenberg HS. Metastatic epidural spinal cord compression. *Neurol Clin*. 1991;9:825–841.
3. Ryu SI, Chang SD, Kim DH, et al. Image-guided hypo-fractionated stereotactic radiosurgery to spinal lesions. *Neurosurgery*. 2001;49(4):838–846.
4. Hatrick NC, Lucas JD, Timothy AR, et al. The surgical treatment of metastatic disease of the spine. *Radiother Oncol*. 2000;56:335–339. 2000.
5. Schaberg J, Gainor BJ. A profile of metastatic carcinoma of the spine. *Spine*. 1985;10:19–20.
6. Ryken TC, Eichholz KM, Gerszten PC, et al. Evidence-based review of the surgical management of vertebral column metastatic disease. *Neurosurg Focus*. 2003;15:E11.
7. Murphy MJ, Jin J-Y. Patient immobilization and movement in spine radiosurgery. Page 38. In: Gerszten PC, Ryu S, eds. Thieme; 2008.
8. Dieterich S, Gibbs IC. The CyberKnife in clinical use: current roles, future expectations. *Front Radiat Ther Oncol*. 2011;43:181–194.
9. Ryken TC, Meeks SL, Traynelis V, et al. Ultrasonographic guidance for spinal extracranial radiosurgery: technique and application for metastatic spinal lesions. *Neurosurg Focus*. 2001;11(6):1–6. 2001.

10. Gerszten PC, Ryu S. Target delineation and dose prescription in spine radiosurgery. Page 43. In Gerszten PC, Ryu S, eds. Thieme; 2008.
11. Tong D, Gillick L, Hendrickson FR. The palliation of symptomatic osseous metastases. Final results of the study of the Radiation Therapy Oncology Group. *Cancer.* 1982;50:893–899.
12. Bone Pain Trial Working Party. 8 Gy single fraction radiotherapy for the treatment of metastatic skeletal pain: randomized comparison with a multifraction schedule over 12 months of patient follow-up. On behalf of the bone pain trial working party. *Radiother Oncol.* 1999;52:111–121.
13. Steenland ES, Leer JW, van Houwelingen H, et al. The effect of a single fraction to multiple fractions on painful bone metastases: a global analysis of the Dutch Bone Metastasis Study. *Radiother Oncol.* 1999;52:101–109.
14. Van Der Kogel AJ. Retreatment tolerance of the spinal cord. *Int J Radiat Oncol Biol Phys.* 1993;26:715.
15. Faul CM, Flickinger JC. The use of radiation in the management of spinal metastases. *J Neurooncol.* 1995;23:149–161, 1995.
16. Emami B, Lyman J, Brown A, et al. Tolerance of normal tissue to therapeutic irradiation. *Int J Radiat Oncol Biol Phys.* 1991;21(1):109–122.
17. Wara WM, Phillips TL, Sheline GE, Schwade JG. Radiation tolerance of the spinal cord. *Cancer.* 1975;35:1558–1562.
18. Schultheiss T. Spinal cord radiation 'tolerance':/? doctrine versus data. *Int J Radiat Oncol Biol Phys.* 1990;19:219–221.
19. Lambert PW, Davis RL. Delayed effects of radiation on the human nervous system. *Neurology.* 1964;14:912–917.
20. Combes PF, Daly N. Late progressive radiation myelopathies:/? a study of 27 cases. *J Radiol Electrol Med Nucl.* 1975;57:815–825.
21. Leibel A, Sheline E. Tolerance of the brain and spinal cord to conventional irradiation. In Gutin P, Leibel S, Sheline G, eds. *Radiation Injury to the Nervous System.* New York, NY: Raven Press; 1991:239–256.
22. Lamy C, Mas JL. Post radiation lower motor neuron syndrome presenting as momomyelix amyotropgy. *J Neurol Neurosurg Psychiatry.* 1991;54:648–649.
23. Ang KK, Price RE, Stephens LC, et al. The tolerance of primate spinal cord to re-irradiation. *Int J Radiat Oncol Biol Phys.* 1993;25:459–464.
24. Ryu S, Gorty S, Kazee Am, et al. 'Full dose' reirradiation of the human cervical spinal cord. *Am J Clin Oncol.* 2002;23:29–31.

Section III

Radiosurgery for Brain Tumors

Section Editors

Jacob Ruzevick and Michael Lim

Chapter 4

Intraparenchymal Tumors

A. Radiosurgery for Primary Brain Tumors

Andy Trang, Marko Spasic, Winward Choy, & Isaac Yang

GLIOBLASTOMA

Glioblastoma multiforme (GBM) is an extremely aggressive tumor that often rapidly infiltrates surrounding normal brain parenchyma (1). Stereotactic radiosurgery (SRS) is an alternative form of treatment for patients with GBM because of its ability to deliver a high dose of radiation accurately, quickly, and noninvasively (2,3). However, well-defined therapy with SRS may leave surrounding cells untreated (4).

Several studies have shown that SRS before radiotherapy, as an upfront treatment or as a boost, provides no appreciable improvement in overall survival (OS) (4–8). Other studies have suggested that SRS may provide a survival advantage when delivered after radiotherapy or at the time of progression (5,7,9,10). However, it is argued that patients treated with SRS for progression may experience improved survival because they have already lived long enough to warrant further therapy, which may only represent selection bias and not therapeutic benefit (11). Nevertheless, the literature suggests there is a trend for increased OS in patients treated with SRS during recurrence (4). Despite the OS benefits of SRS, the rates of recurrence in patients treated with and without SRS were comparable, suggesting that SRS is not effective as upfront therapy but may have a role in recurrence or in postradiotherapy treatment (5). Favorable prognostic factors for SRS include younger patient age, tumor volumes smaller (7) than 10.1 cm^3, and KPS (Karnofsky performance scale) greater than 70 (2).

SRS does not seem to exhibit any benefits when used as an upfront therapy. However, there appears to be prolonged OS in patients who receive SRS at the time of recurrence, especially after radiotherapy (5,6). SRS is especially promising for younger patients with a high KPS (2) and smaller tumors (7,12).

On the other hand, the value of SRS treatment in adjacent peripheral areas of tumors is questionable because of the lower radiation dose administered to those sites (2). This is a major drawback of SRS and in some cases leads to failure of controlling recurrence outside of the central field of therapy (2).

LOW-GRADE ASTROCYTOMA

Because low-grade astrocytomas are relatively well circumscribed, patients harboring these tumors may be good candidates for SRS (13). Patients who would benefit most from the use of SRS include patients with smaller tumors that are either recurrent or unresectable (14–16). Factors associated with better OS for patients undergoing SRS include a KPS score greater than 70, patient age of 18 to 40 years, presence of seizures at presentation, and absence of contrast enhancement on pretreatment computerized tomography or MRI (13,17).

Several studies have reported tumor control rates of 68% to 91.7% for patients with pilocytic astrocytoma and 67% to 87.2% for patients with World Health Organization (WHO) grade II astrocytomas (14,18–23). Although showing good tumor control, reports have noted that radiation-induced side effects may occur in up to 41% in patients with WHO grade II astrocytomas when treated with SRS (14,22).

Radiosurgery may provide an alternative to standard radiotherapy, chemotherapy, and observation in patients with smaller, demarcated tumors. It may also reduce the risk of toxicity by limiting the volume of normal brain irradiated at a high or intermediate dose (14).

EPENDYMOMA

The standard therapeutic approach for primary intracranial ependymomas is surgery followed by postoperative external-beam radiotherapy (EBRT) (24). SRS provides another management option for patients with residual or recurrent ependymoma who have failed surgery and radiotherapy. Predictors of response include smaller tumor volume and homogeneous contrast enhancement on MRI (25). Generally, the outcomes of younger ependymoma patients are significantly worse than those of adult patients (26,27), and supratentorial ependymomas are associated with better survival rates compared with neoplasms of the posterior fossa (25,28).

Patients treated with SRS as a boost after radiotherapy had improved survival compared to those treated with SRS to salvage a radiotherapy failure. Grade II ependymomas with small target volumes (less than 5 cm^3) and homogeneous MRI enhancement are associated with improved progression-free survival (PFS) (25).

The use of SRS as an upfront treatment for very young children (less than 3 years old) has been proposed to delay the use of EBRT to avoid neurotoxicity. Although chemotherapy has often been used in the past for the same purpose, the response of ependymoma to chemotherapy may be suboptimal and progression may still occur during chemotherapy (24). In such cases, SRS provides a new treatment option.

SRS may be a potentially effective salvage therapy when surgery, radiotherapy, and chemotherapy have failed (24,25). SRS provides reasonable local control especially as an SRS boost. However, tumor progression remains an issue, especially for recurrent disease (24). SRS appears to be a feasible and safe modality for patients with ependymomas that are unresectable or for patients with residual tumor after surgery (24).

OLIGODENDROGLIOMA

Oligodendrogliomas are infiltrative in nature (29) and are generally treated by surgical removal followed by radiation therapy and/or chemotherapy. However, the use of SRS as a salvage therapy after treatment failure of oligodendrogliomas may be beneficial, especially if the volume (29) is less than 15 cm^3. Despite SRS, most patients will require postoperative adjuvant management chemotherapy and potentially fractionated radiotherapy (29).

A study by Kano et al. (29) showed that patients who had tumors greater than 15 cm^3 treated with SRS experienced a 5-year PFS of 35.3%, whereas those with tumors less than 15 cm^3 had a 5-year PFS of 84.6%. The 5-year PFS for grade II and III oligodendrogliomas are 38% to 76% and 20% to 40%, respectively (29).

Younger age and smaller overall tumors were favorable prognostic factors for patients who received SRS (29,30). SRS may also benefit newly diagnosed patients who have low-volume grade II oligodendrogliomas with tumors that are not satisfactory for resection (29). Target volumes less than 15 cm^3 and WHO grade II tumors are associated with improvement of PFS (29). Overall, SRS may be a helpful adjunct therapy, compares favorably to other treatments, and is associated with low treatment-associated morbidity as a form of salvage therapy (30).

NEUROCYTOMA

Central neurocytomas (CN) are a rare type of tumor found in the lateral ventricle (near the foramina of Monro) of young adults; they have a good prognosis. CNs are well circumscribed, highly vascularized, and may present with signs of increased intracranial pressure caused by obstruction of the cerebrospinal fluid (CSF) pathway (31–33). These characteristics of neurocytomas—along with evidence that they are well demarcated and relatively radiosensitive—make them a promising target for SRS (31,32,34,35). Currently, resection of the tumor is the main form of upfront treatment and is usually considered curative when total resection is performed; however, tumors in more than half of patients with central neurocytoma cannot be completely resected (32,34–36).

The use of conventional radiation therapy for the treatment of CN has been criticized because of the associated long-term effects on cognitive function (37). However, SRS potentially avoids the side effects with its rapid dose decrease at the target edges (37,38). This has led to the emergence of SRS as an attractive alternative to conventional radiation (32). Many studies have found that patients have relatively good responses to SRS and experience reduction in tumor size with minimal or no toxicity due to the treatment (32,37,39–41).

It is important to delineate a wide margin of safety when planning SRS for CN because the dose falloff for Gamma Knife stereotactic radiosurgery (GKRS) is very steep. Nonenhanced residual tumor may be located outside the margin, which makes SRS insufficient for long-term control of residual tumor growth. Retrospective investigation of SRS planning demonstrated that the tumor recurrence started from the nonenhanced residual tumor that was not considered in the planning of the radiosurgery (32). Patients can develop recurrences outside the targets of prior radiosurgery treatment. Retrospective examination of the imaging studies failed to reveal tumor presence at the site of recurrence; therefore, the value of larger field radiosurgery—as well as cranial spinal axis radiation—needs to be reevaluated in some cases (31).

Although SRS is an effective and safe treatment for residual or recurrent CN (38), it may also be attractive as an initial treatment for CN in the early stages of small size masses located in the lateral ventricle because such lesions can be detected easily by routine MRI.

There is limited data on the use of radiosurgery as an upfront treatment for CN (31), Regular long-term follow-up MRI of at least 5 years should be mandatory to validate the effectiveness of SRS treatment (32). A representative image is shown in Figure 4.A1.

HEMANGIOBLASTOMA

Hemangioblastomas are highly vascular and sharply circumscribed benign, solid tumors that often occur in the posterior fossa. The tumor and associated cysts produce symptoms by exerting mass effect on nearby structures and by increasing intracranial pressure rather than infiltrating the adjacent brain (42–44). Sporadic hemangioblastomas occur predominantly in the cerebellum, whereas Von Hippel–Lindau (VHL)-associated hemangioblastomas are found in the cerebellum, brainstem, and spinal cord (43). Their management frequently requires weighing the benefits and potential complications of therapeutic intervention while considering the slowly progressive nature of the disease (44).

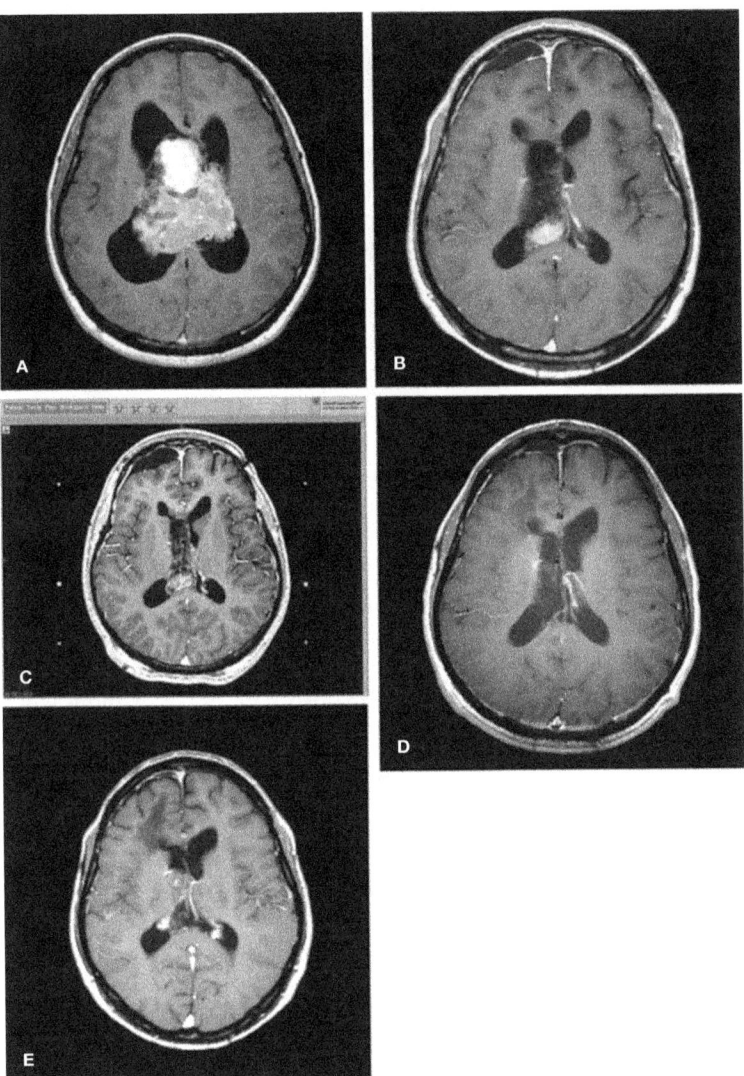

FIGURE 4A.1 Secondary postoperative Gamma Knife SRS was performed on a patient with central neurocytoma after surgical resection and pathological diagnosis. (A) T1-weighted gadolinium-enhanced axial MRI showing a large and heterogeneously enhanced intraventricular mass. (B) A residual mass of 9.2 mL remains near the splenium after an interhemispheric transcallosal approach. (C) The residual mass was treated with Gamma Knife SRS at a dose of 15 Gy, 48% isodose line. The target was a well-enhanced mass of the posterior lateral ventricle. (D) This 37-month follow-up MRI shows a residual intraventricular mass with a volume of 1.2 mL and a rate of reduction in tumor volume of 88%. (E) This 67-month follow-up MRI shows a recurrent mass extending from the anterior thalamus, which was out of the field of the Gamma Knife SRS treatment. Reproduced with permission from John Wiley and Sons and from Kim CY, Paek SH, Jeong SS, et al. Gamma knife radiosurgery for central neurocytoma: primary and secondary treatment. *Cancer*. 2007;110(10):2276–2284.

Small hemangioblastomas are attractive targets for radiosurgery; in many studies, tumor responses correlate significantly with increasing radiosurgery dose (44). However, the management of hemangioblastomas is challenging due to their highly variable nature: solid or cystic, solitary or multiple, and possibly associated with VHL. Approximately 20% of patients with intracranial hemangioblastomas have VHL disease, a rare autosomal dominant trait caused by a defect in the VHL tumor suppressor gene on chromosome 3 (44–46). Surgical resection is the standard treatment for CNS hemangioblastomas; however, their vascularity and sites of origin can make complete resection difficult and postoperative recurrence is common (42,47,48). Hemangioblastomas are amenable to SRS as a minimally invasive option because the tumors are often small, well delineated, and contain susceptible vascular elements (44). SRS may be especially valuable for treatment of multiple and VHL-associated hemangioblastomas (43).

SRS has been shown to be effective in treating the mural nodule of hemangioblastomas but not for the associated cystic component (49). Therefore, patients with a small mural nodule with a large cyst are not suitable for SRS (42,50). Furthermore, the presence of a cystic component at time of SRS is significantly correlated with worse tumor control (42,51,52).

Good outcome and a higher tumor control rate were correlated with higher radiation dose, and there was a trend for tumors above the median size of 1.3 cm^3 to progress (42,44,50,53). A target volume of less than 3.2 cm^3 was significantly associated with better PFS, and a marginal dose of 15 Gy or more was significantly associated with better PFS (43).

Despite the benefits of SRS for multifocal tumors, SRS may not be ideal for treating large symptomatic cystic hemangioblastomas because it does not quickly reduce mass effect; however, it can be useful for patients with limited surgical options (43,44). Overall, better PFS was also associated with smaller tumor volumes, a higher marginal dose, and solid tumor configuration (43).

REFERENCES

1. Crowley RW, Pouratian N, Sheehan JP. Gamma knife surgery for glioblastoma multiforme. *Neurosurg Focus*. 2006;20(4): E17.
2. Masciopinto JE, Levin AB, Mehta MP, et al. Stereotactic radiosurgery for glioblastoma: a final report of 31 patients. *J Neurosurg*. 1995;82(4):530–535.
3. Loeffler JS, Alexander E III, Shea WM, et al. Radiosurgery as part of the initial management of patients with malignant gliomas. *J Clin Oncol*. 1992;10(9):1379–1385.
4. Hsieh PC, Chandler JP, Bhangoo S, et al. Adjuvant gamma knife stereotactic radiosurgery at the time of tumor progression potentially improves survival for patients with glioblastoma multiforme. *Neurosurgery*. 2005;57(4):684–692; discussion 684–692.
5. Pouratian N, Crowley RW, Sherman JH, et al. Gamma Knife radiosurgery after radiation therapy as an adjunctive treatment for glioblastoma. *J Neurooncol*. 2009;94(3):409–418.
6. Mahajan A, McCutcheon IE, Suki D, et al. Case-control study of stereotactic radiosurgery for recurrent glioblastoma multiforme. *J Neurosurg*. 2005;103(2):210–217.

7. Romanelli P, Conti A, Pontoriero A, et al. Role of stereotactic radiosurgery and fractionated stereotactic radiotherapy for the treatment of recurrent glioblastoma multiforme. *Neurosurg Focus.* 2009;27(6):E8.
8. Souhami L, Seiferheld W, Brachman D, et al. Randomized comparison of stereotactic radiosurgery followed by conventional radiotherapy with carmustine to conventional radiotherapy with carmustine for patients with glioblastoma multiforme: report of Radiation Therapy Oncology Group 93–05 protocol. *Int J Radiat Oncol Biol Phys.* 2004;60(3):853–860.
9. Combs SE, Widmer V, Thilmann C, et al. Stereotactic radiosurgery (SRS): treatment option for recurrent glioblastoma multiforme (GBM). *Cancer.* 2005;104(10):2168–2173.
10. Hall WA, Djalilian HR, Sperduto PW, et al. Stereotactic radiosurgery for recurrent malignant gliomas. *J Clin Oncol.* 1995;13(7):1642–1648.
11. Kondziolka D, Flickinger JC, Bissonette DJ, et al. Survival benefit of stereotactic radiosurgery for patients with malignant glial neoplasms. *Neurosurgery.* 1997;41(4):776–783; discussion 783–775.
12. Lederman G, Wronski M, Arbit E, et al. Treatment of recurrent glioblastoma multiforme using fractionated stereotactic radiosurgery and concurrent paclitaxel. *Am J Clin Oncol.* 2000;23(2):155–159.
13. Wang LW, Shiau CY, Chung WY, et al. Gamma Knife surgery for low-grade astrocytomas: evaluation of long-term outcome based on a 10-year experience. *J Neurosurg,* 2006;(105 suppl):127–132.
14. Henderson MA, Fakiris AJ, Timmerman RD, et al. Gamma knife stereotactic radiosurgery for low-grade astrocytomas. *Stereotact Funct Neurosurg.* 2009;87(3):161–167.
15. Suh JHBarnett GH. Stereotactic radiosurgery for brain tumors in pediatric patients. *Technol Cancer Res Treat.* 2003;2(2):141–146.
16. Lo SS, Fakiris AJ, Abdulrahman R, et al. Role of stereotactic radiosurgery and fractionated stereotactic radiotherapy in pediatric brain tumors. *Expert Rev Neurother,* 2008;8(1):121–132.
17. Bauman G, Lote K, Larson D, et al. Pretreatment factors predict overall survival for patients with low-grade glioma: a recursive partitioning analysis. *Int J Radiat Oncol Biol Phys.* 1999;45(4):923–929.
18. Hadjipanayis CG, Kondziolka D, Flickinger JC, et al. The role of stereotactic radiosurgery for low-grade astrocytomas. *Neurosurg Focus.* 2003;14(5):e15.
19. Hadjipanayis CG, Kondziolka D, Gardner P, et al. Stereotactic radiosurgery for pilocytic astrocytomas when multimodal therapy is necessary. *J Neurosurg.* 2002; 97(1):56–64.
20. Hadjipanayis CG, Niranjan A, Tyler-Kabara E, et al. Stereotactic radiosurgery for well-circumscribed fibrillary grade II astrocytomas: an initial experience. *Stereotact Funct Neurosurg.* 2002;79(1):13–24.
21. Somaza SC, Kondziolka D, Lunsford LD, et al. Early outcomes after stereotactic radiosurgery for growing pilocytic astrocytomas in children. *Pediatr Neurosurg.* 1996;25(3):109–115.
22. Kida Y, Kobayashi T, Mori Y. Gamma knife radiosurgery for low-grade astrocytomas: results of long-term follow up. *J Neurosurg.* 2000;(93 suppl 3):42–46.
23. Barcia JA, Barcia-Salorio JL, Ferrer C, et al. Stereotactic radiosurgery of deeply seated low grade gliomas. *Acta Neurochir Suppl.* 1994;62:58–61.
24. Lo SS, Abdulrahman R, Desrosiers PM, et al. The role of Gamma Knife Radiosurgery in the management of unresectable gross disease or gross residual disease after surgery in ependymoma. *J Neurooncol.* 2006;79(1):51–56.

25. Kano H, Niranjan A, Kondziolka D, et al. Outcome predictors for intracranial ependymoma radiosurgery. *Neurosurgery*. 2009;64(2):279–287; discussion 287–278.
26. Healey EA, Barnes PD, Kupsky WJ, et al. The prognostic significance of postoperative residual tumor in ependymoma. *Neurosurgery*. 1991;28(5):666–671; discussion 671–662.
27. Lyons MK, Kelly PJ. Posterior fossa ependymomas: report of 30 cases and review of the literature. *Neurosurgery*. 1991;28(5):659–664; discussion 664–655.
28. Ernestus RI, Schroder R, Stutzer H, et al. Prognostic relevance of localization and grading in intracranial ependymomas of childhood. *Childs Nerv Syst*. 1996;12(9):522–526.
29. Kano H, Niranjan A, Khan A, et al. Does radiosurgery have a role in the management of oligodendrogliomas? *J Neurosurg*. 2009;110(3):564–571.
30. Sarkar A, Pollock BE, Brown PD, et al. Evaluation of gamma knife radiosurgery in the treatment of oligodendrogliomas and mixed oligodendroastrocytomas. *J Neurosurg*. 2002;97(5 suppl):653–656.
31. Yen CP, Sheehan J, Patterson G, et al. Gamma knife surgery for neurocytoma. *J Neurosurg*. 2007;107(1):7–12.
32. Kim CY, Paek SH, Jeong SS, et al. Gamma knife radiosurgery for central neurocytoma: primary and secondary treatment. *Cancer*. 2007;110(10):2276–2284.
33. Hassoun J, Gambarelli D, Grisoli F, et al. Central neurocytoma. An electron-microscopic study of two cases. *Acta Neuropathol*. 1982;56(2):151–156.
34. Kim DG, Paek SH, Kim IH, et al. Central neurocytoma: the role of radiation therapy and long term outcome. *Cancer*. 1997;79(10):1995–2002.
35. Schild SE, Scheithauer BW, Haddock MG, et al. Central neurocytomas. *Cancer*. 1997;79(4):790–795.
36. Hassoun J, Soylemezoglu F, Gambarelli D, et al. Central neurocytoma: a synopsis of clinical and histological features. *Brain Pathol*. 1993;3(3):297–306.
37. Anderson RC, Elder JB, Parsa AT, et al. Radiosurgery for the treatment of recurrent central neurocytomas. *Neurosurgery*, 2001;48(6):1231–1237; discussion 1237–1238.
38. Genc A, Bozkurt SU, Karabagli P, et al. Gamma knife radiosurgery for cranial neurocytomas. *J Neurooncol*. 2011.
39. Bertalanffy A, Roessler K, Dietrich W, et al. Gamma knife radiosurgery of recurrent central neurocytomas: a preliminary report. *J Neurol Neurosurg Psychiatry*. 2001;70(4):489–493.
40. Cobery ST, Noren G, Friehs GM, et al. Gamma knife surgery for treatment of central neurocytomas. Report of four cases. *J Neurosurg*. 2001;94(2):327–330.
41. Tyler-Kabara E, Kondziolka D, Flickinger JC, et al. Stereotactic radiosurgery for residual neurocytoma. Report of four cases. *J Neurosurg*. 2001;95(5):879–882.
42. Sayer FT, Nguyen J, Starke RM, et al. Gamma knife radiosurgery for intracranial hemangioblastomas--outcome at 3 years. *World Neurosurg*. 2011;75(1):99–105; discussion 145-108.
43. Kano H, Niranjan A, Mongia S, et al. The role of stereotactic radiosurgery for intracranial hemangioblastomas. *Neurosurgery*. 2008;63(3):443–450; discussion 450–441.
44. Jawahar A, Kondziolka D, Garces YI, et al. Stereotactic radiosurgery for hemangioblastomas of the brain. *Acta Neurochir (Wien)*. 2000;142(6):641–644; discussion 644–645.
45. Linehan WM, Lerman MI, Zbar B. Identification of the von Hippel-Lindau (VHL) gene. Its role in renal cancer. *JAMA*. 1995;273(7):564–570.
46. Neumann HP, Berger DP, Sigmund G, et al. Pheochromocytomas, multiple endocrine neoplasia type 2, and von Hippel-Lindau disease. *N Engl J Med*. 1993;329(21):1531–1538.

47. Jagannathan J, Lonser RR, Smith R, et al. Surgical management of cerebellar hemangioblastomas in patients with von Hippel-Lindau disease. *J Neurosurg.* 2008;108(2):210–222.
48. Jeffreys R. Clinical and surgical aspects of posterior fossa haemangioblastomata. *J Neurol Neurosurg Psychiatry.* 1975;38(2):105–111.
49. Moss JM, Choi CY, Adler JR Jr, et al. Stereotactic radiosurgical treatment of cranial and spinal hemangioblastomas. *Neurosurgery.* 2009;65(1):79–85; discussion 85.
50. Wang EM, Pan L, Wang BJ, et al. The long-term results of gamma knife radiosurgery for hemangioblastomas of the brain. *J Neurosurg.* 2005;(102 suppl):225–229.
51. Kanno H, Kondo K, Ito S, et al. Somatic mutations of the von Hippel-Lindau tumor suppressor gene in sporadic central nervous system hemangioblastomas. *Cancer Res.* 1994;54(18):4845–4847.
52. Matsunaga S, Shuto T, Inomori S, et al. Gamma knife radiosurgery for intracranial haemangioblastomas. *Acta Neurochir (Wien).* 2007;149(10):1007–1013; discussion 1013.
53. Patrice SJ, Sneed PK, Flickinger JC, et al. Radiosurgery for hemangioblastoma: results of a multiinstitutional experience. *Int J Radiat Oncol Biol Phys.* 1996;35(3):493–499.

Chapter 4
Intraparenchymal Tumors

B. Radiosurgery for Brain Metastases

Lawrence R. Kleinberg

Brain metastasis is a frequent problem in the management of cancer. Brain metastasis is estimated to occur in 170,000 patients each year in the United States, possibly impacting a quarter of all adult solid tumor patients (1,2). This may be a problem of increasing clinical significance as therapies for systemic disease, which frequently do not penetrate the blood–brain barrier, may improve the control of disease elsewhere and thereby increase the importance to survival and quality of life of control of tumor in the brain.

In fact, aggressive management of brain metastasis, often with stereotactic radiosurgery, has indeed been shown to improve quality of life and survival in selected patients in randomized trials carried out in the late 1980s through the 1990s (3,4). Although escalating the dose of whole-brain radiation (1,2,5) has not been demonstrated to be beneficial, surgery and radiosurgery, which substantially intensify therapy for individual lesions in patients with oligometastatic disease, does result in improved outcome. In these trials, surgical resection or radiosurgery was used for control of known gross lesions along with whole-brain radiotherapy (WBRT), which was administered as the standard treatment of the time with the goal of treating undetected small deposits elsewhere in the brain. Because WBRT has short-term and longer term toxicities that might be highly relevant to many patients, there has since been increasing interest in omitting WBRT for selected patients.

There is now strong evidence from randomized trials (6–8) that survival is not adversely affected by omitting WBRT for patients with one to four metastases, and several single-arm reports suggest that this is also an appropriate choice for patients with an even larger number of lesions. In a discussion framed by the reality that survival outcome is similar either way and that the illness will ultimately be fatal due to systemic progression regardless of the intervention used for the brain disease, it is appropriate for patients to themselves make a choice after considering the toxicities and risks of WBRT balanced against reduced incidence of new lesions and need for later treatment with its risks. The most significant available data relevant to physicians and patients in making these decisions are summarized below.

WHOLE-BRAIN RADIOTHERAPY FOR BRAIN METASTASIS: THE HISTORICAL STANDARD FOR ALL PATIENTS

For many years WBRT was the standard and only option for treatment of brain metastasis (1,2), and is still used for many patients for a variety of important reasons: preference by many treating physicians and patients, bulky metastasis, too many lesions to be appropriate candidates for focal treatment, when speed in starting treatment is critical, and when extent of systemic disease or poor condition make it unlikely that the patient will have a favorable enough malignancy outcome to benefit from this more resource intensive intervention. The rationale for omitting whole-brain radiation despite a higher probability of new lesions is described below.

The survival results after WBRT have been analyzed for a large number of patients enrolled in Radiation Therapy Oncology Group (RTOG) clinical trials (9,10). These and subsequent trials did not show a benefit in palliation or survival with increasing doses of WBRT or hyperfractionated therapy (5) in comparison with standard therapy of 30 Gy in 10 fractions. Recursive partitioning analysis (RPA) was used to identify clinically useful prognostic groups based on this database of 1200 patients enrolled on clinical trials, likely a favorable population. Group I includes those patients aged younger than 65, performance score of 70 or greater, controlled primary tumor, and known active disease in the brain only with median survival of 7.3 months; group III includes patients with performance status less than 70 with median survival of 2.3 months; and group II includes all other patients with a median survival of 4.2 months. However, recent trials including WBRT, often along with potential radiosensitizing drugs, have not clearly suggested improved outcome compared with these earlier studies, in the range of 4 to 6 months (11,12) and 7.7 months for the very recently reported RTOG 0614 trial. It is important to recognize that the improved control of brain metastasis may have only limited potential to improve survival as the majority may expire from systemic spread (13).

The toxicities of WBRT may be of important concern to this patient population in which maximizing quality of life in the immediate future may be important for all patients and avoidance of later neurocognitive toxicities may be of great importance as well to the proportion who will become long-term survivors. In the immediate term, WBRT involves a 2- to 3-week time commitment and may cause an interruption of systemic therapy of 3 to 6 weeks that may be an important issue. Short-term toxicities that often are not severe but which may meaningfully affect the quality of life of most patients and may persist for months include: fatigue, malaise, alopecia, decreased hearing, skin reactions, headaches, and cerebral edema with associated neurologic deficits that may require corticosteroids. These toxicities, even when temporary, may interfere with the patients "normal" life and persist for a significant portion of the available survival time.

Recently reported results of a randomized trial (14) conducted by the RTOG demonstrates the impact of WBRT on neurocognitive function during a 1-year period of follow-up. This randomized trial included neurocognitive outcome after prophylactic WBRT for the purpose of preventing metastasis in patients curatively treated for non small cell lung cancer. As a result, the radiation used was less substantial than the doses typically used in the therapy of known metastatic disease, 30 Gy in 15 fractions, and included patients without preexisting tumor-related brain injury. The Mini-Mental State Examination, which may detect gross declines in global function, was significantly more likely to have deteriorated 3 months post-treatment in patients treated with radiation, although this difference did not persist through 6 months and longer follow-up presumably due to recovery from subacute toxicities. However, the more sensitive Hopkins Verbal Learning Test demonstrated a significantly higher proportion of patients with decline at both 3 months and 1 year in both early and delayed recall.

BENEFIT TO AGGRESSIVE MANAGEMENT OF BRAIN METASTASIS: INTENSIFIED LOCAL TREATMENT ALONG WITH WHOLE-BRAIN RADIOTHERAPY

A major stride forward in the management of brain metastasis was a landmark randomized trial organized by Patchell (15), for patients with a single brain metastasis, which convincingly demonstrated for the first time that intensive management of brain metastasis could actually improve survival outcome. This trial, with accrual completed in 1988, demonstrated that resection, when added to standard WBRT, actually improved both survival and function. The results are summarized in Table 4B.1.

A subsequent RTOG trial (3) demonstrated that radiosurgery added to WBRT similarly improved survival for those with a single brain metastasis and quality of life for those with two to three lesions. A single lesion could be up to 4 cm in diameter, if the remainder were less than 3 cm. For patients with one lesion, the median survival improved from 4.9 to 6.5 months ($p = .04$). For two to three lesions, although there was no survival benefit with the addition of radiosurgery, the percentage of patients with stable or improved performance status 6 months after treatment was improved from 27% to 43% ($p = .03$).

These issues are unexplored in randomized trials for those with a larger number of metastases. Although we believe, based on these results, it is appropriate to consider radiosurgery in patients with one to three metastases who have

TABLE 4B.1 Benefit to Surgical Resection

	RT Alone	RT/Surgery
Survival	15 weeks	40 weeks
Local recurrence	52%	20%
Functional independence	8 weeks	38 weeks
Other brain recurrence	13%	20%

Adapted from Patchell RA, Tibbs PA, Walsh JW, et al. A randomized trial of surgery in the treatment of single metastasis to the brain. *N Engl J Med.* 1990;322(8):494–500.

been treated with WBRT, but that for more lesions in the whole-brain treated patient it would be most appropriate to monitor and treat only lesions that may progress later. Moreover, there has been no randomized trial comparing surgery and radiosurgery in the management of brain metastasis.

FOCAL MANAGEMENT WITHOUT WHOLE-BRAIN RADIOTHERAPY: REDUCED TOXICITY WITH GOOD OUTCOME FOR MANY PATIENTS

As a result of the WBRT toxicities described previously there has been increasing interest in eliminating this treatment from the management of patients with oligometastasis. Whole-brain radiation also involves a more significant time commitment and may delay needed systemic therapy. The validity of using radiosurgery alone has now been confirmed in randomized trials with patients with up to four radiosurgery-treatable metastases, demonstrating similar survival with omission of WBRT but greater incidence of new metastasis requiring treatment in the future. Moreover, single institution reports suggest that survival is not meaningfully decreased when even more than 10 metastases are treated with radiosurgery alone without WBRT.

Early studies demonstrated excellent local control of individual metastasis with radiosurgery, suggesting that this is an appropriate alternative to surgical resection (Figure 4B.1). For example, a series reported by Gerosa (16,17) in 2002 demonstrated 93% 1-year actuarial local control for lesions treated this way as well as survival that appeared similar to resection with radiation. It should be noted that radiosurgery has been typically limited to lesions under 3 cm in size (occasionally up to 4 cm), whereas surgical series include larger metastases. Nevertheless, this and similar studies provided motivation to explore further radiosurgery alone without WBRT. Early data from University of California San Francisco (UCSF) also suggested the validity of this approach (17).

Three important randomized trials (6–8) that examined the role of radiosurgery alone versus radiosurgery with WBRT have been reported in the United States, Europe, and Japan. These trials confirmed that there is no suggestion of a survival benefit to adding WBRT to radiosurgery. The important elements of these trials are summarized in Table 4B.2. None of these trials demonstrated a survival benefit to the addition of WBRT even though distant brain failure at previously

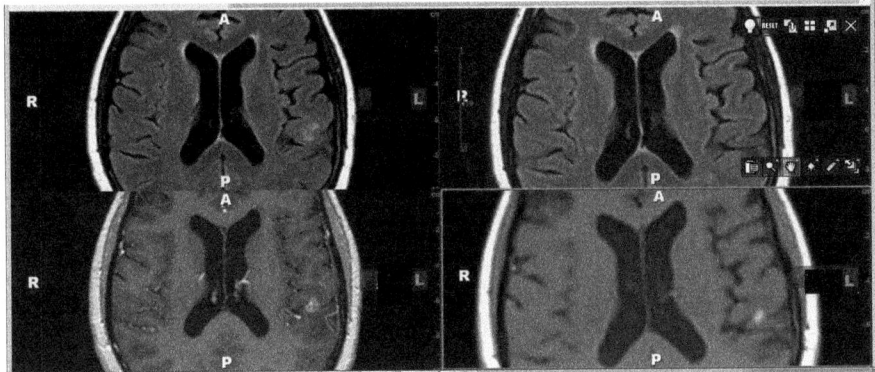

FIGURE 4B.1 63-year-old female with known metastatic breast cancer before (left) and 3 months after stereotactic radiosurgery (right), 18 Gy prescribed to periphery of lesion.

TABLE 4B.2 Postoperative Radiotherapy for Resected Brain Metastasis

	Surg Alone	Surg/RT (5040 Rads)
Survival	43 weeks	48 weeks
Brain recurrence	70%	18%
Original site	46%	10%
Other sites	37%	14%
Neurologic death	44%	14%

Adapted from Patchell RA, Tibbs PA, Regine WF, et al. Postoperative radiotherapy in the treatment of single metastasis to the brain: a randomized trial. *JAMA*. 1998;280(17):1485–1489.

uninvolved sites was higher without WBRT. In contrast, a survival advantage to radiosurgery alone was seen in the single institution trial conducted at M.D Anderson trial reported by Chang, although it should be noted that the primary objective of that trial was not survival but neurocognitive outcome. The trial was closed early due to an observed benefit for the neurocognitive endpoints.

In all three of these randomized studies, distant brain failure, which is potentially preventable, was higher in the absence of WBRT. It ranged from 48% to 64% (6,8) when radiosurgery alone was used. These recurrences generally require treatment when they occur, and this potential need should be considered by patients as they select among treatment options. It is important to note that whole-brain radiation is only partially effective at preventing recurrence elsewhere in the brain, reducing the incidence to 33% to 41% (6–8) in these trials. Thus, to have a survival impact of omission of WBRT an individual patient would need to have brain recurrence, experience a failure of salvage therapy, and not first succumb to the competing risk of systemic disease—therefore we believe either choice is appropriate. Follow-up to screen for new lesions may be important regardless of use of WBRT as new lesions may be symptomatic (18). In general, it is appropriate to discuss with patients selecting this option that there is a much higher chance of needing subsequent treatment that must be traded off against the potential benefits of avoiding WBRT.

TUMOR BED RADIOSURGERY AFTER RESECTION OF BRAIN METASTASIS WITHOUT WHOLE-BRAIN TREATMENT?

The study described previously conducted by Patchell, which demonstrated that a benefit to surgical resection added to whole-brain therapy for a single brain metastasis, was then followed by a trial comparing surgery alone to surgery with or without WBRT (15). The results, summarized in Table 4B.3, indicated similar survival but with high local recurrence rate in the resection bed. As a result of the high local recurrence rate on top of the incidence of new distant lesions, WBRT became the generally accepted standard after resection even in the absence of a survival benefit.

A recently reported European Organisation for Research and Treatment of Cancer (EORTC) (19) randomized trial conducted from 1996 to 2007 confirmed lack of survival benefit (median survival 10.9 months) but substantial local control improvement when WBRT is added in the management. In this randomized trial, the 2-year failure rate in the tumor bed was 59% with surgery alone, reduced to 27% with the addition of conventional radiotherapy with distant brain failure of 42% reduced to 23%.

TABLE 4B.3 Randomized Trials Comparing Radiosurgery, With or Without WBRT

Trial	Patients	Survival	Distant Brain Control
JROSG99–1 (20) Aoyama JAMA 295, 2006, 2483	122 pts 1–4 mets 3 cm maximum diameter KPS > 70	8 versus 7.5 months	1-year actuarial distant brain failure 64% (SRS) versus 41% (WBRT). Neurologic death 19% (SRS) VS. 21% (WBRT)
EORTC (19) 22952–2601 JCO 29, 2010, 134	185 pts 1–3 mets Up to 35 mm diameter for single met Up to 25 mm in diameter for multiple metastasis Performance status 0–2 Able to interrupt chemo for whole-brain RT	10.9 months Whole-brain RT not prognostic	Distant brain failure 33% versus 48%
Chang//MDAH Lancet Oncol 10, 2009, *	58 pts 1–3 mets Up to 4 cm KPS > 70	1-year survival 63% SRS versus 21% WBRT Stopped early due to better cognitive outcome with no WBRT	1-year progression in brain 73% (SRS) versus 27% (WBRT)

As there is not a survival benefit, it is appropriate to either provide whole-brain radiation after surgical resection to reduce the risks of recurrence or omit WBRT to avoid the toxicities described earlier. An appropriate alternative is to stereotactically target the tumor bed, the highest risk area for recurrence. Although not assessed in randomized trials, numerous reports suggest good success at controlling disease in the area at highest risk of need for treatment with a type of radiation unlikely to have the global toxicities of whole-brain treatment. The several single institution trials (21–25) suggest tumor bed recurrence rate varying from 0% to 20% after stereotactic postoperative therapy.

RADIOSURGERY OR SURGERY: WHICH IS OPTIMAL FOR LOCAL MANAGEMENT?

Although both approaches are beneficial, surgery and radiosurgery have not been compared in randomized trials, and any informal comparison of results is fraught with peril as selection criteria for these two therapies may vary widely. In fact, radiosurgery and open surgery may be most applicable to different populations. Surgery is most appropriate when the operative approach is likely to be safe, for large lesions where radiosurgery dose may be limited, for one to two lesions, for symptomatic lesions where removal may immediately relieve symptomatic pressure on normal brain, and when the diagnosis of metastatic cancer is uncertain. Radiosurgery is well suited for lesions under 2 to 3 cm in size as the radiotherapy dose is limited by safety concerns as the size increases beyond this range, for asymptomatic lesions even if steroids are required, lesions not addressable by surgery because of location or quantity, and in patients where medical risks or widespread metastatic diseases decrease the appropriateness of surgery. It is also important to consider that even when surgery is used, radiation is generally necessary to achieve durable local control.

LARGER NUMBERS OF DETECTED BRAIN METASTASES: MAY WHOLE-BRAIN RADIATION BE OMITTED?

Although the validity of focal therapy with radiosurgery without WBRT has been demonstrated for one to three or four lesions in randomized trials, this approach has not been tested when there are more metastases. The potential advantages continue to be the potential for decreased toxicities and decreased time commitment. This therapy may be most appropriate for patients with a favorable performance status and less bulky disease.

Outcome has been described in multiple single institution reports (26–31). The survival appears similar to the outcome expected for therapy with WBRT, and therefore may be beneficial as toxicities may be avoided and systemic therapies may be restarted more quickly. Although survival appears to be somewhat worse with increasing number of metastases, this is also the case when WBRT is used and it should not be assumed that WBRT would have resulted in a meaningfully improved outcome.

Data from UCSF reporting survival after radiosurgery for brain metastasis indicated similar survival regardless of number of lesions up to 16 (32). Amendola from the Miami Neuroscience Center reported median survival of 4.1 months in a group of patients with 10 or more lesions, but survival was substantially better for those with Karnofsky performance status greater than 70 or total tumor volume less than 30 cm^3 (31). Data from our combined experience at Johns Hopkins and the Miami Neuroscience Center also suggests that this therapy is appropriate in patients with four or more lesions, with the observation that poor performance status is a powerful negative prognostic factor for survival as is the total disease volume. In addition, we found that only a modest proportion of patients appeared to expire as a result of the brain metastasis.

This is supported by information from other single institution trials including even more than 10 lesions, which suggest survival that is not appreciably different than what would be expected with WBRT, although there is a general trend observed of lower survival with multiple brain metastases. However, it is not clear that the outcome for patients with a large number of metastases would necessarily be improved with the use of WBRT as number of metastases is associated with poorer survival when that therapy is used as well (9).

Therefore, this approach may be used in selected cases with large number of metastases with the goal of sparing the toxicities of WBRT, where disruptions in needed systemic therapy can be minimized with this approach, and in those who have had prior WBRT, and with careful consideration of the ultimate prognosis and the risk of new lesions in untreated areas. In this situation where both options are appropriate, careful discussion with the patient of the high probability of new lesions requiring treatment inherent in this approach is especially important under the circumstance of known multiple metastases. It is likely that optimal candidates are those with small-volume disease despite the multiplicity of lesions and good performance status. Double contrast and/or thin cut volumetric MRI scan for therapy planning may optimize detection of existing metastasis, which can be treated at the same time thereby minimizing the near-term need for more treatment. We have found this to be an attractive option for patients even with a large number of small metastases given the limited toxicity experienced by most patients.

RADIOSURGERY DOSE SELECTION

The doses used in these randomized trials may provide guidance to dose selection as prescribed to the periphery of the lesion in routine practice. There is no rigorously obtained data to guide optimal selection of radiation dose to balance

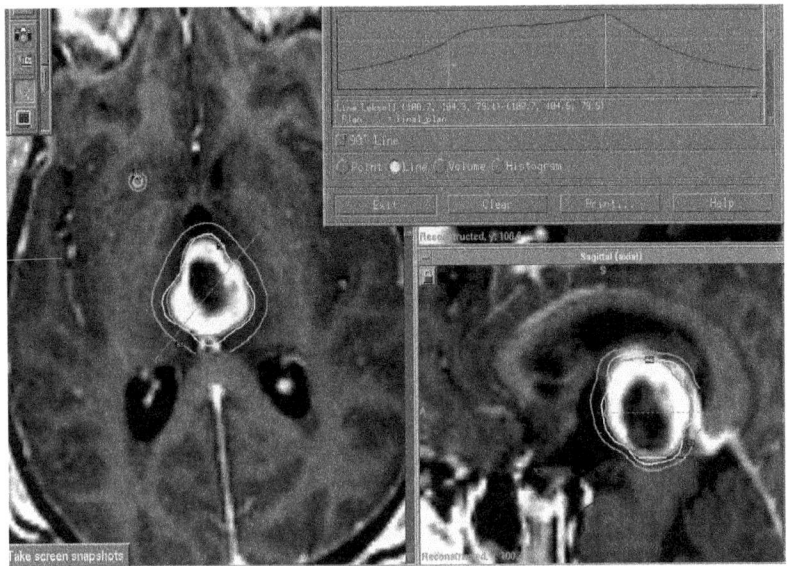

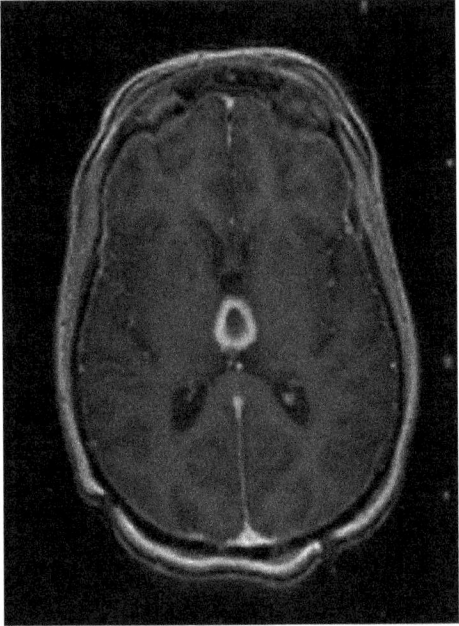

FIGURE 4B.2 Illustrative case. 34-year-old female patient with melanoma. Six months after completing whole-brain radiotherapy she had five growing lesions, including a ventricular mass (A) and four subcentimeter lesions. These were treated with stereotactic radiosurgery 18 Gy prescribed to the periphery. The 4-month follow-up scan is depicted; she expired 8 months later with systemic progression but control of brain disease with intact neurologic function. The 4-month follow-up scan is depicted (B).

control and risks for individual patients. Trial RTOG 90–05 (33) determined maximally tolerated doses of radiosurgery after prior brain radiation. The doses were 24, 18, and 15 Gy, respectively, for tumors less than or equal to 20 mm, 21 to 30 mm, and 31 to 40 mm in maximum diameter. We do not recommend significantly exceeding these guidelines without a compelling rationale even when radiosurgery alone is used as it is useful to preserve the ability to safely add WBRT if needed in the future. In addition, in a disease where cure is not feasible, substantial risk of injury to the brain does not seem justifiable when standard doses already appear effective.

MDAH (34) used dosing according to RTOG 90–05 described earlier, whether or not the patient was randomized to also receive WBRT. In the JROSG trial (20), metastases with a maximum diameter of up to 2 cm were treated with doses of 22 to 25 Gy and those of 2 to 3 cm were treated with doses of 18 to 20 Gy.

A 30% dose reduction was applied when radiosurgery was combined with whole-brain therapy. In the trial conducted by the EORTC (8), minimal peripheral dose of 20 Gy was used for a single lesion with maximal diameter 35 mm for single metastasis and 25 mm maximal diameter for multiple metastases, and not altered if WBRT was also given. Lower doses to individual lesions may be considered, especially when a high number of metastases are treated to ameliorate what may be an increasing cumulative risk of significant toxicity.

In the special case of treatment of a surgical resection cavity, lower doses of 16 to 18 Gy (25) are often used as only subclinical disease is present. Hypofractionated regimens of three to five sessions are also used with little rigorous information to guide selection, which may be safer for large lesions above approximately 3 cm in diameter. Alternatives include 21 to 24 Gy in three fractions and 25 Gy in five fractions. The utility and safety of adding 1–2 mm margin to the target is controversial, but may be especially desirable for postoperative therapy when the goal is treatment of subclinical residual following surgery done several weeks earlier.

CONCLUSION

Aggressive management of brain metastasis can lead to improved survival and quality of life, although the potential impact may be lower in patients with less survival expectancy from systemic disease as measured by poor performance status. Radiosurgery alone without WBRT may be appropriate for many patients, and is associated with decreased toxicity. Although there may be a higher probability of later new lesions requiring treatment, the toxicities affecting quality of life of WBRT is avoided. Radiosurgery alone has been validated by randomized trials for patients with up to four metastases, and there is substantial evidence that it is appropriate for patients with a larger number of lesions. Surgical resection should be considered for patients with a single metastasis, when diagnosis is unclear, for symptomatic lesions, and for larger lesions that might not be well treated with radiosurgery. As local recurrence is common in the resection bed and substantially reduced by treatment, postoperative WBRT or stereotactic tumor cavity boost should be considered.

REFERENCES

1. Tsao MN, Khuntia D, Mehta MP. Brain metastases: what's new with an old problem? *Curr Opin Support Palliat Care*. 2012;6(1):85–90.
2. Platta CS, Khuntia D, Mehta MP, Suh JH. Current treatment strategies for brain metastasis and complications from therapeutic techniques: a review of current literature. *Am J Clin Oncol*. 2010;33(4):398–407.
3. Andrews DW, Scott CB, Sperduto PW, et al. Whole brain radiation therapy with or without stereotactic radiosurgery boost for patients with one to three brain metastases: phase III results of the RTOG 9508 randomised trial. *Lancet*. 2004;363(9422):1665–1672.
4. Patchell RA, Tibbs PA, Walsh JW, et al. A randomized trial of surgery in the treatment of single metastasis to the brain. *N Engl J Med*. 1990;322(8):494–500.
5. Murray KJ, Scott C, Greenberg HM, et al. A randomized phase III study of accelerated hyperfractionation versus standard in patients with unresected brain metastases: a report of the radiation therapy oncology group (RTOG) 9104. *Int J Radiat Oncol Biol Phys*. 1997;39(3):571–574.
6. Aoyama H, Shirato H, Tago M, et al. Stereotactic radiosurgery plus whole-brain radiation therapy vs stereotactic radiosurgery alone for treatment of brain metastases: a randomized controlled trial. *JAMA*. 2006;295(21):2483–2491.
7. Chang EL, Wefel JS, Hess KR, et al. Neurocognition in patients with brain metastases treated with radiosurgery or radiosurgery plus whole-brain irradiation: a randomised controlled trial. *Lancet Oncol*. 2009;10(11):1037–1044.
8. Kocher M, Soffietti R, Abacioglu U, et al. Adjuvant whole-brain radiotherapy versus observation after radiosurgery or surgical resection of one to three cerebral metastases: results of the EORTC 22952–26001 study. *J Clin Oncol*. 2011;29(2):134–141.
9. Sperduto PW, Kased N, Roberge D, et al. Summary report on the graded prognostic assessment: an accurate and facile diagnosis-specific tool to estimate survival for patients with brain metastases. *J Clin Oncol*. 2012;30(4):419–425.
10. Gaspar L, Scott C, Rotman M, et al. Recursive partitioning analysis (RPA) of prognostic factors in three radiation therapy oncology group (RTOG) brain metastases trials. *Int J Radiat Oncol Biol Phys*. 1997;37(4):745–751.
11. Mehta MP, Shapiro WR, Phan SC, et al. Motexafin gadolinium combined with prompt whole brain radiotherapy prolongs time to neurologic progression in non-small-cell lung cancer patients with brain metastases: results of a phase III trial. *Int J Radiat Oncol Biol Phys*. 2009;73(4):1069–1076.
12. Suh JH, Stea B, Nabid A, et al. Phase III study of efaproxiral as an adjunct to whole-brain radiation therapy for brain metastases. *J Clin Oncol*. 2006;24(1):106–114.
13. Kleinberg LR, Batra S, Wolfe A. Survival and brain metastases related mortality: a multicenter review of treatment with gamma knife. Presented at the American Radium Society 94th Annual Meeting, April 28, 2012; Las Vegas, NV.

14. Sun A, Bae K, Gore EM, et al. Phase III trial of prophylactic cranial irradiation compared with observation in patients with locally advanced non-small-cell lung cancer: neurocognitive and quality-of-life analysis. *J Clin Oncol.* 2011;29(3):279–286.
15. Patchell RA, Tibbs PA, Regine WF, et al. Postoperative radiotherapy in the treatment of single metastasis to the brain: a randomized trial. *JAMA.* 1998;280(17):1485–1489.
16. Gerosa M, Nicolato A, Foroni R, et al. Gamma knife radiosurgery for brain metastases: a primary therapeutic option. *J Neurosurg.* 2002;97(5 suppl):515–524.
17. Sneed PK, Lamborn KR, Forstner JM, et al. Radiosurgery for brain metastases: is whole brain radiotherapy necessary? *Int J Radiat Oncol Biol Phys.* 1999;43(3):549–558.
18. Regine WF, Huhn JL, Patchell RA, et al. Risk of symptomatic brain tumor recurrence and neurologic deficit after radiosurgery alone in patients with newly diagnosed brain metastases: results and implications. *Int J Radiat Oncol Biol Phys.* 2002;52(2):333–338.
19. Kocher M, Soffietti R, Abacioglu U, et al. Adjuvant whole-brain radiotherapy versus observation after radiosurgery or surgical resection of one to three cerebral metastases: results of the EORTC 22952-26001 study. *J Clin Oncol.* 2011;29(2):134–141.
20. Aoyama H, Shirato H, Tago M, et al. Stereotactic radiosurgery plus whole-brain radiation therapy vs stereotactic radiosurgery alone for treatment of brain metastases: a randomized controlled trial. *JAMA.* 2006;295(21):2483–2491.
21. Jensen CA, Chan MD, McCoy TP, et al. Cavity-directed radiosurgery as adjuvant therapy after resection of a brain metastasis. *J Neurosurg.* 2011;114(6):1585–1591.
22. Hwang SW, Abozed MM, Hale A, et al. Adjuvant gamma knife radiosurgery following surgical resection of brain metastases: a 9-year retrospective cohort study. *J Neurooncol.* 2010;98(1):77–82.
23. Karlovits BJ, Quigley MR, Karlovits SM, et al. Stereotactic radiosurgery boost to the resection bed for oligometastatic brain disease: challenging the tradition of adjuvant whole-brain radiotherapy. *Neurosurg Focus.* 2009;27(6):E7.
24. Soltys SG, Adler JR, Lipani JD, et al. Stereotactic radiosurgery of the postoperative resection cavity for brain metastases. *Int J Radiat Oncol Biol Phys.* 2008;70(1):187–193.
25. Mathieu D, Kondziolka D, Flickinger JC, et al. Tumor bed radiosurgery after resection of cerebral metastases. *Neurosurgery.* 2008;62(4):817–823; discussion 823–4.
26. Chang WS, Kim HY, Chang JW, Park YG, Chang JH. Analysis of radiosurgical results in patients with brain metastases according to the number of brain lesions: is stereotactic radiosurgery effective for multiple brain metastases? *J Neurosurg.* 2010;(113 suppl):73–78.
27. DiLuna ML, King JT, Jr, Knisely JP, Chiang VL. Prognostic factors for survival after stereotactic radiosurgery vary with the number of cerebral metastases. *Cancer.* 2007;109(1):135–145.
28. Grandhi R, Kondziolka D, Panczykowski D, et al. Stereotactic radiosurgery using the leksell gamma knife perfexion unit in the management of patients with 10 or more brain metastases. *J Neurosurg.* 2012;117(2):237–245.
29. Grandhi R, Kondziolka D, Panczykowski D, et al. Stereotactic radiosurgery using the leksell gamma knife perfexion unit in the management of patients with 10 or more brain metastases. *J Neurosurg.* 2012;117(2):237–245.
30. Hunter GK, Suh JH, Reuther AM, et al. Treatment of five or more brain metastases with stereotactic radiosurgery. *Int J Radiat Oncol Biol Phys.* 2012;83(5):1394–1398.

31. Amendola BE, Wolf A, Coy S, Amendola MA. Radiosurgery as palliation for brain metastases: A retrospective review of 72 patients harboring multiple lesions at presentation. *J Neurosurg*. 2002;97(5 suppl):511–514.
32. Yan ES, Sneed PK, McDermott MW. Number of brain metastases is not an important prognostic factor for survival following radiosurgery for newly diagnosed nonmelanoma brain metastases. *Int J Radiat Oncol Biol Phys.* 2003;57:S131.
33. Shaw E, Scott C, Souhami L, et al. Single dose radiosurgical treatment of recurrent previously irradiated primary brain tumors and brain metastases: final report of RTOG protocol 90–05. *Int J Radiat Oncol Biol Phys*. 2000;47(2):291–298.
34. Chang EL, Wefel JS, Hess KR, et al. Neurocognition in patients with brain metastases treated with radiosurgery or radiosurgery plus whole-brain irradiation: a randomised controlled trial. *Lancet Oncol*. 2009;10(11):1037–1044.

Chapter 5

Skull Base Tumors

A. Radiosurgery for Skull Base Meningioma

Mario Moreno, Timothy Bui, & Gordon Li

GENERAL PRINCIPLES AND OVERVIEW

Meningiomas are typically benign, slow-growing tumors of the central nervous system that account for 15% to 20% of primary brain tumors with an annual incidence of 2.6 in 100,000 (1,2). Meningiomas originate from the meningeal covering of the brain and the spinal cord, emerging from arachnoid cap cells (3). They commonly attach to the dural covering of the brain and the spinal cord and can present a variety of problems to the patient (4).

Meningiomas are classified by the World Health Organization (WHO) into grade 1 (benign), grade 2 (atypical) and grade 3 (anaplastic) which account for 80, 5 to 20, and 1% to 2% of all meningiomas, respectively (5,6). In large clinical series there are strong associations between outcome and grade of the meningiomas, with patients with grade 1 tumors having greater than 80% chance of being progression free at 10 years. For patients with WHO grade 2 meningiomas, only 40% to 60% are progression free at 10 years. The median recurrence-free duration for anaplastic meningioma is 2 years (7).

Meningiomas occur in various intracranial locations with the following distribution: sphenoid ridge (16%), convexity (14%), cerebellopontine angle (13%), parasellar (12%), parasagittal (11%), posterior fossa (8%), olfactory groove (8%), falx (7%), foramen magnum (3%), orbit (3%), and other (6%) (8).

Skull base meningiomas represent a subset of meningiomas and offer one of the biggest challenges in neurosurgery. Meningiomas of the skull base include tumors located in the tentorium, foramen magnum, petrous, clivus, sphenoid wing, suprasellar, paranasal, olfactory, and optic sheath regions.

Gross-total resection of skull base meningiomas are fraught with risks due to lack of accessibility of the tumors and the surrounding critical structures. The use of primary radiosurgical ablation, subtotal resection followed by radiosurgery or radiosurgery for recurrent disease as an alternative to resection is often done safely and has become more common in the treatment paradigm for this difficult-to-treat disease.

EVALUATION AND DIAGNOSIS

Meningiomas are typically slow-growing tumors and are often found incidentally on imaging. If the patient is symptomatic, they may present with headaches, seizures, mental status changes, or focal deficits, which vary with the location and the size of the tumor. On MRI, meningiomas present as an extra-axial mass that is hypointense on T1-weighted images, hyperintense on T2-weighted imaging and uniformly contrast enhanced with gadolinium. Other findings present along with meningiomas include an enhancing dural tail, cerebrospinal fluid/vascular cleft, and hyperostosis of nearby bone. Approximately 10% to 15% of meningiomas exhibit atypical MRI findings that can mimic metastases of primary glial tumors (9).

OVERVIEW OF TREATMENT

The treatment of meningiomas is related to the extent and site of the tumor. If the lesion is asymptomatic and not growing, serial imaging and expectant management are usually the treatments of choice. Surgery is typically the treatment of choice in patients with symptomatic or enlarging resectable meningiomas. Radiation has also been commonly used as a treatment option especially for poor surgical candidates, adjuvant therapy in the case of a subtotal resection, primary treatment for unresectable tumors, or adjuvant therapy in high-grade and recurrent tumors. Chemotherapy for treatment of meningiomas has not been shown to be an effective treatment option for meningiomas although there are ongoing trials studying different regimens (10).

Studies have shown that local control rates of subtotally resected meningiomas treated with conventional external bean radiation could be as effective as gross-total resection (11). These results provided an important basis for the evaluation of techniques for radiation delivery, specifically the application of stereotactic radiosurgery (SRS).

SRS has been increasingly used as an alternative to external-beam radiotherapy for the management of meningiomas. SRS includes conventional linear acceleration, Gamma Knife (GKS), or CyberKnife and the treatments are typically used for recurrent, partially resected, surgically inaccessible tumors or for patients deemed poor surgical candidates. Radiosurgical techniques theoretically have an advantage when compared to conventional external-beam radiation when treating meningiomas as these tumors are slowly proliferating and therapeutic gains may then be achieved for these tumors with larger-sized fractions (2,12,13). In addition, the shortened course of the radiation improves the quality of life during the treatment for the patients.

Skull base meningiomas are often difficult to access surgically, and their location presents a variety of potential risks for complete excision, including cranial nerve dysfunction and cerebrospinal fluid leakage. Because of the increased risk of surgery in this location, radiosurgery is often used as part of the treatment paradigm in these patients.

SKULL BASE MENINGIOMA TREATMENTS

Skull base meningiomas have been treated extensively with SRS since 1990. SRS is a radiation technique delivered in one to five sessions defined by a high degree of spatial accuracy and rapid radiation dose fall at the periphery of the designated target lesion. Since the technique was first conceived in the 1950s, the procedure has advanced with technologic improvements in instrumentation, computing, and imaging. A large series of 972 patients performed at the University of Pittsburgh demonstrated control rates of 93% at 5 years and 87% at 10 and 15 years using a median dose to the tumor margin of 13 Gy for patients with skull base meningiomas who underwent GKS radiosurgery (14). A collection of 18 studies analyzed by Minniti et al. (15) encompassing 2919 skull base meningiomas treated with GKS radiosurgery has reported a 5-year actuarial control of 91%, whereas seven of those studies have also shown a 10-year actuarial control of 87.6% in 1626 skull base meningiomas. Doses of 12 and 18 Gy have been used for the control of skull base meningiomas with an effort to decrease doses in order to minimize toxicity while preserving therapeutic effect.

Starke et al. (16) compiled a database of 255 patients treated at the University of Virginia from 1989 to 2006 with skull base meningiomas. One hundred nine of the patients were treated solely with radiosurgery, whereas the remaining 146 were treated with GKS following resection. After a mean follow-up of 6.5 years (range 2–18), 86% of the patients had no change or displayed a decrease in tumor volume and 90% displayed no change or improvement in their neurological condition. The review determined the use of GKS for the control of tumors and neurological preservation in patients with skull base meningiomas.

CyberKnife radiosurgery provides an alternative radiosurgical treatment in which a frameless system uses image guidance provided by the patient's bony anatomy. In CyberKnife radiosurgery, the radiation is delivered from a 6 MV linear accelerator, which is mounted on a robotic manipulator. The system is then capable of focusing beams from greater than 1200 directions allowing for optimized dose delivery. CyberKnife image guidance provides a high degree of accuracy without the need of rigid fixation, as x-ray images are continuously being obtained in real time during the extent of the procedure. The images are then collected and analyzed with software and minute adjustments are made by the robotic apparatus. The frameless image-guide system provides a means to perform radiosurgery in a single dose or spread out over various sessions, which is especially important when treating lesions near radiation-sensitive structures such as in skull base meningiomas. Delivery of biologically greater radiation doses can be achieved while minimizing damage to surrounding structures (Figure 5A.1). A recent series of 199 patients with skull base meningiomas treated with CyberKnife radiosurgery in which 63 of those patients received multi-session radiosurgery demonstrated decrease in tumor size in 36 patients, stable tumor size in 148 patients, and tumor growth in seven patients (17). In a study by Mahadevan et al. (18), 16 patients with skull base meningiomas were treated with a 5-fraction regimen with a dose of 5 Gy per fraction for a total of 25 Gy.

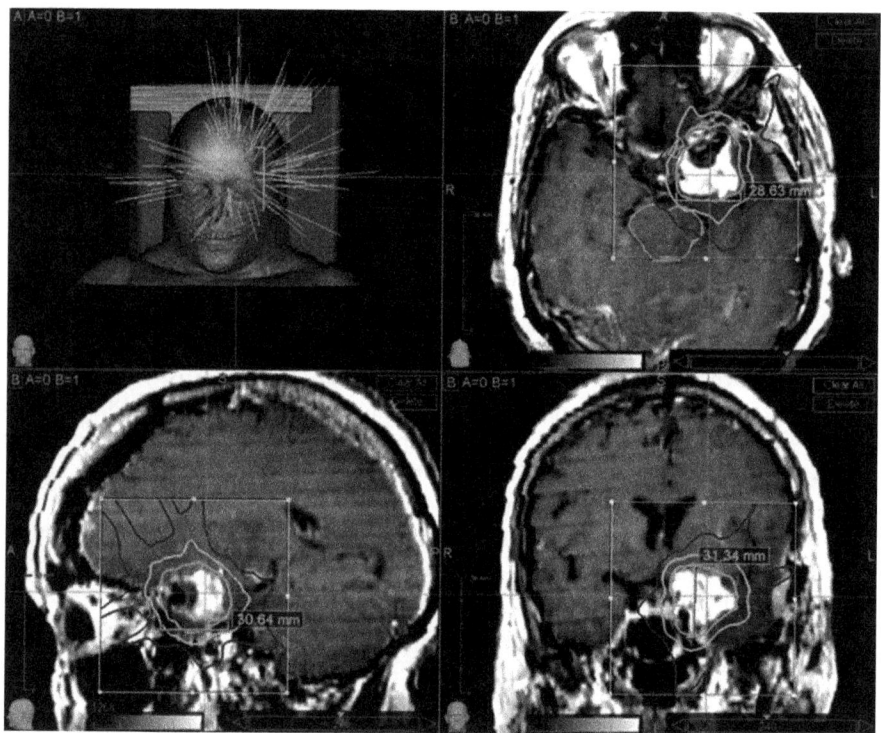

FIGURE 5A.1 CyberKnife planning for a residual left-sided medial sphenoid wing meningioma.

Radiological assessment after treatment showed local control in all tumors and no deficit in cranial nerve function.

COMPLICATIONS

Radiosurgical ablation of meningiomas is well tolerated with symptomatic complication rates ranging from 2.5% to 14% (19–21). As techniques and technologies have improved, doses to normal anatomy have been reduced and the risk of post radiosurgical complications has decreased (22–24). Patients treated since 1991 experience less toxicity (5.3% vs. 22.9%), largely because radiosurgery prescription doses were gradually decreased from a median marginal dose of 17 Gy (range 10–20) between 1987 and 1991 to 14 Gy (range 8.9–20 Gy) between 1991 and 2000 (25). Cranial nerve damage, particularly optic neuropathy, is a well-documented complication of all skull base irradiation, including SRS with one study reporting an incidence of 26.7% of optic neuropathy in patients treated with larger doses (10–15 Gy). Tishler et al. (26) studied the risk of injury to cranial nerves II to VI in 62 patients with radiosurgical doses between 10 and 40 Gy near the cavernous sinus. With a median follow-up of 19 months, 12 patients developed cranial nerve injury 3 to 41 months after treatment. Injury to cranial nerves III to VI was not related to dose. But in four patients with optic nerve injury, there was an increased risk in patients receiving greater than 8 Gy to any portion of the optic apparatus as compared to those receiving less than 8 Gy (24% vs. 0%). These risks were demonstrated with single-fraction GKS radiosurgery. A study of 49 patients (27 with meningiomas) at Stanford University using multisession CyberKnife radiosurgery for tumors within 2 mm of the optic apparatus showed 46 patients with unchanged or improved vision after two to five sessions at an average dose of 20.3 Gy (27).

Vascular complications occur in approximately 1% to 2% of patients treated with SRS. Stafford et al. (28) reported on 190 patients with meningioma (77% skull base tumors) treated with GKS. Two patients (1%) developed symptomatic carotid stenosis, 35 and 60 months after doses greater than 25 Gy to the carotid.

With larger skull base meningiomas, greater than 3.5 cm in diameter, the possible complications of SRS are significant enough to prevent the use of the treatment under most circumstances. In such instances, the risks of radiosurgery include major cranial nerve deficits, radiation necrosis, or peritumoral edema, as well as less common artery stenosis and hypothalamic dysfunction. A strategy that is typically used for managing such tumors is to combine conservative microsurgical resection with radiosurgical ablation of the smaller tumor remnant. This approach may be complicated in many elderly or medically infirm patients who are poor patients for any open surgery. Multisession radiosurgery theoretically allows for a smaller number of fractions delivered with a biologically greater radiation dose while simultaneously minimizing the risk of adjacent structures. At our institution, we are currently studying this hypothesis.

With any radiation exposure, the risk of secondary malignancies is an important consideration when comparing surgical and radiotherapeutic options. Although there have been case reports of secondary complications after SRS (29), a large retrospective study demonstrated no increased risk (30).

CONCLUSION

SRS represents a safe and highly effective treatment option for the management of skull base meningiomas. Radiosurgery provides a noninvasive method for treating lesions of the brain, such as skull base meningiomas that are critically located. The low rate of complications, either transient or permanent, have an acceptable incidence and the localized irradiation of the lesions also limits the structures exposed. Radionecrosis of the brain and cranial nerve deficits may be minimized by lowering the delivered dose or through multisession therapy.

REFERENCES

1. Wara WM, Bauman GS, Sneed PK, et al., Brain, brain stem, and cerebellum. In: Perez CA, Brady LW, eds. *Principles and Practice of Radiation Oncology*. 3rd ed. Philadelphia, PA: Lippincott-Raven; 1997:777–828.
2. Monte F, De. Current management of meningiomas. *Oncology*. 1995;9:83–96.
3. Cushing H. The meningiomas (dural endotheliomas). Their source and favoured seats of origin. *Brain*. 1922;45:282–316.
4. Rockhill J, Mrugala M, Chamberlain MC. Intracranial meningiomas: an overview of diagnosis and treatment. *Neurosurg Focus*. 2007;23(4):E1.
5. Simon M, Boström JP, Hartmann C. Molecular genetics of meningiomas: from basic research to potential clinical applications. *Neurosurgery*. 2007;60(5):787–98; discussion 787.
6. Louis DN, Ohgaki H, Wisteler OD, Cavenee WK. *WHO Classification of Tumours of the Central Nervous System*. Geneva, Switzerland: World Health Organization; 2007.
7. Rogers L, Mehta M. Role of radiation therapy in treating intracranial meningiomas. *Neurosurg Focus*. 2007;23(4):E4.
8. Mendenhall WM, Friedman WA, Amdur RJ, Foote KD. Management of benign skull base meningiomas: a review. *Skull Base*. 2004;14(1):53–60; discussion 61.
9. Buetow MP, Buetow PC, Smirniotopoulos JG. Typical, atypical, and misleading features in meningioma. *Radiographics*. 1991;11(6):1087–1106.
10. Chamberlain MC, Tsao-Wei DD, Groshen S. Temozolomide for treatment-resistant recurrent meningioma. *Neurology*. 2004;62(7):1210–1212.
11. Goldsmith BJ, Wara WM, Wilson CB, Larson DA. Postoperative irradiation for subtotally resected meningiomas. A retrospective analysis of 140 patients treated from 1967 to 1990. *J Neurosurg*. 1994;80(2):195–201.
12. Withers HR, Thames HD Jr, Peters LJ. Biological bases for high RBE values for late effects of neutron irradiation. *Int J Radiat Oncol Biol Phys*. 1982;8(12):2071–2076.

13. Thames HD Jr, Withers HR, Peters LJ, Fletcher GH. Changes in early and late radiation responses with altered dose fractionation: implications for dose-survival relationships. *Int J Radiat Oncol Biol Phys.* 1982;8(2):219–226.
14. Kondziolka D, Mathieu D, Lunsford LD, et al. Radiosurgery as definitive management of intracranial meningiomas. *Neurosurgery.* 2008;62(1):53–8; discussion 58.
15. Minniti G, Amichetti M, Enrici RM. Radiotherapy and radiosurgery for benign skull base meningiomas. *Radiat Oncol.* 2009;4:42.
16. Starke RM, Williams BJ, Hiles C, Nguyen JH, Elsharkawy MY, Sheehan JP. Gamma knife surgery for skull base meningiomas. *J Neurosurg.* 2012;116(3):588–597.
17. Colombo, F. Casentini, L. Cavedon, C. Scalchi, P. Cora, S. Franceson, P. Cyberknife radiosurgery for benign meningiomas: short-term results in 199 patients. *Neurosurgery.* 2008;62(suppl 2):733–743.
18. Mahadevan A, Floyd S, Wong E, Chen C, Kasper E. Clinical outcome after hypofractionated stereotactic radiotherapy (HSRT) for benign skull base tumors. *Comput Aided Surg.* 2011;16(3):112–120.
19. Kreil W, Luggin J, Fuchs I, Weigl V, Eustacchio S, Papaefthymiou G. Long term experience of gamma knife radiosurgery for benign skull base meningiomas. *J Neurol Neurosurg Psychiatr.* 2005;76(10):1425–1430.
20. Chang JH, Chang JW, Choi JY, Park YG, Chung SS. Complications after gamma knife radiosurgery for benign meningiomas. *J Neurol Neurosurg Psychiatr.* 2003;74(2):226–230.
21. Kobayashi T, Kida Y, Mori Y. Long-term results of stereotactic gamma radiosurgery of meningiomas. *Surg Neurol.* 2001;55(6):325–331.
22. Kreil W, Luggin J, Fuchs I, Weigl V, Eustacchio S, Papaefthymiou G. Long term experience of gamma knife radiosurgery for benign skull base meningiomas. *J Neurol Neurosurg Psychiatr.* 2005;76(10):1425–1430.
23. Chang JH, Chang JW, Choi JY, Park YG, Chung SS. Complications after gamma knife radiosurgery for benign meningiomas. *J Neurol Neurosurg Psychiatr.* 2003;74(2):226–230.
24. Kobayashi T, Kida Y, Mori Y. Long-term results of stereotactic gamma radiosurgery of meningiomas. *Surg Neurol.* 2001;55(6):325–331.
25. Flickinger JC, Kondziolka D, Maitz AH, Lunsford LD. Gamma knife radiosurgery of imaging-diagnosed intracranial meningioma. *Int J Radiat Oncol Biol Phys.* 2003;56(3):801–806.
26. Tishler RB, Loeffler JS, Lunsford LD, et al. Tolerance of cranial nerves of the cavernous sinus to radiosurgery. *Int J Radiat Oncol Biol Phys.* 1993;27(2):215–221.
27. Adler JR Jr, Gibbs IC, Puataweepong P, Chang SD. Visual field preservation after multi-session cyberknife radiosurgery for perioptic lesions. *Neurosurgery.* 2006;59(2):244–54; discussion 244.
28. Stafford SL, Pollock BE, Foote RL, et al. Meningioma radiosurgery: tumor control, outcomes, and complications among 190 consecutive patients. *Neurosurgery.* 2001;49(5):1029–37; discussion 1037.
29. Balasubramaniam A, Shannon P, Hodaie M, Laperriere N, Michaels H, Guha A. Glioblastoma multiforme after stereotactic radiotherapy for acoustic neuroma: case report and review of the literature. *Neuro-oncology.* 2007;9(4):447–453.
30. Rowe J, Grainger A, Walton L, Silcocks P, Radatz M, Kemeny A. Risk of malignancy after gamma knife stereotactic radiosurgery. *Neurosurgery.* 2007;60(1):60–5; discussion 65.

Chapter 5

Skull-Base Tumors

B. Role of Radiosurgery for Hemangiopericytomas

Bowen Jiang, Anand Veeravagu, & Steven D. Chang

Hemangiopericytomas (HPCs) are highly vascular tumors arising from capillary-associated pericytes. Clinically and radiographically, HPCs resemble meningiomas but are distinctive due to their aggressiveness, rapid growth, high recurrence rates, and propensity for extracranial metastasis. In one series, 50% of patients with HPCs developed extracranial metastasis, with bone and liver being the most common sites (1). Local recurrence has been cited to be as high as 91% within 5 years (2). Overall, central nervous system (CNS) HPCs are rare and account for 0.4% of primary CNS tumors and 2.4% of meningiomas (3,4).

RATIONALE FOR RADIOSURGERY

Surgical resection is the initial treatment of choice for the management of HPCs and carries an operative mortality of 9% to 24% (5,6). Given the proposed cellular origin, dural sinus invasion, anatomic inaccessibility, and high vascularity of HPCs, gross total resection is often insufficient to manage these lesions. The primary challenge with surgical resection alone is the high rate of postoperative recurrence, which has been reported to occur within a median of 12 months post initial resection (1). Although multiple resections are feasible, the morbidity associated with each intervention makes this option unattractive. Adjuvant radiosurgery combines the efficacy of resection with the more minimal rate of radiotherapy-induced morbidity. Conventional radiotherapy has been proposed for postsurgical treatment of HPCs, but the focal, well-defined nature of these lesions on MR imaging makes them attractive targets for stereotactic radiosurgery (SRS). SRS is particularly beneficial for skull-base HPCs, which usually present as reasonably small as a result of their proximity to cranial nerves, whose dysfunction often signals the presence of tumor (7). Although conventional radiotherapy of skull-base HPCs may include critical skull-base structures, such as the pituitary, optic nerves, and brainstem, the steep dose gradient that can be achieved using SRS minimizes the radiation delivered to these areas. The role of external-beam radiotherapy (EBRT), Gamma Knife (GKS), and CyberKnife (CK) in the management of HPCs will be further discussed in this chapter.

RADIOSURGERY PLANNING AND TECHNIQUES

For patients undergoing linear accelerator (LINAC)-based SRS, a technique modeled after that of Winston and Lutz could be used (8). First, localization should be performed using CT images fused to thinly sliced contrast-enhanced MR. Multiple noncoplanar arc radiation could be used with the appropriate circular secondary collimators, the diameters of which ranged from 7.5 to 25 mm (mean 12.8 mm) in the authors' experience (7).

In the case of CK-based SRS, patients should be first placed on a treatment couch and have a thermoplastic mask constructed. CT imaging at 1.25-mm slice thickness administered with Omnipaque contrast should be obtained, fused with corresponding MR scans, and transferred to the treatment planning computer. A radiosurgeon will then outline and contour the tumor volume. The authors recommend an inverse treatment planning strategy, which will achieve a highly conformal treatment plan that minimizes the dose to critical structures. For extracranial HPCs, the Xsight spine tracking system is now the standard of practice, because this technology has obviated the use of fiducial implantation and can localize spinal targets by directly referencing adjacent vertebral structures (9).

Patients who undergo GKS SRS require placement of a Leksell stereotactic frame (Elekta AB) under monitored anesthesia with the supplement of a local anesthetic. Contrast-enhanced T1-weighted axial MR images with 1.3-mm-thick slices are often used for contouring and dose planning.

TREATMENT DOSE

The treatment dose is often determined on the basis of tumor size, location, proximity of critical neurological structures, number of isocenters (tumors with complex geometric shapes should be treated with multiple isocenters), and history of prior conventional radiotherapy. In the most recent series from the authors' institution, 14 patients with 24 tumors (mean volume 9.16 cm^3) were followed for a median of 37 months. The marginal dose ranged from 16 to 30 Gy and the maximum dose ranged from 22 to 37 Gy (9). The marginal dose was prescribed to the 78% isodose contour at the edge of tumor (range 72%–89%). Sixteen tumors were treated with one fraction, four with two fractions, and four with three fractions or more. There were no radiation-induced injuries or complications in this series. Between the years of 1987 and 2010, 11 published studies on the use of SRS (LINAC, CK, GKS) for recurrent and residual HPCs reported that a mean prescription dose was 16.2 Gy to the tumor margin (1,5,7,9–16). One of these studies concluded that a marginal dose of less than 14 Gy is associated with considerable lack of tumor control (50% progression) as opposed to marginal doses of more than 14 Gy (19% progression) (12). Marginal doses of more than 14 Gy resulted in progression-free survival rates of 93.3% and 75.4% at 1 and 5 years, respectively. Doses of less than 14 Gy had progression-free survival of 75.0% and 56.3% at 1 and 5 years (12) (Figure 5B.1).

CK was used to treat a 47-year-old male with a 56.7 cm^3 hemangiopericytoma in the posterior fossa. A single fraction at marginal dose of 21 Gy and maxi-

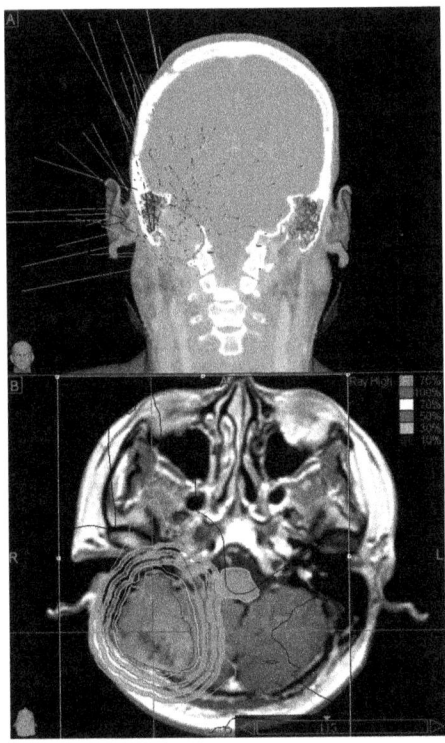

FIGURE 5B.1 Sample treatment plan.

mum dose of 27.6 Gy was used. The isodose line was 76% and the conformity index was 1.19. At 15-months follow-up, the tumor was stable.

RADIOSURGERY OUTCOMES

Generally, radiosurgery is associated with favorable tumor control, both in terms of tumor volume reduction and delaying the time to recurrence. Both conventional fractionated radiotherapy and SRS have been used in the management of HPCs. Patients with more widespread, diffuse tumors are usually candidates for fractionated therapies, whereas patients with smaller, focal lesions are better suited for SRS.

EXTERNAL-BEAM RADIOTHERAPY

EBRT has been used as adjuvant therapy for the treatment of local recurrences, often following surgical resection. At a focal fractionated dose of 50 Gy, studies have shown a significant increase in the length of time to tumor recurrence (3,17). Dufour et al. (17) demonstrated that postoperative EBRT decreased the local recurrence rate to 12.5% compared to 88% with surgery alone. Guthrie et al. (3) reported that radiation therapy after surgical resection extended the mean time to recurrence from 34 to 75 months and extended survival from 62 to 92 months. More recently, Schiariti et al. (18) reported on 39 patients who underwent microsurgical resection with a mean follow-up period of 123 months. EBRT extended the disease-free interval from 154 to 254 months but was not effective in preventing metastasis. In those patients with EBRT and complete resection, the mean recurrence-free interval was found to be 126.3 months longer and overall survival 126 months longer than without EBRT. However, data to suggest that EBRT after excision does not significantly improve overall survival, progression-free survival, or recurrence-free intervals are also available (12).

STEREOTACTIC RADIOSURGERY—GAMMA KNIFE

The authors reviewed all 11 published studies between 1987 and 2010 on the use of SRS (LINAC, GKS, and CK) for recurrent and residual HPCs. There were 137 patients with 241 lesions; the mean follow-up period was 37.2 months and the mean tumor control rate was 81.3% at last follow-up (Table 5B.1) (1,5,7,9–16).

The first preliminary SRS report for the treatment of HPCs was provided by Coffey et al. (10). Five patients with 11 tumors were treated with GKS. At a

TABLE 5B.1 Published Studies on SRS for Recurrent and Residual Hemangiopericytoma

Series	Institution	Study Period	No. of Patients/ Lesions	Mean Marginal Dose (Gy)	Mean Follow-Up (Months)	Tumor Control at Last FU (%)
Coffey et al. (1993) (10)	Mayo Clinic	1990–1992	5/11	15.5	14.8	81.8
Galanis et al. (1998) (1)	Mayo Clinic	1976–1996	10/20	12–18	6–36	100[a]
Payne et al. (2000) (14)	U of Virginia	1991–1999	10/12	14	24.8	75
Sheehan et al. (2002) (15)	U of Pittsburgh	1987–2001	14/15	15	31.3	80
Chang and Sakamoto (2003) (7)	Stanford	1992–2002	8/8	20.5	44	75
Ecker et al. (2003) (11)	Mayo Clinic	1980–2000	15/45	16	45.6	93[b]
Kano et al. (2008) (12)	U of Pittsburgh	1989–2006	20/29	15	37.9	72.4
Sun et al. (2009) (16)	Beijing Neu. Ins.	1994–2006	22/58	13.5	26	89.7
Iwai (2009) (19)	Osaka City Hosp	1994–2003	8/13	15.1	61	100
Olson et al. (2010) (13)	U of Virginia	1989–2008	21/28	17	69	46.4
Veeravagu et al. (2010) (9)	Stanford	2002–2009	14/22	21.2	37	81.8

[a]Tumors responded to GKS with decrease or stability in volume, but effect lasted less than 1 year in majority of patients. Study also includes the five patients from Coffey et al. (1993) (10) manuscript.

[b]Also includes five patients from Coffey et al. (1993) (10) manuscript.

FU = Follow up

Adapted from Veeravagu A, Jiang B, Patil CG, Lee M, Soltys SG, Gibbs IC, Chang SD. CK SRS for recurrent, metastatic, and residual HPCs. *J Hematol Oncol.* 2011;4(26).

mean marginal dose of 15.5 Gy and a mean follow-up period of 14.8 months, the authors reported a tumor control rate of 81.8%. Galanis et al. (1) added five more patients to the Coffey series for a total of 20 HPCs. Seven of the ten patients had previously undergone radiotherapy and all ten had undergone at least one prior surgical resection. Fourteen of the HPCs decreased in size, four disappeared radiographically, and two were stable in size. However, these effects lasted no more than 1 year and at 5 years, the distant metastasis rate was 33%.

Payne et al. (14) reported on ten patients with 12 lesions who had undergone treatment with GKS. Nine of the patients had undergone prior craniotomies and four patients received prior fractionated radiotherapy. With a range of peripheral doses from 14 to 37 Gy and a mean follow-up period of 24.8 months, the authors demonstrated a 75% tumor control rate. Local control was 67% at 22 months. Four of the nine tumors that decreased in size, however, subsequently increased in size after a mean of 22 months post radiosurgery.

Reasonable tumor control was presented by Sheehan et al. (15) in a series on 14 patients with 15 HPCs treated with GKS. Seven patients had previously undergone conventional radiotherapy (range 30–61 Gy). The marginal radiosurgery doses ranged from 11 to 20 Gy and the mean follow-up period was 31.3 months. At last follow-up, tumor regression was demonstrated in 80% of the 15 tumors. However, 29% of the patients developed remote lesions, indicating that radiosurgery provided little protection from metastatic spread. In a study by Sun et al. (16), 22 patients with 58 foci underwent GKS at a mean tumor margin dose of 13.5 Gy. Even though the overall tumor control rate was 89.7% at 26-month follow-up, intracranial metastases eventually developed in seven patients (31.8%) and extracranial metastases developed in three patients (13.6%). Similarly, other studies have indicated that metastatic disease is diagnosed between 63 and 99 months after the initial diagnosis (1,17). The incidence of distant metastasis increases with time and has been reported as 13%, 33%, and 64% at 5, 10, and 15 years, respectively (3).

Studies from Ecker et al. (11) and Kano et al. (12) resonated previous reports in terms of dosage used, tumor control, and rate of distal metastasis. In the Ecker series, 15 patients with 45 lesions were treated with GKS (11). In total, nine patients eventually died due to metastatic disease and five patients died from tumor burden. Kano et al. (12) published a series consisting of 20 patients who had undergone GKS for 29 tumors. A tumor control rate of 72.4% was reported at a mean follow-up period of 37.9 months. Eight patients (40%) had died at an average of 62.6 months following GKS therapy.

Recently, Olson et al. (13) showed a tumor control rate of 46.4% in a series with 21 patients and 28 lesions treated with GKS at a mean marginal dose of 17 Gy. Even though this tumor control rate is low compared with other series, the mean follow-up time of 69 months is much greater than those previously reported. The longer follow-up time potentially provided a greater chance for HPCs, even those previously well-controlled with SRS, to recur and/or metastasize (20).

STEREOTACTIC RADIOSURGERY—CYBERKNIFE

The authors for this chapter have had success using CK as the SRS device in the management of HPCs. Chang and Sakamoto's series in 2003 demonstrated tumor control in 75% of the HPCs treated during a mean 44-month follow-up period (7). In this series, a LINAC-based radiosurgery system was used to treat four tumors and CK radiosurgery was used to treat four tumors in a total of eight patients. The mean dose rates to tumor periphery in this series were 20.5 Gy, higher compared with those in other series (16.2 Gy). The higher prescription dose, however, did not translate to increased tumor control rates or radiosurgery-related complications.

Veeravagu et al. (9) used CK to treat 24 tumors. A tumor control rate of 81.8% was achieved with a mean follow-up of 37 months. Adverse effects of radiation were not observed. Progression-free survival rate was 95%, 71.5%, and 71.5% at 1, 3, and 5 years after multiple CK treatments. The 5-year survival rate after SRS was 81%. As is the case in other series, all patients had previously undergone either single or multiple craniotomies for attempted gross total resection.

Conclusions from the CK studies are similar to those made by other groups. SRS is a focal, localized treatment modality and does not prevent metastases, intracranial or otherwise (20). Metastases outside the treatment area often developed within a few years after initial treatment, but in one case was reported to appear after 22 years (5). Due to the aggressive nature of HPCs, initial decreases in tumor size or even disappearance can be followed by regrowth (14). Therefore, close clinical and radiographic follow-up is mandatory in this patient population.

LONG-TERM PROGNOSIS

A recent systematic review identified 563 patients with intracranial HPCs in the published literature (21). The overall median survival was 13 years, with 1-, 5-, 10-, and 20-year survival rates of 95%, 82%, 60%, and 23%, respectively. Gross total resection alone was associated with a median survival of 13 years, whereas subtotal resection resulted in a median survival of 9.75 years. Patients with tumors of the posterior fossa had a median survival of 10.75 versus 15.6 years for those with tumors located elsewhere. Interestingly, in this report, postoperative adjuvant radiation was not associated with a superior survival benefit, with patients receiving greater than 50 Gy of radiation having worse survival outcomes. However, as previously reviewed, there is evidence that adjuvant radiation with GKS and CK SRS is associated with increased tumor control and survival (1,5,7,9–16).

CONCLUSION

HPCs are known for their aggressive pathology, high recurrence rate, and propensity for distant metastasis. Surgical resection remains the initial treatment option; however, postoperative SRS with LINAC, GKS, and CK has been shown to be effective in increasing time to recurrence as well as patient survival. Close clinical and radiographic follow-up is necessary due to the high probability of local recurrence and distant metastases. Because radiosurgery is a focal treatment, it does not eliminate the possibility of regional or distant metastases, which remain sources of significant morbidity and mortality for these patients.

REFERENCES

1. Galanis E, Buckner JC, Scheithauer BW, Kimmel DW, Schomberg PJ, Piepgras DG. Management of recurrent meningeal hemangiopericytoma. *Cancer.* 1998; 82(10):1915–1920.
2. Vuorinen V, Sallinen P, Haapasalo H, Visakorpi T, Kallio M, Jääskeläinen J. Outcome of 31 intracranial haemangiopericytomas: poor predictive value of cell proliferation indices. *Acta Neurochir (Wien).* 1996;138(12):1399–1408.
3. Guthrie BL, Ebersold MJ, Scheithauer BW, Shaw EG. Meningeal hemangiopericytoma: histopathological features, treatment, and long-term follow-up of 44 cases. *Neurosurgery.* 1989;25(4):514–522.
4. Kleihues P, Louis DN, Scheithauer BW, et al. The WHO classification of tumors of the nervous system. *J Neuropathol Exp Neurol.* 2002;61(3):215–25; discussion 226.
5. Suzuki H, Haga Y, Oguro K, Shinoda S, Masuzawa T, Kanai N. Intracranial hemangiopericytoma with extracranial metastasis occurring after 22 years. *Neurol Med Chir (Tokyo).* 2002;42(7):297–300.
6. Pitkethly DT, Hardman JM, Kempe LG, Earle KM. Angioblastic meningiomas; clinicopathologic study of 81 cases. *J Neurosurg.* 1970;32(5):539–544.
7. Chang SD, Sakamoto GT. The role of radiosurgery for hemangiopericytomas. *Neurosurg Focus.* 2003;14(5):e14.
8. Winston KR, Lutz W. Linear accelerator as a neurosurgical tool for stereotactic radiosurgery. *Neurosurgery.* 1988;22(3):454–464.
9. Veeravagu A, Jiang B, Patil CG, et al. CyberKnife stereotactic radiosurgery for recurrent, metastatic, and residual hemangiopericytomas. *J Hematol Oncol.* 2011;4:26.
10. Coffey RJ, Cascino TL, Shaw EG. Radiosurgical treatment of recurrent hemangiopericytomas of the meninges: preliminary results. *J Neurosurg.* 1993;78(6):903–908.
11. Ecker RD, Marsh WR, Pollock BE, et al. Hemangiopericytoma in the central nervous system: treatment, pathological features, and long-term follow up in 38 patients. *J Neurosurg.* 2003;98(6):1182–1187.
12. Kano H, Niranjan A, Kondziolka D, Flickinger JC, Lunsford LD. Adjuvant stereotactic radiosurgery after resection of intracranial hemangiopericytomas. *Int J Radiat Oncol Biol Phys.* 2008;72(5):1333–1339.
13. Olson C, Yen CP, Schlesinger D, Sheehan J. Radiosurgery for intracranial hemangiopericytomas: outcomes after initial and repeat Gamma Knife surgery. *J Neurosurg.* 2010;112(1):133–139.
14. Payne BR, Prasad D, Steiner M, Steiner L. Gamma surgery for hemangiopericytomas. *Acta Neurochir (Wien).* 2000;142(5):527–36; discussion 536.
15. Sheehan J, Kondziolka D, Flickinger J, Lunsford LD. Radiosurgery for treatment of recurrent intracranial hemangiopericytomas. *Neurosurgery.* 2002;51(4):905–10; discussion 910.
16. Sun S, Liu A, Wang C. Gamma knife radiosurgery for recurrent and residual meningeal hemangiopericytomas. *Stereotact Funct Neurosurg.* 2009;87(2):114–119.

17. Dufour H, Metellus P, Fuentes S, et al. Meningeal hemangiopericytoma: a retrospective study of 21 patients with special review of postoperative external radiotherapy. *Neurosurgery*. 2001;48(4):756–762; discussion 762–753.
18. Schiariti M, Goetz P, El-Maghraby H, Tailor J, Kitchen N. Hemangiopericytoma: long-term outcome revisited. Clinical article. *J Neurosurg*. 2011;114(3):747–755.
19. Iwai Y, Yamanaka K. Gamma knife radiosurgery for other primary intra-axial tumors. *Prog Neurol Surg*. 2009;22:129–141
20. Sheehan J, Marchan E. Intracranial hemangiopericytoma: Gamma Knife surgery. In: Hayat M, ed. *Tumors of the Central Nervous System, Volume 3: Brain Tumors, Part 1*. New York, NY: Springer; 2010:273–278.
21. Rutkowski MJ, Sughrue ME, Kane AJ, et al. Predictors of mortality following treatment of intracranial hemangiopericytoma. *J Neurosurg*. 2010;113(2):333–339.

Chapter 5

Skull-Base Tumors

C. Stereotactic Radiosurgery for Glomus Jugulare Tumors

Zachary D. Guss, Anubhav G. Amin, & Michael Lim

The glomus body was first recognized by Guild in 1941 as a small structure found within the jugular bulb adventitia in the floor of the middle ear (1). Histologically, it is composed of epithelioid cells within a capillary network surrounded by a fibrous capsule (2). Glomus bodies serve as chemoreceptors, similar to ciliary, carotid, and aortic bodies (3). The first case report of a glomus jugulare tumor was published in 1945 by Rosenwasser (4). These tumors arise from paraganglionic tissue of cranial nerves IX and X (5).

Glomus jugulare tumors are rare, with an incidence of one per 1.3 million people (6). Incidental glomus jugulare tumors occur more frequently in women; however, pedigree studies of familial glomus tumors indicate that tumors with an inherited component are passed along the paternal line, most likely via genetic imprinting (7,8). Familial glomus jugulare tumors display different traits than incidental cases, with a younger median age at diagnosis, a higher propensity for multicentric and bilateral tumors, and no gender overrepresentation (9,10).

Although glomus jugulare tumors are highly vascular, they typically display benign features (Figure 5C.1). Less than an estimated 4% of glomus jugulare tumors are metastatic, and these patients have a significantly higher rate of local recurrence and death compared to patients with nonmetastatic disease (11).

Symptoms are typically a consequence of mass effect and compression of lower cranial nerves. Patients frequently present with ear pain, loss of hearing,

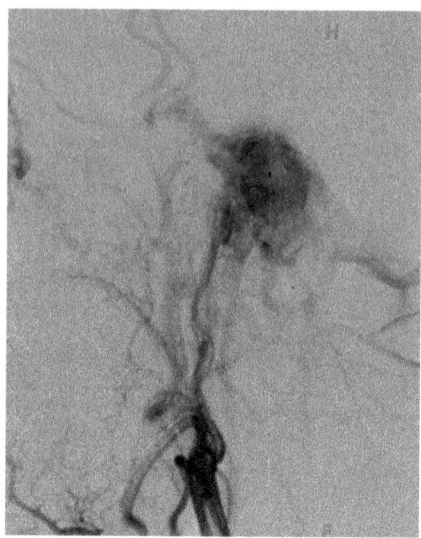

FIGURE 5C.1 Angiogram of a glomus jugulare tumor reveals tumoral blush within the left jugular foramen predominantly fed by branches of the ascending pharyngeal and posterior auricular arteries. These branches are amenable to endovascular embolization.

vertigo, headache, and tinnitus (12,13). Rarely, patients may present with an endocrinological syndrome, as 1% to 3% of these tumors are secretory (14,15).

METHODS

Radiation therapy has long been used in the management of glomus jugulare tumors. In the 1960s and 1970s, cobalt or megavoltage radiation therapy emerged as a primary intervention or adjunct to surgery (16–18). Given the unsatisfactory accuracy and precision of the radiation therapy devices of that era, surgery demonstrated superior outcomes (19).

Since then, however, stereotactic radiosurgery (SRS) has emerged as an appealing radiation therapy modality for glomus jugulare tumors. SRS technologies are precise, allowing for dose escalation (Figure 5C.2). SRS technologies include CyberKnife, Gamma Knife, and linear accelerators. A meta-analysis that we conducted at Johns Hopkins Hospital of SRS for glomus jugulare tumors revealed a single-fraction approach with a median dose of 15 Gy (range of median across all included studies 12–20.4 Gy) to be the most common (5). Special considerations are warranted for large tumors or those that abut critical structures such as the brainstem. At our institution, such cases receive 500 cGy for five fractions.

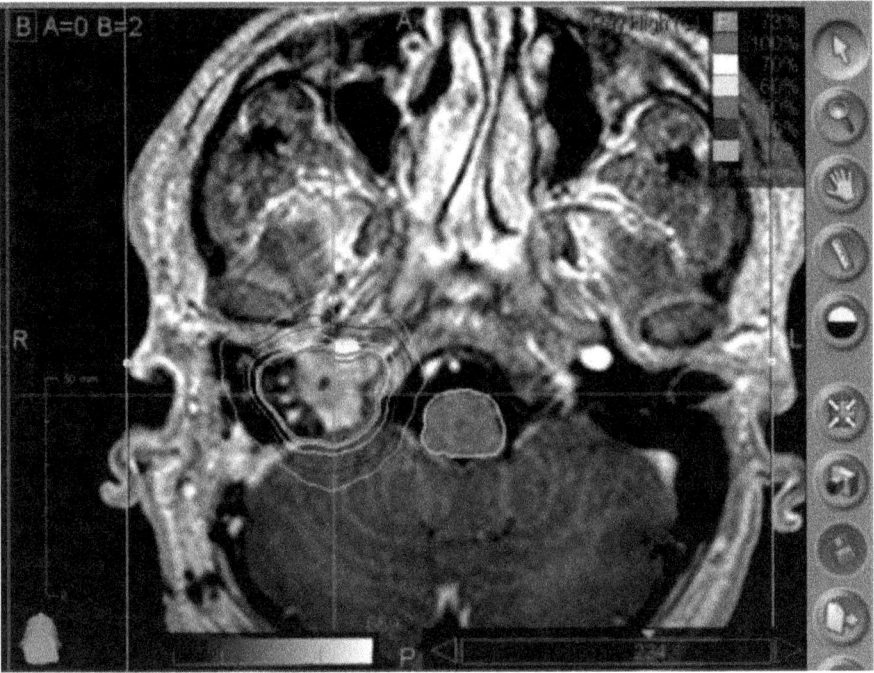

FIGURE 5C.2 CyberKnife treatment plan for a glomus jugulare tumor. The precision of SRS helps avoid nearby critical structures.

OUTCOMES

Two meta-analyses published in 2010 and 2011, by Johns Hopkins Hospital and the University of California at San Francisco (UCSF), shed insight on the outcomes of patients with SRS who receive radiosurgery (2,5). The UCSF study demonstrated that patients who receive SRS alone have a higher tumor control rate (95%) than those who receive a subtotal resection (69%), gross total resection (86%), or combined resection and radiosurgery (71%). SRS was associated with fewer cranial nerve (CN) IX–XI deficits than surgery, whereas CN XII deficits were similar.

The Johns Hopkins Hospital study focused solely on SRS outcomes. Across all studies, patients who received SRS for glomus jugulare tumors experienced a tumor control rate of 97% and a clinical control rate of 95%. Several studies reported no toxicities, whereas some reported low rates of nausea and vomiting, vertigo, and CN deficits. Although the conclusions from both meta-analyses should be limited, the literature suggests SRS offers excellent tumor control and acceptable toxicity. A prospective trial assessing SRS and surgery would address lingering questions of comparative effectiveness and safety.

Several more recent reports have added to the credibility of SRS as a valuable modality for treating glomus jugulare tumors. A report from the Taipei

Veterans General Hospital in Taiwan analyzed the results of 11 patients with glomus jugulare tumors who received Gamma Knife SRS with a median follow-up time of 40.3 months (20). All patients experienced tumor control, whereas none developed CN toxicities. A study from Hacettepe University in Turkey recently published the results of 14 patients with unresectable glomus jugulare tumors who received CyberKnife SRS. All patients either exhibited tumor control or tumor regression, and no patient experienced toxicity.

CONCLUSION

Radiation therapy has long been used for the management of glomus jugulare tumors, and developments in radiation therapy technologies have made it a compelling treatment option. Recent meta-analyses and case series have demonstrated that SRS can adequately manage most glomus jugulare tumors with equal or even superior clinical results relative to surgery with less invasiveness. Prospective trials are necessary to definitively compare SRS and surgery, although the current retrospective results are very favorable for SRS.

REFERENCES

1. Ruben RJ. The history of the glomus tumors—nonchromaffim chemodectoma: a glimpse of biomedical Camelot. *Acta Otolaryngol*. 2007;127(4):411–416.
2. Ivan ME, Sughrue ME, Clark AJ, et al. A meta-analysis of tumor control rates and treatment-related morbidity for patients with glomus jugulare tumors. *J Neurosurg*. 2011;114(5):1299–1305.
3. Ghani GA, Sung YF, Per-Lee JH. Glomus jugulare tumors–origin, pathology, and anesthetic considerations. *Anesth Analg*. 1983;62(7):686–691.
4. Rosenwasser H. Glomus jugularis tumor of the middle ear; carotid body tumor, tympanic body tumor, nonchromaffin paraganglioma. *Laryngoscope*. 1952;62(6):623–633.
5. Guss ZD, Batra S, Limb CJ, et al. Radiosurgery of glomus jugulare tumors: a meta-analysis. *Int J Radiat Oncol Biol Phys*. 2011;81(4):e497–e502.
6. Moffat DA, Hardy DG. Surgical management of large glomus jugulare tumours: infra- and trans-temporal approach. *J Laryngol Otol*. 1989;103(12):1167–1180.
7. Alford BR, Guilford FR. A comprehensive study of tumors of the glomus jugulare. *Laryngoscope*. 1962;72:765–805.
8. van der Mey AG, Maaswinkel-Mooy PD, Cornelisse CJ, Schmidt PH, van de Kamp JJ. Genomic imprinting in hereditary glomus tumours: evidence for new genetic theory. *Lancet*. 1989;2(8675):1291–1294.
9. Sugarbaker EV, Chretien PB, Jacobs JB. Bilateral familial carotid body tumors: report of a patient with an occult contralateral tumor and postoperative hypertension. *Ann Surg*. 1971;174(2):242–247.
10. Guss ZD, Batra S, Li G, et al. Radiosurgery for glomus jugulare: history and recent progress. *Neurosurg Focus*. 2009;27(6):E5.

11. Brewis C, Bottrill ID, Wharton SB, Moffat DA. Metastases from glomus jugulare tumours. *J Laryngol Otol*. 2000;114(1):17–23.
12. Lattes R, Waltner JG. Nonchromaffin paraganglioma of the middle ear; carotid-body-like tumor; glomus-jugulare tumor. *Cancer*. 1949;2(3):447–468.
13. Larson TC III, Reese DF, Baker HL Jr, McDonald TJ. Glomus tympanicum chemodectomas: radiographic and clinical characteristics. *Radiology*. 1987;163(3):801–806.
14. Azzarelli B, Felten S, Muller J, Miyamoto R, Purvin V. Dopamine in paragangliomas of the glomus jugulare. *Laryngoscope*. 1988;98(5):573–578.
15. Netterville JL, Jackson CG, Miller FR, Wanamaker JR, Glasscock ME. Vagal paraganglioma: a review of 46 patients treated during a 20-year period. *Arch Otolaryngol Head Neck Surg*. 1998;124(10):1133–1140.
16. Grubb WB Jr, Lampe I. The role of radiation therapy in the treatment of chemodectomas of the glomus jugulare. *Laryngoscope*. 1965;75(12):1861–1871.
17. Silverstone SM. Radiation therapy of glomus jugulare tumors. *Arch Otolaryngol*. 1973;97(1):43–48.
18. Gardner G, Cocke EW Jr, Robertson JT, Trumbull ML, Palmer RE. Combined approach surgery for removal of glomus jugulare tumors. *Laryngoscope*. 1977;87(5 Pt 1):665–688.
19. Spector GJ, Fierstein J, Ogura JH. A comparison of therapeutic modalities of glomus tumors in the temporal bone. *Laryngoscope*. 1976;86(5):690–696.
20. Lee CC, Pan DH, Wu JC, et al. Gamma knife radiosurgery for glomus jugulare and tympanicum. *Stereotact Funct Neurosurg*. 2011;89(5):291–298.

Chapter 5

Skull-Base Tumors

D. Radiosurgery for Vestibular Schwannomas

Jacob Ruzevick, Michael Lim, & Daniele Rigamonti

Vestibular schwannomas (VSs) arise from aberrant growth and proliferation of schwann cells surrounding the vestibular nerve. Their incidence and prevalence is approximately 1/100,000 and 2–7/10,000, respectively, with most developing between 30 and 60 years of age (1–3). VSs represent 6-10% of all intracranial tumors and approximately 80% of all cerebellopontine angle tumors. If left untreated, VSs can lead to compression of the brainstem and cerebellum (4). VSs are usually slowly progressive, with most patients presenting with gradual sensori-neural hearing loss with any combination of tinnitus, unsteadiness, trigeminal nerve dysfunction, or facial nerve dysfunction. At a later stage, increased intracranial pressure, or brainstem or cerebellar symptoms may occur (3).

INDICATIONS FOR RADIOSURGERY

Radiosurgery is indicated in patients with newly diagnosed unequivocally growing VS and recurrent VS following surgery. The location and size of the VS should influence the decision to pursue radiosurgery. Tumors located in the intracanalicular space and tumors that are small (18× more likely to progress as compared to large tumors) and without brainstem compression are most amenable to radiotherapy (5). One method of grading VSs, and influencing radiosurgery versus microsurgery is the Koos criteria (Table 5D.1), which takes into

TABLE 5D.1 Koos Criteria for Grading VSs

Grade	Tumor size
1	0–10 mm, Intracanalicular
2	10–20 mm Total, 0–10 mm extrameatal
3	20–30 mm Total
4	>30 mm Total, brain stem deformation

account size, location, and mass effect on the brain stem. Koos grade I–III are highly treatable with radiosurgery, whereas Koos grade IV tumors, due to brainstem deformation, are best treated using microsurgical approaches.

DIAGNOSTIC IMAGING AND PRE-TREATMENT WORK-UP

In a patient who presents with gradual unilateral hearing loss with any combination of tinnitus, unsteadiness, or trigeminal nerve dysfunction, VS should be considered in the differential diagnosis. Gadolinium-enhanced MRI is the gold standard of imaging for detection of VSs as this modality can detect tumors as small as 1 to 2 mm in diameter. Some groups have reported using fast spin echo T2 MRI; however, in a study of 1233 patients, up to 44% of VSs were not confidently identified using this modality. Fast spin echo T2 MRI in combination with gadolinium-enhanced MRI would yield a sensitivity of 100% and negative predictive value of 100% and be able to identify other disease processes whose symptoms are similar to that of VS (6). In patients with implanted pacemakers or other ferromagnetic devices, contrast CT or unique 1.5T MRI protocols can be used to visualize the tumor.

Audiological studies are used to determine the degree of auditory dysfunction. They most commonly include pure tone average, speech reception threshold, and speech discrimination score. Finally, in patients with symptomatic hydrocephalus, a shunt can be placed prior to radiotherapy if patients are not strong candidates for microsurgery.

CONSIDERATIONS FOR PATIENTS WITH NEUROFIBROMATOSIS 2

Neurofibromatosis type 2 (NF2) has an incidence of 1/30,000 to 50,000 live births and is characterized by bilateral VSs. Patients with NF2 warrant special consideration because of the risk of complete deafness due to bilateral VSs. Growth patterns of tumors in NF2 patients differ from sporadically arising tumors in that they tend to engulf or even invade the cochlear nerve. In several case series', hearing preservation, trigeminal nerve function, and tumor control rate are adequate when treatment is initiated while the patient still has functional hearing (7,8). Finally, due to the genetic alterations in NF2, these patients may carry an increased risk of radiation-induced de novo tumor formation due to normal cells' inability to repair radiation-induced DNA damage, although this has not been confirmed.

RADIATION FOR PATIENTS WITH VESTIBULAR SCHWANNOMA

Radiation treatment options for VS include conventional radiation, fractionated stereotactic radiosurgery (FSR), and stereotactic radiosurgery (SRS). Today, most patients receive SRS or FSR. The most common devices for SRS are the Gamma Knife, linear accelerator LINAC; including CyberKnife, or proton beam. Gamma Knife is a frame-based approach that uses a three-dimensional MRI. Gamma Knife is thought to be the most precise with a published accuracy of 0.25 mm. Treatment with LINAC or proton beam system often involves CT imaging that is fused to an MRI. The appeal for LINAC machines such as the CyberKnife is that patients do not need to be placed into a stereotactic frame and thus can have all guidance planning completed on the day of treatment.

Although treatment planning requires complete coverage of the tumor, special attention must be paid to sparing the facial, cochlear, and trigeminal nerve. Planning for Gamma Knife radiosurgery includes outlining the tumor volume, multiple isocenters, beam weighting, and plug patterns. To optimize tumor conformality, especially in tumor regions residing next to or on the facial and cochlear nerves, multiple collimators can be used to increase accuracy. Centers using LINAC systems can achieve similar results using multileaf collimators.

Radiation to the tumor margin is typically 12 to 13 Gy when using Gamma Knife and is associated with low rates of toxicity. In patients with NF2, lower doses or a longer fractionation schedule may be prescribed for the tumor margin to account for the likely damaged auditory apparatus.

Stereotactic radiation therapy using the CyberKnife system is another option for treatment of VSs; however, data on long-term follow-up is not currently available.

CLINICAL RESULTS OF RADIOSURGERY FOR VESTIBULAR SCHWANNOMAS

Published case series by many groups have shown Gamma Knife, LINAC, proton beam therapy, and stereotactic radiotherapy to be efficacious in terms of tumor control, hearing preservation, and surrounding cranial nerve preservation. A summary of clinical efficacy of these radiation delivery systems is provided in Table 5D.2.

TABLE 5D.2 Selected Outcomes of Radiosurgery for VSs

Reference	Patients	Follow-Up	Modality	Tumor Control Rate (%)	Miscellany
Kondziolka et al. (1998) (9)	162	—	GK	98	Preservation of normal facial function (79%), normal trigeminal function (73%), and baseline hearing (51%). No new neurologic deficits.
Litvack et al. (2003) (10)	134	31.7 months	GK	96.7	Functional hearing preserved (61.7%). No long-term facial weakness reported.
Niranjan et al. (1999) (11)	29	—	GK	100	Serviceable hearing preservation in 100% of patients receiving marginal tumor doses ≤ 14 Gy or less but 20% in patients who received greater than14 Gy. No patient developed a facial or trigeminal neuropathy.
Flickinger et al. (2001) (12)	190	30 months	GK	97.1	New facial weakness (1.1%), facial numbness (2.6%), preservation of speech discrimination (91%).
Kondziolka et al. (2003) (13)	157	10 years	GK	98.5	—
Suh et al. (2000) (14)	29	49 months	LINAC	94	New or progressive trigeminal (15%) or facial nerve (32%) deficits. Subjective hearing loss in 74% of patients.
Spiegelman et al. (2001) (15)	44	32 months	LINAC	98	Hearing preserved in 71% of patients. New facial neuropathy in 24% of patients and persisted in 8%.
Weber et al. (2003) (16)	88	38.7 months	Proton Beam	93.6	Serviceable hearing preserved in 33% of patients. Facial nerve and trigeminal nerve preserved in 91.1% and 93.6% of patients, respectively.
Ishihara et al. (2004) (17)	38	27 months	SRT	94	Facial paresis (2.6%), trigeminal neuropathy (2.6%).
Fuss et al. (2000) (18)	51	42 months	SRT	95	Transient facial nerve paralysis (2%), trigeminal dysesthesias (4%).
Sawamura et al. (2003) (19)	101	45 months	FSRT	91.4	Hearing preserved in 71% of patients. Complications included transient facial nerve palsy (4%), trigeminal neuropathy (14%), balance disturbance (17%).
Kapoor et al. (2011) (5)	496	52.6 months	FSRT	88	Three percent required salvage microsurgical treatment. Tumors with baseline volumes less than 1 cm^3 were 18.02 times more likely to progress than those greater than 1 cm^3 or greater. Complications include facial weakness (1.6%), trigeminal paresthesias (2.8%), hydrocephalus (0.9%), possible radiation-induced neoplasia (0.5%).

Using Gamma Knife, control of tumor growth is reported in greater than 93% of patients, with follow-up extending up to 10 years. Similarly, pretreatment hearing can be preserved in 60% to 70% of patients. However, if hearing loss occurs, it is generally noted 6 to 24 months following treatment. Damage to surrounding cranial nerves is greatly minimized with the facial and trigeminal nerve being preserved in greater than 95% of patients, especially when a marginal dose of 12 to 13 Gy is used. Marginal doses greater than 14 Gy are associated with a 2.5% risk of facial weakness and a 3.9% risk of facial numbness (20).

Case reports using LINAC radiosurgery report similar tumor control rates as Gamma Knife. Tumor control rates in several published series are greater than 94%. However, follow-up in these series was limited to less than 5 years. Hearing preservation was highly variable, ranging from 26% to 71% (14,15).

Studies using proton beam therapy reported tumor control in greater than 93% of patients when followed for 39 months and 84% when followed for 5 years. Hearing was preserved in 33% of patients and facial and trigeminal nerve function was preserved in 91.1% and 89% of patients, respectively (16,21).

In published series, fractionated radiotherapy has shown acceptable results with tumor control reported as greater than 90% when using a total dose of 40 to 50 Gy in 20 to 25 fractions (19). One study comparing single fraction and FSR did not report a significant difference in tumor control after 33 months follow-up (22). Kapoor et al. (5) report in a series of 496 patients that 3% required salvage microsurgical treatment and 30% showed radiographic progression, of which 9% of total patients demonstrated growth rate that doubled from baseline. Furthermore, small tumors (less than 1 cm^3) were 18 times more likely to progress in size following treatment, which corroborates findings from Lederman et al., who reported only 61% of small VSs shrank in size following treatment as compared to 81% of larger tumors (23).

RADIOSURGERY FOLLOWING MICROSURGERY

In patients who do not have a complete resection following microsurgery for VS, radiosurgery is an effective option for follow-up treatment. Tumor control rates are reported in greater than 93% of patients. However, identification of residual tumor prior to radiotherapy is a notable challenge. Prior to retreating unequivocal growth, adequate follow-up must be obtained.

MICROSURGERY FOLLOWING RADIOSURGERY

Microsurgery following radiosurgery is indicated in patients with progressive tumor growth with neurologic deterioration following initial radiosurgery.

Several groups have shown that when microsurgery is necessary following failed radiosurgery (tumor progression leading to neurologic symptoms), these cases are more technically difficult due to radiation-induced scarring (24,25). Furthermore, because tumor expansion following radiosurgery can occur up to 18 months following treatment, careful and prolonged observation is required to confirm that the growth is due to actual tumor progression.

FOLLOW-UP

Following radiation therapy, all patients should be followed with gadolinium-enhanced MRI and audiological examinations. Serial imaging should be scheduled at 6 months, 1 year, and then at 2- to 4-year intervals following treatment. Of note, up to 18 months following radiosurgery, up to 10% tumors may appear to enlarge, due to true neoplastic growth (2%–5%) or necrotic death of the tumor core with expansion of the tumor margins. In the latter case, tumor volume may expand 1 to 2 mm despite losing central contrast enhancement with the majority of tumors regressing in size after 12 months.

ASSESSING SUCCESS OF RADIOSURGERY FOR VESTIBULAR SCHWANNOMAS

Currently, treatment for VSs is considered successful if no additional treatment (radiation or salvage surgery) is needed. Notable populations of patients fall into the category of radiographically confirmed tumor progression without apparent clinical symptoms. Kapoor et al. (5) report in a series of 496 patients that 30% of patients showed some tumor progression. Of this group, 35 patients (9% of total) had significant tumor progression in which the tumor volume more than doubled during the follow-up period. Under the classic definition of treatment success, these patients would be considered successful despite obvious radiographic failure. Nonetheless, despite 30% of patients showing radiographic progression after at least 5 years, only 3% of patients required microsurgery.

An important variable related to tumor control is follow-up time. Fuss et al. (24) reported that tumor control decreased over time with 100% tumor control at 2 years but 95% at 5 years. Kapoor et al. (5) report in their series that the vast majority of failures will occur within 5 years of treatment with few failures emerging following this time period. Due to these findings, much of the patient data within the literature have inadequate follow-up periods, and thus inaccurate success rates. It is imperative that determining success of radiosurgery treatment for VSs requires serial imaging for at least 5 years to not only document possible tumor growth, but to correlate clinical findings with radiographic progression following initial treatment (Figure 5D.1).

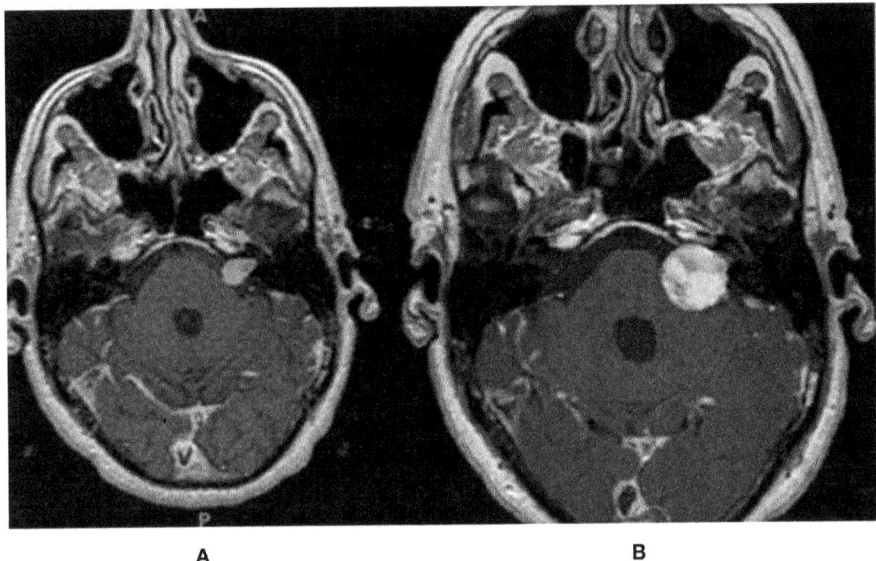

FIGURE 5D.1 (A) Vestibular Schwannoma in a 65-year-old man at time of treatment (approximate baseline volume of 800 mm³). (B) The same tumor after 32 months of follow-up has undergone a five fold growth (approximate volume is 4080 mm³). With "freedom from surgical intervention" used as a criterion, this obvious radiologic failure would be considered a success.

Reprinted from Kapoor et al., Long-term outcomes of VS treated with fractionated stereotactic radiotherapy: an institutional experience. *Int. J Radiat Oncol Biol Phys.* 2011;81(3):647–653 with permission from Elsevier.

COMPLICATIONS

Complications following radiosurgery for VSs are hearing loss, facial numbness, weakness, or pain, and temporary unsteadiness. A rare complication following radiosurgery is radiation-induced neoplasia, which occurs with an incidence of approximately 3/200,000 treated cases. This can be induction of a secondary neoplasm (26) or malignant transformation of a previously benign VS (27). Both possibilities have previously been reported as very rare complications in patients without NF2 and in the general patient population due to precise mapping of target radiation. However, Kapoor et al. (5) report 0.5% of patients with possible radiation-induced neoplasia suggesting long-term surveillance may increase the reported incidence of radiation-induced neoplasia.

CONCLUSION

VSs are slow-growing neoplasms arising in Schwann cells that surround the vestibular or cochlear nerve and usually cause clinical symptoms of unilateral hearing loss with any combination of tinnitus, vertigo, trigeminal or facial nerve dysfunction, among others. Radiosurgery (Gamma Knife, LINAC, proton beam, and stereotactic radiotherapy) has emerged as an effective treatment modality for the treatment of certain VSs, including primary tumors, and tumors requiring salvage therapy following microsurgery. Although published series have shown each radiosurgery modality to be efficacious, most published series do not report data beyond a 5-year follow-up, which has been shown to effect treatment success.

For patients who present with a VS, either primary or recurrent, that does not compress the brainstem, a period of observation prior to radiosurgery is recommended. Only after tumor growth has been documented through serial MRI should treatment be pursued. Radiosurgery may also be used following failed microsurgery; however, identification of residual tumor, while sparing the surrounding trigeminal and facial nerves, has been shown to be difficult.

In conclusion, due to the risks of microsurgical removal for small tumors, radiosurgery can be considered a first-line therapy in patients with VSs, on the premise that documented tumor progression is confirmed and radiographic follow-up to assess for tumor growth is routinely monitored.

REFERENCES

1. Anderson TD, Loevner LA, Bigelow DC, Mirza N. Prevalence of unsuspected acoustic neuroma found by magnetic resonance imaging. *Otolaryngol Head Neck Surg.* 2000;122(5):643–646.
2. Lin D, Hegarty JL, Fischbein NJ, Jackler RK. The prevalence of "incidental" acoustic neuroma. *Arch Otolaryngol Head Neck Surg.* 2005;131(3):241–244.
3. Ho SY, Kveton JF. Acoustic neuroma. Assessment and management. *Otolaryngol Clin North Am.* 2002;35(2):viii, 393–404.
4. Springborg J, Poulsgaard L, Thomsen J. Nonvestibular schwannoma tumors in the cerebellopontine angle: A structured approach and management guidelines. *Skull Base.* 2008 July; 18(4):217–227.
5. Kapoor S, Batra S, Carson K, et al. Long-term outcomes of vestibular schwannomas treated with fractionated stereotactic radiotherapy: an institutional experience. *Int J Radiat Oncol Biol Phys.* 2011;81(3):647–653.
6. Zealley IA, Cooper RC, Clifford KM, et al. MRI screening for acoustic neuroma: a comparison of fast spin echo and contrast enhanced imaging in 1233 patients. *Br J Radiol.* 2000;73(867):242–247.
7. Rowe JG, Radatz MW, Walton L, Soanes T, Rodgers J, Kemeny AA. Clinical experience with gamma knife stereotactic radiosurgery in the management of vestibular schwannomas secondary to type 2 neurofibromatosis. *J Neurol Neurosurg Psychiatr.* 2003;74(9):1288–1293.
8. Subach BR, Kondziolka D, Lunsford LD, Bissonette DJ, Flickinger JC, Maitz AH. Stereotactic radiosurgery in the management of acoustic neuromas associated with neurofibromatosis Type 2. *J Neurosurg.* 1999;90(5):815–822.
9. Kondziolka D, Lunsford LD, McLaughlin MR, Flickinger JC. Long-term outcomes after radiosurgery for acoustic neuromas. *N Engl J Med.* 1998;339(20):1426–1433.

10. Litvack ZN, Norén G, Chougule PB, Zheng Z. Preservation of functional hearing after gamma knife surgery for vestibular schwannoma. *Neurosurg Focus.* 2003;14(5):e3.
11. Niranjan A, Lunsford LD, Flickinger JC, Maitz A, Kondziolka D. Dose reduction improves hearing preservation rates after intracanalicular acoustic tumor radiosurgery. *Neurosurgery.* 1999;45(4):753–762; discussion 762–755.
12. Flickinger JC, Kondziolka D, Niranjan A, Lunsford LD. Results of acoustic neuroma radiosurgery: an analysis of 5 years' experience using current methods. *J Neurosurg.* 2001;94(1):1–6.
13. Kondziolka D, Nathoo N, Flickinger JC, Niranjan A, Maitz AH, Lunsford LD. Long-term results after radiosurgery for benign intracranial tumors. *Neurosurgery.* 2003;53(4):815–821; discussion 821–812.
14. Suh JH, Barnett GH, Sohn JW, Kupelian PA, Cohen BH. Results of linear accelerator-based stereotactic radiosurgery for recurrent and newly diagnosed acoustic neuromas. *Int J Cancer.* 2000;90(3):145–151.
15. Spiegelmann R, Lidar Z, Gofman J, Alezra D, Hadani M, Pfeffer R. Linear accelerator radiosurgery for vestibular schwannoma. *J Neurosurg.* 2001;94(1):7–13.
16. Weber DC, Chan AW, Bussiere MR, et al. Proton beam radiosurgery for vestibular schwannoma: tumor control and cranial nerve toxicity. *Neurosurgery.* 2003;53(3):577–586; discussion 586–578.
17. Ishihara H, Saito K, Nishizaki T, et al. CyberKnife radiosurgery for vestibular schwannoma. *Minim Invasive Neurosurg.* 2004;47(5):290–293.
18. Fuss M, Debus J, Lohr F, et al. Conventionally fractionated stereotactic radiotherapy (FSRT) for acoustic neuromas. *Int J Radiat Oncol Biol Phys.* 2000;48(5):1381–1387.
19. Sawamura Y, Shirato H, Sakamoto T, et al. Management of vestibular schwannoma by fractionated stereotactic radiotherapy and associated cerebrospinal fluid malabsorption. *J Neurosurg.* 2003;99(4):685–692.
20. Flickinger JC, Kondziolka D, Niranjan A, Maitz A, Voynov G, Lunsford LD. Acoustic neuroma radiosurgery with marginal tumor doses of 12 to 13 Gy. *Int J Radiat Oncol Biol Phys.* 2004;60(1):225–230.
21. Harsh GR, Thornton AF, Chapman PH, Bussiere MR, Rabinov JD, Loeffler JS. Proton beam stereotactic radiosurgery of vestibular schwannomas. *Int J Radiat Oncol Biol Phys.* 2002;54(1):35–44.
22. Meijer OW, Vandertop WP, Baayen JC, Slotman BJ. Single-fraction vs. fractionated LINAC-based stereotactic radiosurgery for vestibular schwannoma: a single-institution study. *Int J Radiat Oncol Biol Phys.* 2003;56(5):1390–1396.
23. Lederman G, Lowry J, Wertheim S, Fine M, Lombardi E, Wronski M, Artbit E. Acoustic neuroma: potential benefits of fractionated stereotactic radiosurgery. *Stereotact Funct Neurosurg.* 1997;69(1-4 Pt2): 175–182.
24. Lee DJ, Van Dyke GS, Kim J. Update on pathogenesis and treatment of acne. *Curr Opin Pediatr.* 2003;15(4):405–410.
25. Pollock BE, Lunsford LD, Kondziolka D, et al. Vestibular schwannoma management. Part II. Failed radiosurgery and the role of delayed microsurgery. *J Neurosurg.* 1998;89(6):949–955.
26. Shamisa A, Bance M, Nag S, et al. Glioblastoma multiforme occurring in a patient treated with gamma knife surgery. Case report and review of the literature. *J Neurosurg.* 2001;94(5):816–821.
27. Shin M, Ueki K, Kurita H, Kirino T. Malignant transformation of a vestibular schwannoma after gamma knife radiosurgery. *Lancet.* 2002;360(9329):309–310.

Chapter 5

Skull-Base Tumors

E. Stereotactic Fractionated Radiation Therapy for Optic Nerve Sheath Meningiomas

Neil R. Miller

Optic nerve sheath meningiomas (ONSMs) account for one third of primary optic nerve tumors, are the second most common optic nerve tumors after gliomas, and are the most common tumors of the optic nerve sheath. Although ONSMs are said to comprise 1% to 2% of all meningiomas, their reported incidence has increased since the development of more advanced neuroimaging techniques, which also have contributed significantly to earlier recognition of the disease. The mean age at presentation for ONSMs is 41 years (range 3–80 years), with women being affected more frequently than men (3:2) (1). Patients with neurofibromatosis have a higher incidence of ONSM compared with the general population. Almost all cases are unilateral.

ONSMs may be primary or secondary. Secondary ONSMs arise intracranially from dura on or near the planum sphenoidale and spread anteriorly within the confines of the optic nerve sheath through the optic canal to surround the orbital portion of the nerve, whereas primary ONSMs arise from arachnoid cap cells within the dural sheath surrounding the orbital or, less commonly, the canalicular portion of the optic nerve.

Independent of the primary site of origin, ONSMs usually spread around the optic nerve through the subdural and subarachnoid spaces, following pathways of least resistance such as vessels and dural septae. As they spread, they compromise the function of the nerve by impairing blood supply to the nerve and by compressing nerve fibers, thus interfering with axon transport. In addition, because these tumors are interposed between the nerve substance and its extradurally derived blood supply, most ONSMs are not amenable to resection with preservation of vision. In addition, there are no medications that will stop or reverse the growth of these lesions. Accordingly, radiation therapy has become the treatment of choice when treatment is needed to protect or restore vision.

CLINICAL MANIFESTATIONS

The majority of patients with ONSMs present with a slowly progressive optic neuropathy characterized by a variable loss of visual acuity. In a study by Dutton (1), 45% of patients had a visual acuity of 20/40 or better, whereas fewer than 25% had counting fingers or worse. Even patients who do not have significant reduction in visual acuity at presentation often have disturbances of color vision and visual field. Less common symptoms in patients with ONSMs include periocular or retrobulbar pain or discomfort, double vision, and transient visual obscurations. The obscurations of vision are very brief, lasting only a few seconds, almost always associated with optic disc swelling, and in some cases exacerbated or induced by eye movement.

Almost all patients with a unilateral ONSM have an ipsilateral relative afferent pupillary defect, and most have optic disc swelling without peripapillary hemorrhages or soft or hard exudates. Other ophthalmoscopic findings include macular swelling contiguous with a swollen optic disc, choroidal folds, and acquired retinochoroidal shunt vessels (Figure 5E.1). Indeed, the triad of visual loss, optic disc pallor, and retinochoroidal shunts is almost pathognomonic for ONSM, although Hollenhorst et al. (2) observed that this triad tends to occur relatively late in the course of the disorder. Orbital signs such as proptosis are present in 30% to 65% of patients with ONSMs, depending on the series. Mechanical restriction of ocular motility is found in 39% of patients but usually is asymptomatic.

IMAGING

The diagnosis of an ONSM may be made by a variety of imaging studies, most often high-resolution computed tomographic scanning, thin-section MRI, or ultrasonography. These studies obviate the need for tissue biopsy in most cases, making an early diagnosis possible without potentially damaging the optic nerve during surgery.

ONSMs have three main morphologic patterns on imaging: tubular, fusiform, and globular. CT scanning typically shows enlargement of the optic nerve with an increased density peripherally and decreased density centrally (the "tram-track" sign; Figure 5E.2). These changes are particularly well seen after intravenous injection of iodinated contrast material. In addition, in some cases

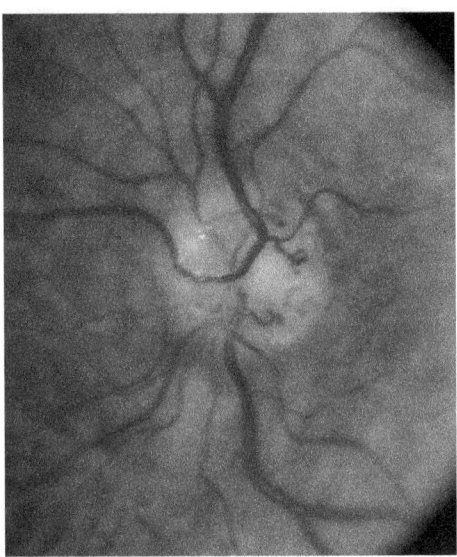

FIGURE 5E.1 Optic disc appearance in advanced optic nerve sheath meningioma showing mild pallid swelling with retinochoroidal collateral vessels.

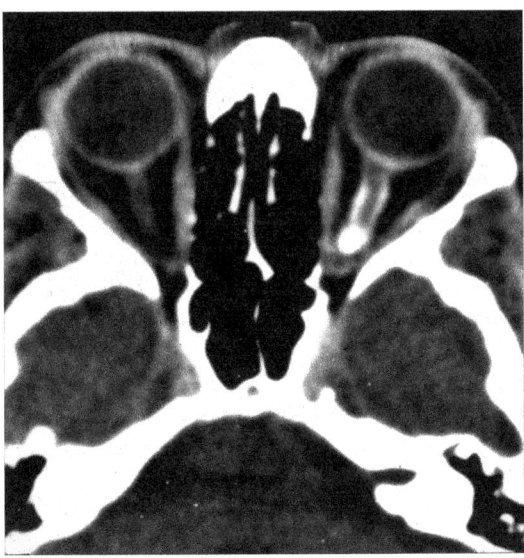

FIGURE 5E.2 Axial CT scan showing tram-track appearance of left optic nerve in a patient with a presumed left optic nerve sheath meningioma.

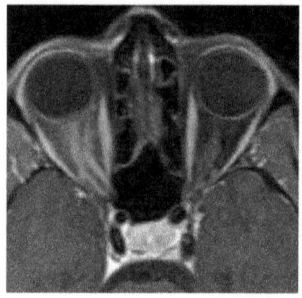 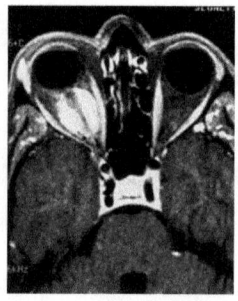 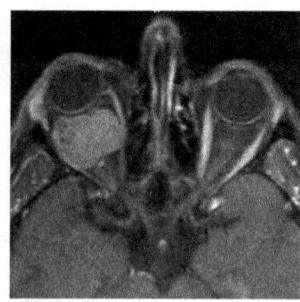

FIGURE 5E.3 MRI appearance of primary ONSMs. (A) T1-weighted, contrast-enhanced axial MRI of a diffuse right ONSM showing "tram-track" sign. (B) T1-weighted, contrast-enhanced, axial MRI of a fusiform right ONSM. (C) T1-weighted, unenhanced, axial MRI of an ONSM that presented as a well-circumscribed globular mass adjacent to the right optic nerve.

of ONSM, calcifications surrounding the nerve are present on CT scanning, although they may be masked by contrast enhancement and thus are best identified on precontrast soft-tissue and bone-windowed images. The presence of such calcifications is thought to indicate slow growth.

MRI provides somewhat better detail of ONSMs than does CT scanning (Figure 5E.3). In particular, the soft-tissue component of the tumor is readily visible, particularly in T1-weighted, contrast-enhanced, fat-saturated images. The appearance of the optic nerve on enhanced coronal MRI images is most often that of a hypodense area (the optic nerve) surrounded by an enhancing thin, fusiform, or globular ring of tissue (the tumor). Careful examination of these images discloses that, rather than having a perfectly smooth outline, all forms of ONSMs have very fine extensions into the adjacent orbital fat (Figure 5E.4). MRI also provides superb tissue detail that allows an assessment of intracranial extension.

In addition to CT scanning and MRI, ultrasonography of the orbit can be helpful in the diagnosis of an ONSM. The typical echographic characteristics of an ONSM were described by Byrnes and Green (3) and consist of an enlargement in the diameter of the nerve with predominantly medium-high reflectivity and an irregular acoustic structure. There may be shadowing from internal calcification. In many cases, performance of a 30-degree test reveals solid thickening of the nerve, whereas in others, the tumor is located more posteriorly, and the 30-degree test is negative or shows changes consistent with anterior nerve enlargement due to cerebrospinal fluid trapped by the tumor.

MANAGEMENT

The threshold for radiation damage to the optic nerve and the optic chiasm is estimated to be 8 to 10 Gy for a single dose. Because doses of radiation in this

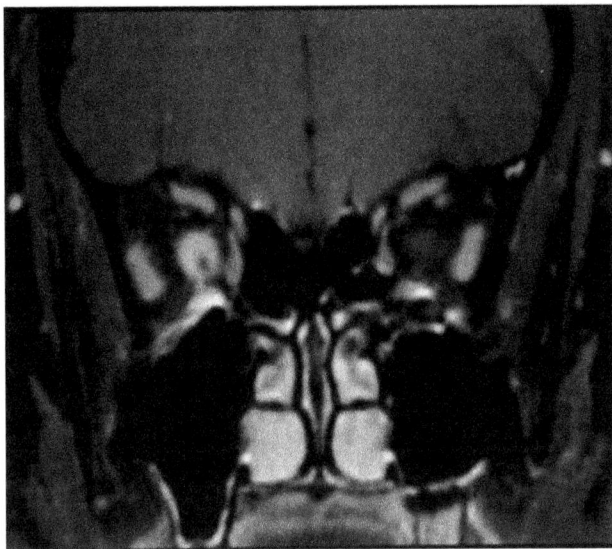

FIGURE 5E.4 Magnetic resonance image, coronal view, enhanced, showing typical features of a right optic nerve sheath meningioma. Note that there is a ring of diffuse enhancement surrounding the right optic nerve, which is hypointense. Note also the fine extensions of the mass into the surrounding orbital tissue.

low range are unlikely to be sufficient for long-term meningioma control, and because a high, single dose of radiation is associated with a high risk of tissue damage, single-dose stereotactic radiosurgery (SRS) is not widely used to treat ONSMs; however, a 5- to 6-week course of fractionated stereotactic radiotherapy (FSR) can deliver a sufficient amount of radiation to an ONSM in a manner more focused than that of conventional fractionated radiation therapy, thus providing the requisite amount of radiation to control the tumor while, one hopes, minimizing the complications from exposure of the surrounding tissue to high doses of radiation. Although a 5- to 6-week course of therapy, 50 to 54 Gy at 1.8 to 2 Gy per day, is inconvenient for the patient compared with single-dose or very short-course (3–5 days) treatment, it is the most validated regimen for minimizing the risk of severe damage to the visual sensory pathway, with respect to both short- and long-term outcome.

FSR requires complex planning that is facilitated by sophisticated software and three-dimensional imaging. A specially configured and stabilized treatment machine that can deliver validated imaging and precisely target the radiation based on three-dimensional stereotactic spatial coordinates is used. Depending on the machine to be used, the pretreatment imaging (CT scanning, MRI, or both) and the radiation delivery require the patient to be immobilized repeatedly, although some linear accelerator (LINAC) units such as the CyberKnife use a tracking and/or noninvasive mask system that eliminates the need for invasive immobilization that historically has been used for single-dose SRS. Using this technique, every beam is size and shape adjusted by a variety of different devices, microleaf collimators being the most advanced method of achieving a high-degree of conformality to the tumor, thus minimizing potentially damaging irradiation of surrounding tissue. Although class 1 data are not available to confirm better long-term tumor control and visual outcome with the use of stereotactic technology compared with what is achieved with conventional fractionated radiation therapy, it is logical to assume that the increased accuracy in targeting and dose delivery should result in better treatment of the tumor. In addition, the added confidence in physical and dose accuracy reduces the need to expand the high-dose region to create a margin of error for positioning and targeting uncertainty. This allows reduction of dose to important unaffected tissues at risk for toxicity such as the retina and optic nerve and allows for the use of radiation plans where confidence in targeting permits use of dose distributions with sharp reduction beyond the intended target.

Fractionated intensity-modulated radiotherapy (IMRT) is a high-precision technique that can be used instead of FSR for both planning and administering radiation to ONSMs. With this technology, not only can the shape of the beam of radiation be altered to enhance dose conformity, but the intensity at various positions within the beam can be modulated to reduce high-dose volumes or enhance low-dose areas and, thus, enhance the ability of the radiation to target the tumor and protect unaffected adjacent normal tissue.

Patients with presumed ONSMs treated with both FSR or IMRT generally have an excellent short-term and long-term prognosis characterized by sustained visual improvement or at least stability with minimal complications (Figures 5E.5 and 5E.6; 4–11). Combining the data from published studies, it would appear that about 95% of patients with presumed or, rarely, biopsy-proven ONSMs treated with one of these techniques experience improvement in or stability of visual function in the affected eye. Improvement in visual function generally begins within 3 months after treatment in the majority of the cases and, in some cases, within a few weeks after completion of radiation (12). Posttreatment imaging generally shows no change in tumor size or extent, although some tumors, particularly those with a fusiform or globular appearance, demonstrate a slight reduction in volume over time.

Acute effects of both FSR and IMRT may include headache, nausea, local erythema, and focal alopecia. None of these complications tends to be severe or permanent. Patients rarely experience a worsening of vision during treatment; however, this tends to be transient and usually responds dramatically to treatment with systemic corticosteroids.

FSR and IMRT are not without potential permanent visual complications. Radiation retinopathy is the most common, usually developing between 14 months and 4 years following treatment with at least 45 to 50 Gy of radiation. Patients in whom this complication occurs may be asymptomatic, but some authors have reported loss of vision ranging from 20/25 to light perception (13,14). We believe that patients with ONSMs involving the proximal part of the

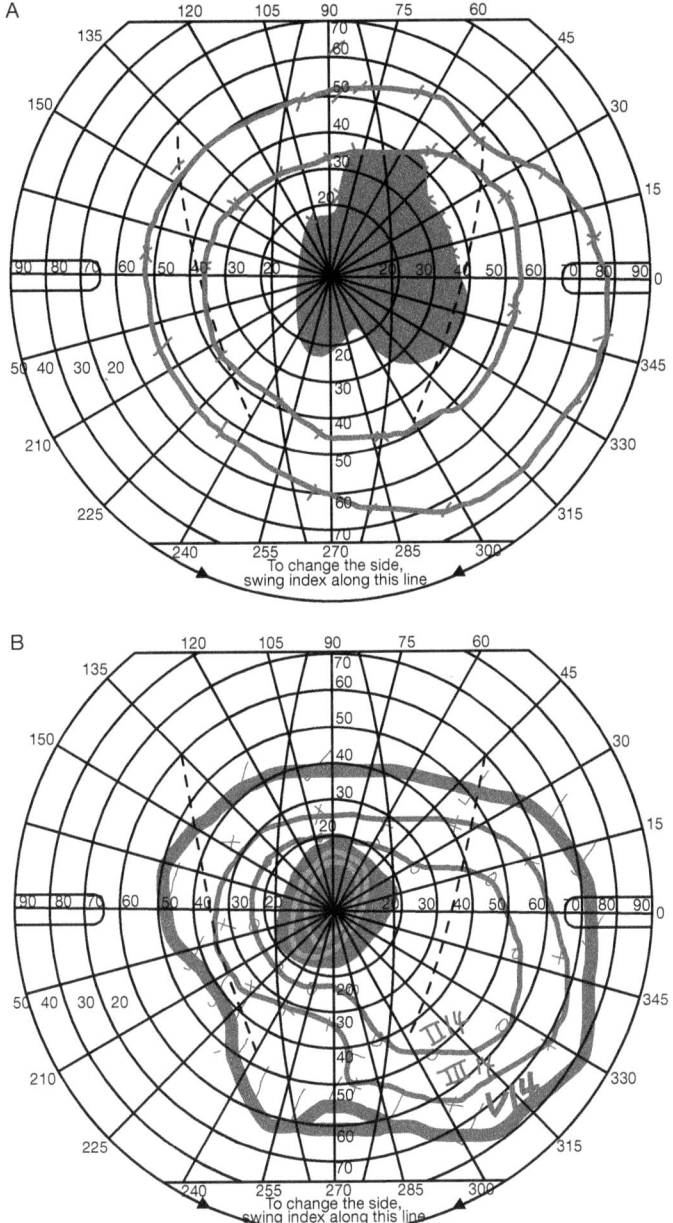

FIGURE 5E.5 Visual fields obtained before (A) and 15 years after (B) SRS for a presumed right optic nerve sheath meningioma. Before treatment, the patient had a slightly constricted peripheral field and a very large central scotoma. After treatment, the patient has a full peripheral field and a persistent but somewhat smaller central scotoma.

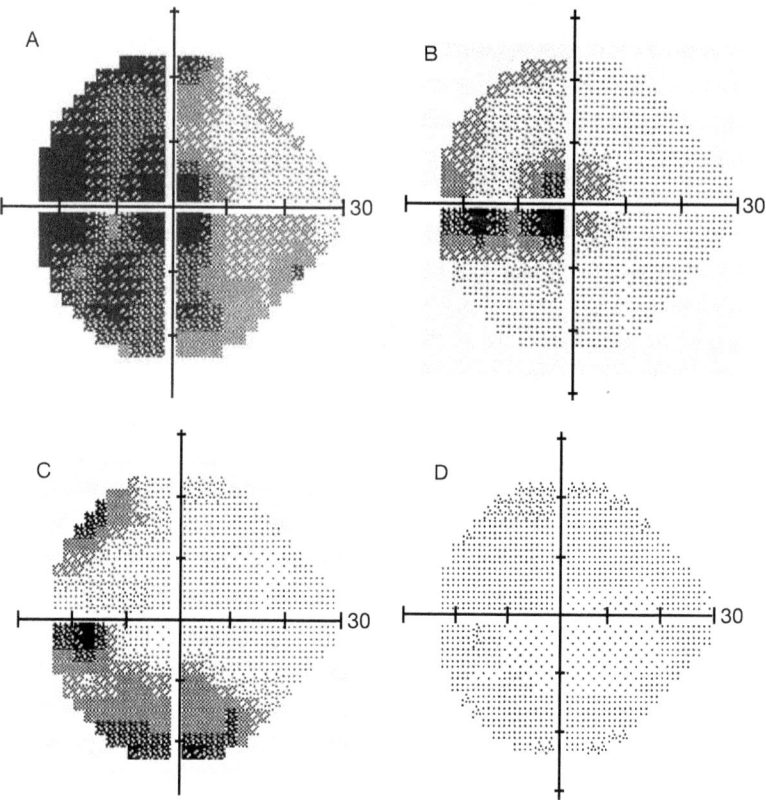

FIGURE 5E.6 Pre (A and C) and post (B and D) visual fields of two patients before and more than 5 years after FSR for presumed ONSMs.

optic nerve adjacent to the globe are at the greatest risk of developing radiation-induced retinopathy, and this potential complication thus should be considered when deciding whether or not to treat such patients.

Other late ophthalmic complications of FSR/IMRT include cataract, dry eye, and iritis. Although radiation optic neuropathy is a potential complication, it appears to occur rarely; we have never seen a case. Indeed, it has been estimated that the risk of damage to the visual sensory system with FSR/IMRT is 3% with a total fractionated dose less than 55 Gy, 3% to 7% with a total dose of 55 to 60 Gy, and 7% to 20% with doses of 60 Gy or higher (15). Finally, some patients continue to lose vision from tumor progression despite FSR/IMRT, although this should not be considered a complication of the treatment.

Late nonocular side effects of FSR/IMRT include pituitary dysfunction and punctate white-matter lesions in the cerebral hemispheres sometimes associated with cognitive dysfunction. Dose tolerance for the pituitary gland is not precisely known, but clinically meaningful reductions in one or more hormone levels may become reduced years after treatment. Thus, limiting the dose to the pituitary and hypothalamus is desirable. The volume of normal brain receiving near the prescribed dose of radiation also should be limited, with the goal being to protect cognitive function, although this complication should be uncommon with the volumes generally used to treat ONSMs unless there is substantial intracranial extension of the tumor. Nevertheless, interval monitoring of both pituitary function and cognitive status in this setting is appropriate.

In the final analysis, adherence to dose guidelines for normal tissues, consistent with the primary objective of effectively treating the tumor, can limit the risk of long-term complications in patients with ONSMs. Such patients generally can be expected to retain useful vision in both their affected and unaffected eyes, retain normal neurologic function, and have a normal life expectancy.

CONCLUSION

The main goals in the management of ONSMs are ensuring a favorable visual outcome, establishing local control of the tumor, and minimizing the risks of treatment-related morbidity. Limitations for any treatment study of ONSMs include both the rarity and usually very slow course of the disease, the fact that there often is no tissue diagnosis so that some patients in a treatment trial could have lesions other than an ONSM (e.g. sarcoidosis), the necessity of pooling data from multiple different treatment centers, and the need for a long (greater than 10 years) follow-up period to detect late recurrences and late side effects of the treatment.

In the studies described so far, the long-term efficacy of FSR in preserving or improving vision appears to be excellent, with more than half of the patients having an improvement within 3 months following treatment. The results also suggest that earlier treatment might offer a better chance of preserving useful vision. Based on the results of published studies, we believe that FSR is the best option for most cases of progressive or advanced disease; however, because of improved imaging, patients with presumed ONSMs associated with mild progressive or stable visual loss are being diagnosed earlier, and the choice between observation and radiation has become more difficult.

REFERENCES

1. Dutton JJ. Optic nerve sheath meningiomas. *Surv Ophthalmol.* 1992;37:167–183.
2. Hollenhorst RW Jr, Hollenhorst RW Sr, MacCarty CS. Visual prognosis of optic nerve sheath meningiomas producing shunt vessels on the optic disk: the Hoyt-Spencer syndrome. *Trans Am Ophthalmol Soc.* 1977;75:141–163.
3. Byrne SF, Green RL. *Ultrasound of the Eye and Orbit.* 2nd ed. St. Louis, MO: Mosby; 2002.

4. Andrews DW, Faroozan R, Yang BP, et al. Fractionated stereotactic radiotherapy for the treatment of optic nerve sheath meningiomas: preliminary observations of 33 optic nerves in 30 patients with historical comparison to observation with or without prior surgery. *Neurosurgery*. 2002;51:890–902.
5. Liu JK, Forman S, Hershewe GL, Moorthy CR, Benzil DL. Optic nerve sheath meningiomas: visual improvement after stereotactic radiotherapy. *Neurosurgery*. 2002;50:950–955.
6. Pitz S, Becker G, Schiefer U, et al. Stereotactic fractionated irradiation of optic nerve sheath meningioma: a new treatment alternative. *Br J Ophthalmol*. 2002;86(11):1265–1268.
7. Baumert BG, Villa S, Studer G, Mirimanoff RO, Davis JB, Landau K. Early improvements in vision after fractionated stereotactic radiotherapy for primary optic nerve sheath meningioma. *Radiother Oncol*. 2004;72:169–174.
8. Arvold ND, Lessell S, Bussiere M, et al. Visual outcome and tumour control after conformal radiotherapy for patients with optic nerve sheath meningioma. *Int J Radiation Oncol Biol Phys*. 2009;75(4):1166–1172.
9. Lesser RL, Knisely JP, Wang SL, Yu JB, Kupersmith MJ. Long-term response to fractionated radiotherapy of presumed optic nerve sheath meningioma. *Br J Ophthalmol*. 2010;94(5):559–563.
10. Metellus P, Kapoor S, Kharkar S, et al. Fractionated conformal radiotherapy for management of optic nerve sheath meningiomas: long-term outcomes of tumor control and visual function at a single institution. *Int J Radiat Oncol Biol Phys*. 2011;80(1):185–192; Epub ahead of print.
11. Saeed P, Rootman J, Nugent RA, White VA, Mackenzie IR, Koornneef L. Optic nerve sheath meningiomas. *Ophthalmology*. 2003;110:2019–2030.
12. Vaghefi MR, Larson DA, Horton JC. Optic nerve sheath meningioma: visual improvement during radiation treatment. *Am J Ophthalmol*. 142(2):343–344.
13. Narayan S, Cornblath WT, Sandler HM, Elner V, Hayman JA. Preliminary visual outcomes after three-dimensional conformal radiation therapy for optic nerve sheath meningioma. *Int J Radiat Oncol Biol Phys*. 2003;56:537–543.
14. Subramanian PS, Bressler NM, Miller NR. Radiation retinopathy after fractionated stereotactic radiotherapy for optic nerve sheath meningioma. *Ophthalmology*. 2004;111:565–567.
15. Marks LB, Yorke ED, Jackson A, et al. Use of normal complication probability models in the clinic. *Int J Radiat Oncol Biol Phys*. 2010;76(3 suppl):S10–19.

Chapter 5

Skull-Base Tumors

F. Role of Radiosurgery for Sellar Lesions

Bowen Jiang, Wendy Hara, & Gordon Li

GENERAL PRINCIPLES AND OVERVIEW

The sella turcica is an anatomically and pathologically important depression of the sphenoid bone at the skull base. This region is bound superiorly by the pituitary stalk and optic chiasm, inferiorly by the sphenoid sinus, and medial/laterally by the cavernous sinus and carotid arteries. Mass lesions that affect the sellar and parasellar regions include an array of tumors, cysts, vascular malformations, and inflammatory/infectious etiologies. The most common neoplastic lesions in this area are pituitary adenomas, craniopharyngiomas, skull-base meningiomas, and metastasis. Despite being generally histologically benign, sellar neoplasms can cause severe and often permanent damage to nearby hypothalamic, visual, and endocrine apparatus. The presentation of these tumors may include symptoms related to endocrine derangement of the hypothalamic–pituitary axis, secretion of hormones by functional tumors, increased intracranial pressure, and/or visual field defects due to mass effect on the optic chiasm.

PITUITARY ADENOMAS

Pituitary adenomas account for 15% to 20% of primary intracranial neoplasms. They can be classified broadly as hormone secreting (75%) or nonsecretory (25%). The most common secretory pituitary tumor is the prolactinoma, which can lead to galactorrhea, amenorrhea, infertility, and/or impotence. Somatotrophic adenomas such as a growth-hormone-secreting tumor can result in acromegaly. Nonsecretory adenomas tend to grow progressively and cause mass effect, including compression of the optic chiasm leading to bitemporal hemianopsia.

Craniopharyngiomas

Craniopharyngiomas are benign extra-axial epithelial tumors arising from remnants of the Rathke pouch, near the pituitary gland. Although craniopharyngiomas are rare, they are the most common suprasellar tumor in the pediatric age group, accounting for as many as 5% of all intracranial tumors or up to 10% of pediatric brain tumors. The incidence has been estimated to be approximately 1.5 per million people per year.

Meningiomas

Meningiomas are the second most common primary central nervous system (CNS) neoplasm and arise from arachnoid meningothelial cells of the meninges. Most meningiomas are diagnosed in the sixth or seventh decades of life and are more common in women; these tumors are mostly benign and exhibit indolent growth patterns. Parasellar and medial sphenoid meningiomas collectively make up roughly 12% of all intracranial meningiomas.

Metastasis

The sellar region is often affected by metastasis, with series demonstrating a 1.8% to 6% incidence in autopsied cancer patients. Breast cancer is the most frequent primary cancer to metastasize to this region, followed by lung, gastrointestinal (GI), and nasopharyngeal cancers. Lymphomas, leukemias, and multiple myeloma have also been known to affect the sellar region. Most patients are asymptomatic, but among those with symptoms diabetes insipidus is the most common presentation.

EVALUATION AND DIAGNOSIS

Imaging

Thin-slice MRI of the sella with and without gadolinium is the gold standard. CT can be used to evaluate degree of sinus aeration and bone erosion.

Endocrine

All facets of the hypothalamic–pituitary–adrenal axis should be accessed in a suspected pituitary adenoma. Evaluation of hypo or hyperpituitary could include serum adrenocorticotropic hormone (ACTH), cortisol, thyroid-stimulating hormone (TSH), free T4, luteinizing hormone (LH), follicle-stimulating hormone (FSH), growth hormone (GH), insulin-like growth factor 1 (IGF-1), prolactin, and estradiol/testosterone. Levels of prolactin greater than 200 ng/ml suggests a prolactinoma as opposed to stalk effect.

Ophthalmological Evaluation

Patients should undergo visual field and acuity testing. A dilated fundoscopic exam should be completed to evaluate for nerve edema.

RADIOSURGERY MANAGEMENT STRATEGIES

Radiation therapy has been used as both an initial step in the management of sellar lesions and as an adjuvant therapy to surgical resection. Conventional or fractionated radiotherapy refers to the repeated administration of smaller doses, with fractionation schemes consisting of 1.5 to 2 Gy daily up to a cumulative dose of 30 to 54 Gy. Stereotactic radiosurgery is able to deliver large doses of radiation to a small and precisely defined target. As such, stereotactic radiosurgery can deliver larger doses over conventional radiotherapy while sparing nearby structures like the optic apparatus. In recent years, stereotactic radiosurgery has blossomed under two radiation-delivery technologies, a multiple cobalt60 gamma radiation-emitting source such as the Gamma Knife and a modified linear accelerator such as the CyberKnife. Both stereotactic systems can deliver a radiation beam to within approximately 1 mm of the lesion and will be the subject of further discussion in this chapter.

TREATMENT GOALS AND INDICATIONS

- An important goal in managing sellar lesions is to remove mass effect on the surrounding neurocritical structures, including the optic nerve, optic chiasm, and cavernous sinus. Patients with secretory pituitary adenomas also benefit from normalization of hormonal function. The primary therapy for sellar neoplastic lesions remains surgical resection, most frequently via transsphenoidal or transcranial approach. However, stereotactic radiosurgery remains an important management modality,

particularly in treating residual disease, inoperable lesions, or medically/surgically refractory lesions. Indications for stereotactic radiosurgery include: residual tumor status post surgical resection or tumor present in the cavernous sinus
- Pituitary function and hormonal function not normalized with optimal medical and surgical management.
- Patient is a high-risk surgical candidate.

RADIOSURGICAL PLANNING AND TECHNIQUE

Stereotactic radiosurgery in the form of the Gamma Knife (GKS) and CyberKnife are frequently used in the management of sellar lesions. With the Gamma Knife, a fixed-head frame using four pins that penetrate the outer table of the skull is usually done under local anesthesia. The CyberKnife machine uses a compact linear accelerator mounted on a robotic arm. Patients are kept relatively immobile with the use of a noninvasive head restraint, such as the molded Aquaplast mask. X-rays are taken frequently throughout the treatment course to track any movement of the skull and the robotic arm adjusts the position of the linear accelerator accordingly. For both Gamma Knife and CyberKnife, therapeutic effectiveness involves the delivery of multiple pencil beams to converge on a target. Small collimators are used to ensure that energy deposition drops off steeply just beyond the target volume. Prior to initiation of therapy a treatment planning session involving creation of the immobilization devices, and a thin-slice contrast-enhanced CT (1.25 mm) and MR scan are done. The images are fused and the target is then delineated on computer software and a radiation plan created with the aid of a radiation physicist. Reports have shown that conformational contouring could allow for a treatment plan for sellar lesions to be within 0.1 mm accuracy with the Gamma Knife (1).

In terms of managing secretory pituitary adenomas, there is evidence that stopping antisecretory medications at the time of radiosurgery is associated with better endocrine normalization (2,3). The authors also recommend using a fractionation scheme (i.e., with CyberKnife) when the single-fraction dose exceeds 13 Gy to more than 20% of the brainstem, as is often encountered in sellar lesions such as craniopharyngiomas (4).

DOSING

There are several assumptions that contribute to dosimetry calculations for stereotactic radiation delivery. In a review by Timmerman et al. (5) the authors outlined three requirements necessary for a successful treatment: (a) the ability to describe the location of the target, (b) the ability to shape the prescription isodose surface to the surface of the target volume, and (c) the ability to construct radiation dose distributions with very rapid falloff dose to spare surrounding healthy tissue. In a review of the current literature, the dosage ranges for specific tumors are described below.

Pituitary Adenoma (Secretory)

To avoid injury to the optic apparatus, the radiation dose for the optic nerve should be less than 8 to 12 Gy (6). The degree of hormone normalization is associated with amount of radiation, with less normalization correlated with lower marginal doses. A dose of 15 Gy is considered reliable for early tumor growth control (7). For patients with GH-secreting adenomas, a review of 22 studies before 2003 shows a marginal dose range of 15 to 34 Gy. In the 23 published studies from 2003 to 2010, a marginal dose range of 10 to 32 Gy has been reported (8). In practice, 20 to 25 Gy is commonly prescribed. Prolactinomas are treated with a marginal dose range of 14 to 33 Gy based on 17 studies (9). Higher doses appear to have a faster response. ACTH-secreting adenomas are commonly treated with 20 to 25 Gy (range 15–30 Gy) with faster biochemical response with SRS as compared to fractionated treatment (10,11). Most of these studies used Gamma Knife as the radiosurgery device. For both secretory and nonsecretory pituitary adenomas, the 50% isodose is the most common prescription isodose line in the GKS series because this line is where the slope of the radiation falloff is the steepest (11).

Pituitary Adenoma (Nonsecretory)

In general, nonsecretory pituitary adenomas can be treated with a smaller radiosurgical dose, optimally between 14 and 18 Gy with the goal of stabilization or shrinkage of the tumor. A review of 13 series showed that marginal doses ranged from 14 to 25 Gy (11,12).

Craniopharyngiomas

Ten Gamma Knife studies have reported marginal doses ranging from 8 to 25 Gy, with most prescribing 10 to 15 Gy (4). Three CyberKnife series have reported larger marginal doses, which ranged from 21 to 40 Gy, treated to an isodose curve of 75% (13,14). The CyberKnife series used fractionation in order to minimize toxicity to the optic apparatus and brainstem.

Meningiomas

Median marginal doses of 12 to 16 Gy have been reported in the literature for skull-base lesions (15,16). Larger lesions (greater than 10 cm^3 in volume) could be adequately controlled with approximately 15 Gy (17).

SAMPLE TREATMENT PLAN

A 32-year-old female patient initially presented with headache and visual field deficits and was diagnosed with a craniopharyngioma. She underwent three prior surgical resections. Prior to the radiosurgical treatment, the residual disease was 1.4 cm^3. A treatment dose of 18 Gy was delivered in three fractions to the 75% isodose curve, with a maximum dose of 22.5 Gy. At last follow-up, the tumor was decreased in size and the patient's symptoms were improved.

CLINICAL OUTCOMES AND PROGNOSIS

There are two main therapeutic goals in treating sellar lesions with stereotactic radiosurgery. The first is to limit or decrease tumor volume, thus reducing the amount of mass/compressive effect on nearby structures. The second goal, particularly for secretory pituitary adenomas, is to normalize hormone profiles. In nearly all published series, stereotactic radiosurgery is associated with excellent tumor control. For nonsecretory pituitary adenomas, the mean tumor control rate has been reported to be around 93%, with a range of 68% to 100% (18). For secretory pituitary adenomas, there is a lack of consistency in the current literature in presenting final outcomes, with many studies reporting different ranges of "cure" for endocrine normalization. In 20 series for GH-secreting pituitary adenomas, endocrine cure rates vary from 0% to 96% with improvement shown in an additional 0% to 67% of patients (11). The overall tumor control in GH adenoma series ranges from 92% to 100% in 23 studies (8). The endocrine remission rate for prolactinomas is approximately 15% to 50% after SRS and can increase to 40% to 80% with the addition of medical therapy (19–22). The published studies for craniopharyngiomas demonstrate an average control rate of 90% for solid tumors, 88% for cystic tumors, and 60% for mixed tumors. Tumor control was achieved with a mean marginal dose of 12 Gy and recurrence of tumor was observed in 85% of cases that received a marginal dose less than 6 Gy (4). External-beam radiotherapy is often used initially with SRS for local recurrences. For meningiomas, 15 studies with a total 2,734 patients were reviewed; 77.1% were classified as skull base and/or sellar. Overall disease stabilization rate was 89%, on par with reported averages for pituitary adenomas and craniopharyngiomas (23).

COMPLICATIONS

According to a systematic review by Witt et al. of more than 1,255 patients who underwent stereotactic radiosurgery for pituitary adenomas, radiation-induced optic neuropathy was found in 11 patients (0.9%; 11). Several sources have indicated 10 to 12 Gy as the upper limit for radiation to the optic apparatus without neuropathy, and most radiosurgeons have in fact used 8 Gy or less to avoid such complications. Interestingly, the cranial nerves in the cavernous sinus (CN III, IV, V, VI) are highly tolerant to radiation, with only 0.4% (5 of 1,255) patients showing permanent neurological deficits (11). Furthermore, according to two studies on sellar meningiomas, tumor volume, tumor margin dose, and a history of previous external-beam radiotherapy were not correlated with radiation-related complications (24,25).

Vascular injury is rare following stereotactic radiosurgery to the sella, with some series indicating that internal carotid artery (ICA) dosage should be limited to less than 30 Gy (26). Stereotactic radiation-induced neoplasms are also rare, with zero cases reported by Sheehan et al. in a review of 35 series with 1,621 patients (27), and eight cases reported in over 200,000 patients worldwide who have been treated with Gamma Knife. Finally, pituitary insufficiency has been reported in 1.5% to 72% of patients; this large range may be associated with variations in standards for hormone normalization, length of follow-up, tumor volume, and other treatment modalities.

REFERENCES

1. Takakura K, Hayashi M, Izawa M. Pituitary tumors. In: Chin L, Regine W, eds. *Principles and Practice of Stereotactic Radiosurgery*. New York, NY: Springer; 2008:299–307.
2. Landolt AM, Haller D, Lomax N, et al. Octreotide may act as a radioprotective agent in acromegaly. *J Clin Endocrinol Metab*. 2000;85(3):1287–1289.
3. Landolt AM, Lomax N. Gamma knife radiosurgery for prolactinomas. *J Neurosurg*. 2000;93(suppl 3):14–18.
4. Veeravagu A, Lee M, Jiang B, Chang SD. The role of radiosurgery in the treatment of craniopharyngiomas. *Neurosurg Focus*. 2010;28(4):E11.
5. Timmerman R, Papiez L, Suntharalingam M. Extracranial stereotactic radiation delivery: expansion of technology beyond the brain. *Technol Cancer Res Treat*. 2003;2(2):153–160.
6. Adler JR Jr, Gibbs IC, Puataweepong P, Chang SD. Visual field preservation after multi-session CyberKnife radiosurgery for perioptic lesions. *Neurosurgery*. 2006;59(2):244–54; discussion 244.
7. Lunsford LD. Stereotactic radiosurgery for patients with pituitary adenomas. In: *Radiosurgery Practice Guideline Initiative*. IRSA;2004:1–12.
8. Stapleton CJ, Liu CY, Weiss MH. The role of stereotactic radiosurgery in the multimodal management of growth hormone-secreting pituitary adenomas. *Neurosurg Focus*. 2010;29(4):E11.

9. Tanaka S, Link MJ, Brown PD, Stafford SL, Young WF Jr, Pollock BE. Gamma knife radiosurgery for patients with prolactin-secreting pituitary adenomas. *World Neurosurg.* 2010;74(1):147–152.
10. Mitsumori M, Shrieve DC, Alexander E III, et al. Initial clinical results of LINAC-based stereotactic radiosurgery and stereotactic radiotherapy for pituitary adenomas. *Int J Radiat Oncol Biol Phys.* 1998;42(3):573–580.
11. Witt TC. Stereotactic radiosurgery for pituitary tumors. *Neurosurg Focus.* 2003;14(5):e10.
12. Jagannathan J, Yen CP, Pouratian N, Laws ER, Sheehan JP. Stereotactic radiosurgery for pituitary adenomas: a comprehensive review of indications, techniques and long-term results using the Gamma Knife. *J Neurooncol.* 2009;92(3):345–356.
13. Iwata H, Tatewaki K, Inoue M, et al. Single and hypofractionated stereotactic radiotherapy with CyberKnife for craniopharyngioma. *J Neurooncol.* 2012;106(3):571–577.
14. Lee M, Kalani MY, Cheshier S, Gibbs IC, Adler JR, Chang SD. Radiation therapy and CyberKnife radiosurgery in the management of craniopharyngiomas. *Neurosurg Focus.* 2008;24(5):E4.
15. Igaki H, Maruyama K, Koga T, et al. Stereotactic radiosurgery for skull base meningioma. *Neurol Med Chir (Tokyo).* 2009;49(10):456–461.
16. Sheehan JP, Williams BJ, Yen CP. Stereotactic radiosurgery for WHO grade I meningiomas. *J Neurooncol.* 2010;99(3):407–416.
17. Bledsoe JM, Link MJ, Stafford SL, Park PJ, Pollock BE. Radiosurgery for large-volume (> 10 cm^3) benign meningiomas. *J Neurosurg.* 2010;112(5):951–956.
18. Jagannathan J, Schlesinger DJ, Oskouian RJ Jr, et al. Stereotactic radiosurgery for pituitary adenomas. In: Lunsford LD, Sheehan JP, eds. *Intracranial Stereotactic Radiosurgery.* New York, NY:Thieme;2009:Chapter 9.
19. Pan L, Zhang N, Wang EM, Wang BJ, Dai JZ, Cai PW. Gamma knife radiosurgery as a primary treatment for prolactinomas. *J Neurosurg.* 2000;93(suppl 3):10–13.
20. Sheehan J, Rainey J, Nguyen J, Grimsdale R, Han S. Temozolomide-induced inhibition of pituitary adenoma cells. *J Neurosurg.* 2011;114(2):354–358.
21. Sheehan JM, Vance ML, Sheehan JP, Ellegala DB, Laws ER Jr. Radiosurgery for Cushing's disease after failed transsphenoidal surgery. *J Neurosurg.* 2000;93(5):738–742.
22. Tsang RW, Brierley JD, Panzarella T, Gospodarowicz MK, Sutcliffe SB, Simpson WJ. Role of radiation therapy in clinical hormonally-active pituitary adenomas. *Radiother Oncol.* 1996;41(1):45–53.
23. Pannullo SC, Fraser JF, Moliterno J, Cobb W, Stieg PE. Stereotactic radiosurgery: a meta-analysis of current therapeutic applications in neuro-oncologic disease. *J Neurooncol.* 2011;103(1):1–17.
24. Kondziolka D, Levy EI, Niranjan A, Flickinger JC, Lunsford LD. Long-term outcomes after meningioma radiosurgery: physician and patient perspectives. *J Neurosurg.* 1999;91(1):44–50.
25. Stafford SL, Pollock BE, Foote RL, et al. Meningioma radiosurgery: tumor control, outcomes, and complications among 190 consecutive patients. *Neurosurgery.* 2001;49(5):1029–37; discussion 1037.
26. Shin M, Kurita H, Sasaki T, et al. Stereotactic radiosurgery for pituitary adenoma invading the cavernous sinus. *J Neurosurg.* 2000;93(Suppl 3):2–5.
27. Sheehan JP, Niranjan A, Sheehan JM, et al. Stereotactic radiosurgery for pituitary adenomas: an intermediate review of its safety, efficacy, and role in the neurosurgical treatment armamentarium. *J Neurosurg.* 2005;102(4):678–691.

Chapter 6

Imaging Changes Following Radiosurgery for Metastatic Intracranial Tumors: A Review of Differentiating Radiation Effects From Tumor Recurrence

Jacob Ruzevick & Lawrence R. Kleinberg

Stereotactic radiosurgery (SRS) has become standard adjuvant treatment for patients with primary and metastatic intracranial lesions. Recently, there has been a growing appreciation for imaging changes following radiation therapy that can be difficult or impossible to distinguish from the imaging findings of true reoccurrence, which may require intervention. Pseudoprogression, the term used to describe this phenomenon, was originally applied to such changes related to conventional radiotherapy for patients with malignant glioma. In these patients, follow-up MRI demonstrated progression in a substantial proportion of patients, which after surgical biopsy or maintenance of original therapy, proved to be a benign process.

An understanding of pseudoprogression is especially important in the setting of SRS for metastatic disease, both because of the high initial dose of radiation and because the probability of actual early reoccurrence is low as compared to malignant glioma, for which reoccurrence is universal and rapidly fatal. Several groups have reported on pseudoprogression in different intracranial pathologies, showing the incidence of at least temporary tumor enlargement following SRS to be at least 30%, which in many cases exceeds the probability of actual treatment failure after the first year following treatment (1–13).

Pseudoprogression has been well documented for intracranial pathologies that are often treated with SRS, which include vestibular schwannoma, meningioma, brain metastases, and in select cases of malignant glioma. Such changes can also be observed after therapy of arterial venous malformations where it is clear that imaging changes are treatment induced, as bleeding is the only result of treatment failure.

Pseudoprogression is indistinguishable from true progression in a single imaging study and as such, can be considered a retrospective assessment. Although advanced imaging techniques are currently being studied to differentiate between pseudoprogression, radiation necrosis, and true progression, the Neuro-Oncology Working Group concluded that these studies continue to require rigorous validation studies before they are incorporated into widespread use (4).

The gold standard for monitoring treatment success after SRS is serial magnetic resonance imaging. Currently, there is no clinically reliable method for distinguishing treatment effects from progression of the underlying pathology. However, mistakenly assuming treatment effect as progression of the underlying illness can lead to unnecessary and/or risky interventions. For example, if pseudoprogression is mistaken for treatment failure (a) further radiation may be recommended when the imaging changes merely represent a radiation-related change or injury; (b) surgery, which carries its own risks, may proceed as salvage treatment and/or; (c) systemic therapies, which are still aiding the patient, may be altered with the presumption that the mistaken failure represents failure of the systemic chemotherapy. As such, it is important to consider pseudoprogression when early, localized imaging changes are encountered in managing patients who underwent SRS for intracranial pathologies.

IMAGING CHANGES AFTER RADIOSURGERY FOR INTRACRANIAL TUMORS

The incidence of metastatic disease to the brain is estimated to be greater than 170,000 new cases per year in the United States (15) with lung, breast, melanoma, renal, and colon cancers being the predominant primary pathologies. The predominant response to radiation treatment is a gradual decrease or stability of the tumor over a period of months to years. As such, evaluation of posttreatment imaging studies is paramount in determining whether further treatments are necessary. However, this can be complicated by the fact that posttreatment contrast enhancement or a transient increase in size are often nonspecific and may not be a true marker of disease progression. In tumors treated with SRS, approximately 1/3 to 1/2 of patients will experience transient growth as seen by imaging abnormalities up to 2 or more years following initial treatment. Furthermore, during this time period, homogenous ring enhancement may also occur. Several groups have reported on this phenomenon. Ross et al. (16) report that 73% of malignant gliomas and 23% of metastatic intracranial tumors were larger after a mean follow-up of 13 weeks following SRS. In a study of 28 child patients with low-grade astrocytoma, 43% showed an increase in lesion size, gadolinium-enhancement, and edema. Confirmation of radiation effect was made as patients were followed due to a lack of clinical symptoms (17). A summary of selected studies noting imaging changes is shown in Table 6.1.

In a comprehensive review of one institutional experience with brain metastasis patients, Patel et al. (18) report that increases in lesion size began as early as 6 weeks following Gamma Knife treatment, but that this was observed up to 15 months later. Furthermore, the average percent change in lesion volume from the initial pre-SRS treatment imaging was +3.6% and +11.6% at 12 and 15 months, respectively. At all other follow-up periods (up to 36 months), the average lesion volume had decreased from pretreatment size, definitively showing that the increase in lesion size was transient. Radiosensitive tumors showed the greatest flux in tumor volume with multiple episodes of transient growth over the 36-month follow-up period. Radiosensitive lesions (defined as lung, breast, or colon) were more likely to change than radio-resistant tumors (melanoma or renal). Kaplan–Meier analysis of this phenomenon found that patients with pseudoprogression following SRS had better survival as compared to those patients who did not show pseudoprogression of their lesions. Furthermore, in patients undergoing resection or biopsy for an increasing lesion on MRI, suspicious spectroscopy, diffusion weighted imaging, and/or 18 F-fluorodeoxyglucose positron emission tomography (FDG-PET) scan, 96% (22 of 23) had pathology consistent with radiation necrosis.

The most common imaging change following radiosurgery is perilesional edema, with or without increased contrast enhancement, and is the most likely source for changes in neurological status following radiation treatment. The time course of edema following radiosurgery typically peaks in 6 to 8 months, although it has been reported as far out as 23 months (19,20). The presence of post-treatment edema has been correlated with pretreatment peritumoral edema, sagittal sinus occlusion, larger tumor volumes, doses greater than 16 Gy delivered in a single fraction, marginal doses of radiation, and location of the

TABLE 6.1 Summary of Studies Reporting Pseudoprogression in Intracranial Pathologies

Study	Pathology	Total # of Patients	Early Progression	Pseudoprogression (% of Early Progression)
Multiple authors (1–13)	Glioblastoma multiforme	1179	39% (Weighted average)	36% (Weighted average)
Hayhurst et al. (2011) (21)	Vestibular schwannoma	75	49/75 (65%)	17/75 (23%)
Patel et al. (2011) (18)	Multiple metastases	120	NA	32%
Valanne et al. (1996) (22)	Cavernous angioma	1 (Case report)	1/1 (100%)	1/1 (100%)
Miyatake et al. (2009) (23)	Meningioma	13	NA	3/13 (21%)

primary pathology. Mechanisms of radiation-induced edema are thought to be the release of toxins from damaged tumor cells, in conjunction with disruption of the leptomeninges, leading to the spread of vasogenic fluid into the brain parenchyma. Furthermore, normal brain surrounding a tumor may receive high enough doses of radiation to cause radiation-induced injury due to the infiltrative nature of some tumors, as compared to those that are encapsulated in a connective tissue core.

In attempts to discern the difference between radiation effects and tumor progression, other imaging modalities, such as positron emission tomography and single-photon emission computed tomography (SPECT), have been evaluated although these modalities do not appear promising (24–26). FDG-PET scanning is approximately 40% sensitive in determining tumor progression from radiation necrosis. For hexamethylpropyleneamine oxime (HMPAO) SPECT imaging, low uptake of both thallium and HMPAO is associated with radiation effects, whereas increased uptake of both agents are associated with tumor progression. However, due to lack of widespread clinical availability and feasibility of serial imaging, as well as high false-positive rates, both FDG-PET and HMPAO are unlikely to offer an efficacious method of determining radiation effect.

IMAGING CHANGES SEEN AFTER RADIOSURGERY FOR ARTERIOVENOUS MALFORMATIONS

Radiosurgery is an effective method for treating arteriovenous malformations (AVMs) that are less than 3 mL and in difficult to resect brain regions. Hemorrhage remains the most catastrophic event following radiosurgery, but is usually unrelated to the SRS itself. Other imaging changes that have been described include parenchymal changes and uniform or irregular enhancement of the lesion after gadolinium-enhanced MRI in upward of 30% of patients. The majority of patients with imaging changes not due to hemorrhage do not show neurological deficits (27). Levegrün et al. report that imaging changes (edema or blood–brain barrier breakdown) were not dependent on the prescribed radiation dose. Rather, the total volume receiving at least 12 Gy as well as the 20 cm^3 of brain tissue receiving the highest dose were significantly associated with imaging changes following radiation treatment, suggesting single dose and volume parameters can be predictive of radiation-induced imaging changes following treatment.

Interestingly, patients who undergo SRS for AVM could be a useful population to more rigorously study SRS-related imaging changes as the underlying pathology rarely causes similar imaging changes and radiation rarely causes hemorrhage.

BIOLOGY OF IMAGING CHANGES AFTER RADIOSURGERY

The goal of radiosurgery is to induce tumor-cell-specific, double-stranded DNA damage irrespective of cell cycle phase. By delivering many foci of radiation, which converge at the site of the intracranial pathology, irreversible damage can be inflicted on tumor cells while sparing normal brain parenchyma. In the case of AVMs, the likely mechanism of nidus obliteration is endothelial damage, which starts a cascade of intimal smooth muscle proliferation, collagen deposition, and sclerosis. In metastatic lesions, Patel et al. (18) reported that specific changes on MRI correlated with coagulative necrosis (central T1 hypointensity), reactive gliosis and demyelination (surrounding T1 hypointensity), and vascular hyalinization (T1 ring-enhancing portion).

The mechanism of pseudoprogression is not well understood, although general hypotheses have been proposed and include a pronounced tissue reaction to inflammation, edema, and abnormal vessel permeability leading to new or enhanced contrast uptake. Second, because the brain is thought to be devoid of lymphatics, it may take longer to clear cellular debris, leading to an increased inflammatory reaction. Further evidence for this consists of correlations between pseudoprogression and increased survival, suggesting that an inflammatory component may be involved (28).

Imaging changes after radiation treatment can also correlate with clinical symptoms. Side effects following radiation treatment can be distinguished based on time and are categorized into acute (less than 6 weeks), subacute (less than 6 months), and longterm (greater than 6 months). The physiologic mechanism of these changes in the acute and subacute setting are likely due to secondary treatment effects such as vasodilation, disruption of the blood–brain barrier, and edema, rather than direct DNA damage. The presence of long-term side effects may be caused by cellular toxicity caused by direct radiation damage, although it has been proposed that necrosis, secondary to capillary blood vessel damage, may be the cause (29).

DIAGNOSING AND MANAGING PSEUDOPROGRESSION

Correctly diagnosing pseudoprogression versus tumor recurrence has major effects on treatment decisions for patients with intracranial pathologies and allows for continuation of primary adjuvant therapies instead of moving toward secondary or experimental treatments (1). Diagnosing pseudoprogression is made by serial imaging studies that show initial growth and eventual regression. Slow, continued growth over time without any signs of regression is considered to have a high probability of being tumor progression rather than pseudoprogression.

A second challenge is distinguishing pseudoprogression from radiation necrosis. Although pseudoprogression can represent a mild form of radiation necrosis, pseudoprogression often occurs earlier and is self-limiting. In contrast, radiation necrosis typically occurs 18 to 24 months following treatment and may be either self-limited or progressive, thus requiring intervention (29).

Clinical decision making following the spectrum of imaging changes following treatment with SRS can range from maintenance on the primary adjuvant treatment in the setting of metastatic cancer to reoperation for tumor debulking. If imaging changes suggest complete or partial response, continuation of the primary treatment is obvious. Asymptomatic patients with suspected or confirmed pseudoprogression may also be kept on their primary adjuvant therapy, which may still be effective, although continued imaging studies at shorter intervals are critical.

For serial imaging that is suggestive of continued tumor progression, especially in the setting of neurologic symptoms, surgery should be considered when feasible, even in the face of uncertainty, as invasive procedures may be warranted against the possibility that a growing tumor will cause worsening brain injury. If there are substantial clinical symptoms, surgery is generally the optimal treatment choice as it is therapeutic if recurrent tumor is the actual cause and in the case of progressive radiation necrosis, may improve the patient's condition by removing the potentially advancing nidus of necrotic tissue.

ILLUSTRATIVE CASE

Illustrated here is an example case of a 37-year-old female with intracranial metastatic breast cancer. Her initial breast cancer diagnosis was made in 1998 and confirmed to be ER/PR+ with 3+ grading for HER-2/Neu positivity. In 2000, 10 intracranial metastases were identified on volumetric MRI (Figure 6.1). SRS and whole-brain radiation therapy were then administered (Figure 6.2). MRI at 4 months post SRS showed a decrease in the size of one of the intracranial metastases. However, at 16 months posttreatment, a transient ring-enhancing growth was noted (Figure 6.3). Because of the increase in lesion size, a biopsy sample was obtained and the final pathology report was brain with inflammation and necrosis with no tumor identified. In the setting of pseudoprogression, imaging studies at more regular intervals may have suggested the increase in lesional size was a result of pseudoprogression rather than the suspected tumor growth.

RECOMMENDATIONS

The diagnostic algorithm for deciding between conservative management versus a change in treatment in patients with suspected progression should be influenced by the typical behavior of the underlying pathology. For example, malignant glioma has a high rate of local recurrence after radiation and may progress rapidly, suggesting that imaging changes are more likely due to disease

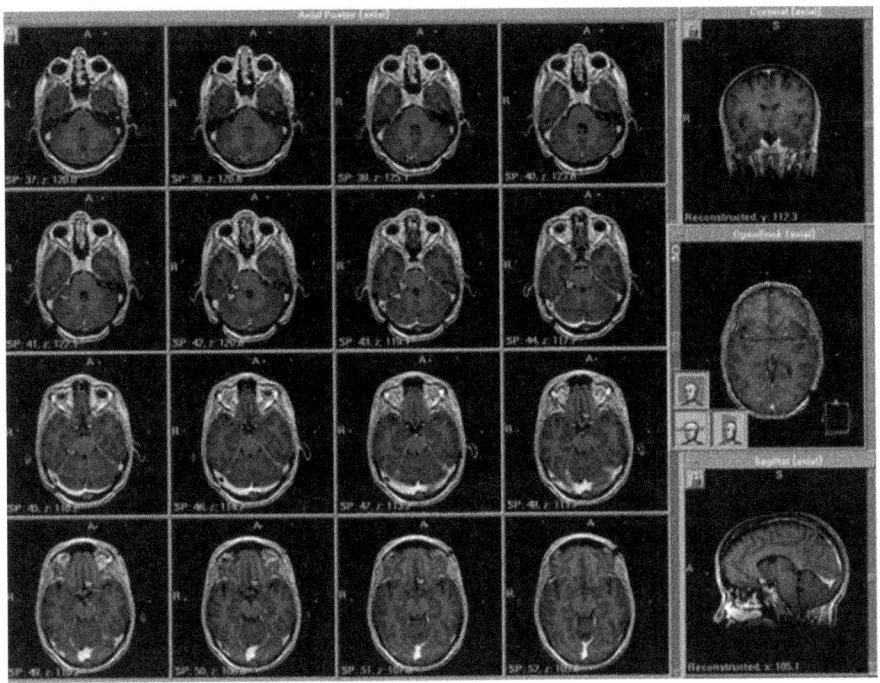

FIGURE 6.1 Pretreatment volumetric MRI showing the presence of 10 intracranial metastases from a primary breast cancer lesion.

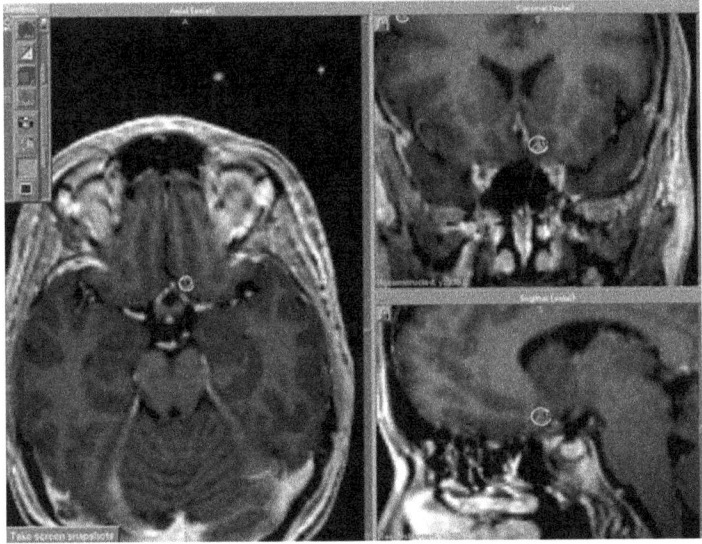

FIGURE 6.2 Representative image of planning for Gamma Knife treatment for 1 of 10 confirmed intracranial metastases.

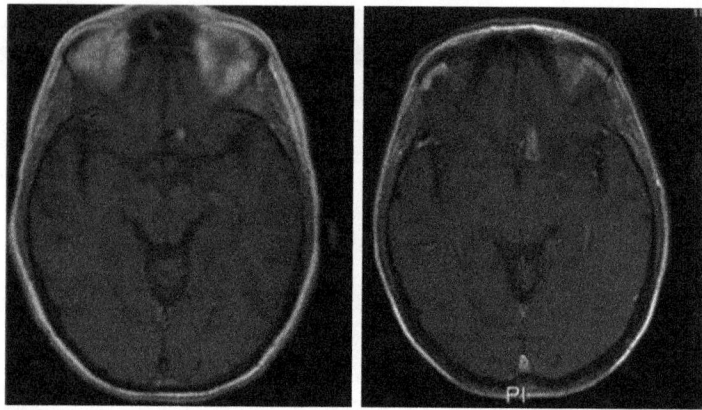

FIGURE 6.3 MRI imaging showing a small lesion at 4 months post SRS *(left)* and 16 months post SRS *(right)*. Following a biopsy, the increase in size and ring-enhancement was confirmed to be inflammation and necrosis due pseudoprogression, rather than actual tumor progression.

progression. In contrast, meningiomas and vestibular schwannomas have a high probability of long-term control after radiation, indicating that imaging changes following radiation are likely to be an effect of treatment. Brain metastases treated with SRS also have a significant probability of demonstrating later imaging changes related to therapy, although the probability of true recurrence and imaging changes may be roughly equivalent.

In patients with evidence of disease progression, especially in those with neurological symptoms that do not resolve on steroids, there is greater rationale for intervention for symptomatic relief. In this setting, surgical intervention is an appropriate therapy because it will: (a) provide symptomatic relief from recurrent tumor; (b) provide diagnostic information to guide future management; (c) decrease the effects from mass effect due to radiation; and (d) arrest an expanding nidus of radiation necrosis.

CONCLUSION

Pseudoprogression is a common imaging finding following SRS for intracranial pathologies. Because no current imaging modality can accurately detect tumor progression from pseudoprogression, the current gold standard for differentiating between the two is made by serial imaging studies. Because secondary adjuvant treatments or surgery carry significant risks to the patient, conservative management in the setting of asymptomatic pseudoprogression or frank necrosis following radiation treatment is suggested, even though the possibility of disease progression is possible.

REFERENCES

1. Sanghera P, Perry J, Sahgal A, et al. Pseudoprogression following chemoradiotherapy for glioblastoma multiforme. *Can J Neurol Sci.* 2010;37(1):36–42.
2. Pouleau HB, Sadeghi N, Baleriaux D, Melot C, De Witte O, Lefranc F. High levels of cellular proliferation predict pseudoprogression in glioblastoma patients. *Int J Oncol.* 2012;40(4):923–928.
3. Young RJ, Gupta A, Shah AD, et al. Potential utility of conventional MRI signs in diagnosing pseudoprogression in glioblastoma. *Neurology.* 2011;76(22):1918–1924.
4. Topkan E, Topuk S, Oymak E, Parlak C, Pehlivan B. Pseudoprogression in patients with glioblastoma multiforme after concurrent radiotherapy and temozolomide. *Am J Clin Oncol.* 2012;35(3):284–289.
5. Hoffman WF, Levin VA, Wilson CB. Evaluation of malignant glioma patients during the postirradiation period. *J Neurosurg.* 1979;50(5):624–628.
6. de Wit MC, de Bruin HG, Eijkenboom W, Sillevis Smitt PA, van den Bent MJ. Immediate post-radiotherapy changes in malignant glioma can mimic tumor progression. *Neurology.* 2004;63(3):535–537.
7. Chamberlain MC, Glantz MJ, Chalmers L, Van Horn A, Sloan AE. Early necrosis following concurrent Temodar and radiotherapy in patients with glioblastoma. *J Neurooncol.* 2007;82(1):81–83.
8. Brandes AA, Franceschi E, Tosoni A, et al. MGMT promoter methylation status can predict the incidence and outcome of pseudoprogression after concomitant radiochemotherapy in newly diagnosed glioblastoma patients. *J Clin Oncol.* 2008;26(13):2192–2197.
9. Perry A, Schmidt RE. Cancer therapy-associated CNS neuropathology: an update and review of the literature. *Acta Neuropathol.* 2006;111(3):197–212.
10. Taal W, Brandsma D, de Bruin HG, et al. Incidence of early pseudo-progression in a cohort of malignant glioma patients treated with chemoirradiation with temozolomide. *Cancer.* 2008;113(2):405–410.
11. Gerstner ER, McNamara MB, Norden AD, Lafrankie D, Wen PY. Effect of adding temozolomide to radiation therapy on the incidence of pseudo-progression. *J Neurooncol.* 2009;94(1):97–101.
12. Chaskis C, Neyns B, Michotte A, De Ridder M, Everaert H. Pseudoprogression after radiotherapy with concurrent temozolomide for high-grade glioma: clinical observations and working recommendations. *Surg Neurol.* 2009;72(4):423–428.
13. Mangla R, Singh G, Ziegelitz D, et al. Changes in relative cerebral blood volume 1 month after radiation-temozolomide therapy can help predict overall survival in patients with glioblastoma. *Radiology.* 2010;256(2):575–584.
14. Wen PY, Macdonald DR, Reardon DA, et al. Updated response assessment criteria for high-grade gliomas: response assessment in neuro-oncology working group. *J Clin Oncol.* 2010;28(11):1963–1972.
15. Suh JH. Stereotactic radiosurgery for the management of brain metastases. *N Engl J Med.* 2010;362(12):1119–1127.
16. Ross DA, Sandler HM, Balter JM, Hayman JA, Archer PG, Auer DL. Imaging changes after stereotactic radiosurgery of primary and secondary malignant brain tumors. *J Neurooncol.* 2002;56(2):175–181.
17. Bakardjiev AI, Barnes PD, Goumnerova LC, et al. Magnetic resonance imaging changes after stereotactic radiation therapy for childhood low grade astrocytoma. *Cancer.* 1996;78(4):864–873.

18. Patel TR, McHugh BJ, Bi WL, Minja FJ, Knisely JP, Chiang VL. A comprehensive review of MR imaging changes following radiosurgery to 500 brain metastases. *Am J Neuroradiol.* 2011;32(10):1885–1892.
19. Cai R, Barnett GH, Novak E, Chao ST, Suh JH. Principal risk of peritumoral edema after stereotactic radiosurgery for intracranial meningioma is tumor-brain contact interface area. *Neurosurgery.* 2010;66(3):513–522.
20. Kondziolka D, Mathieu D, Lunsford LD, et al. Radiosurgery as definitive management of intracranial meningiomas. *Neurosurgery.* 2008;62(1):53–58; discussion 58–60.
21. Hayhurst C, Zadeh G. Tumor pseudoprogression following radiosurgery for vestibular schwannoma. *Neuro-oncology.* 2011.
22. Valanne LK, Ketonen LM, Berg MJ. Pseudoprogression of cerebral cavernous angiomas: the importance of proper magnetic resonance imaging technique. *J Neuroimaging.* 1996;6(3):195–196.
23. Miyatake S, Kawabata S, Nonoguchi N, et al. Pseudoprogression in boron neutron capture therapy for malignant gliomas and meningiomas. *Neuro-oncology.* 2009;11(4):430–436.
24. Schwartz RB, Carvalho PA, Alexander E 3rd, Loeffler JS, Folkerth R, Holman BL. Radiation necrosis vs high-grade recurrent glioma: differentiation by using dual-isotope SPECT with 201TI and 99mTc-HMPAO. *Am J Neuroradiol.* 1991;12(6):1187–1192.
25. Schwartz RB, Holman BL, Polak JF, et al. Dual-isotope single-photon emission computerized tomography scanning in patients with glioblastoma multiforme: association with patient survival and histopathological characteristics of tumor after high-dose radiotherapy. *J Neurosurg.* 1998;89(1):60–68.
26. Carvalho PA, Schwartz RB, Alexander E 3rd, et al. Detection of recurrent gliomas with quantitative thallium-201/technetium-99m HMPAO single-photon emission computerized tomography. *J Neurosurg.* 1992;77(4):565–570.
27. Blamek S, Boba M, Larysz D, et al. The incidence of imaging abnormalities after stereotactic radiosurgery for cerebral arteriovenous and cavernous malformations. *Acta Neurochir Suppl.* 2010;106:187–190.
28. Brandsma D, Stalpers L, Taal W, Sminia P, van den Bent MJ. Clinical features, mechanisms, and management of pseudoprogression in malignant gliomas. *Lancet Oncol.* 2008;9(5):453–461.
29. Hygino da Cruz LC Jr, Rodriguez I, Domingues RC, Gasparetto EL, Sorensen AG. Pseudoprogression and pseudoresponse: Imaging challenges in the assessment of posttreatment glioma. *Ame J Neuroradiol.* 2011;32(11):1978–1985.

Section IV

Radiosurgery for Intracranial Vascular Lesions

Section Editor

Daniele Rigamonti

Chapter 7

Radiosurgery for Arteriovenous Malformations

*Jacob Ruzevick, Sachin Batra,
Michael Lim, & Daniele Rigamonti*

Arteriovenous malformations (AVMs) are a rare, typically congenital condition characterized by shunts between arterial and venous blood vessels. The incidence of AVMs is estimated at 1.1/100,000 (1) with a prevalence estimated at 18/100,000 (2). AVMs are most often found in the supratentorial compartment and usually involve the distribution of the middle cerebral artery (3). AVMs can also exist within the dura and thus are known as dural venous fistulas. Although the cause of AVMs is unclear, treatment remains a necessity, particularly for symptomatic patients as failure to intervene could lead to potentially catastrophic hemorrhage within one or several of the intraparenchymal, subarachnoid, or intraventricular compartments (4). AVMs typically present before age 40, affect males and females equally (5), and are responsible for approximately 2% of all hemorrhagic strokes, 3% of strokes in young adults, and 9% of all subarachnoid hemorrhages (3,6; Figure 7.1).

Current treatment strategies for obliteration of AVMs include surgery, endovascular embolization, and radiosurgery (Gamma Knife [GK], proton beam radiation, or linear accelerators). The goal of all treatment modalities is complete occlusion or excision of the AVM nidus to prevent future hemorrhage and its associated neurological deficits.

The use of radiation therapy for AVMs has classically been considered useful for small (less than 3 mL) AVMs with obliteration rates reported between 54% and 92% (4,7–20) with complete obliteration of AVMs using radiation therapy occurring after 1 to 3 years (15,16,21). Evidence for radiation therapy in larger AVMs (greater than 10 mL) suggests radiation therapy fails to cure a significant percentage of patients (22) and may be associated with long-term adverse events (23–26).

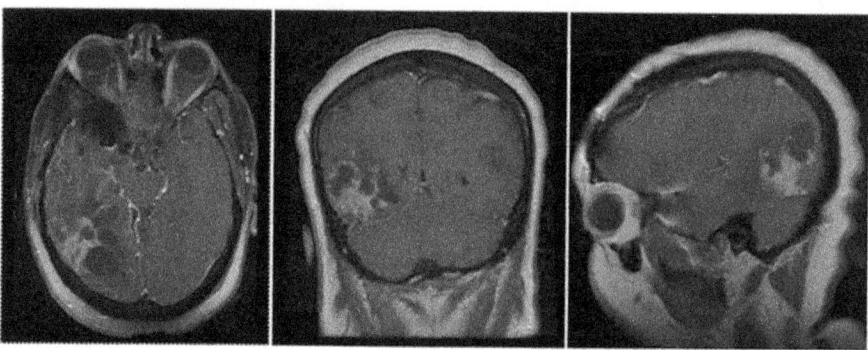

FIGURE 7.1 Axial *(left)*, coronal *(middle)*, and sagittal *(right)*, gadolinium-enhanced T1-weighted MRI showing an AVM located in the right posterior temporal lobe.

CLASSIFICATION OF AVM

Over the past 20 years, determining which treatment strategy is best for obliteration of AVMs was traditionally based on the Spetzler–Martin (SM) surgical 5-tier grading system (Table 7.1; 27). Stratification of lesions using size, location, and venous drainage, although not universally accepted for radiosurgery, is generally predictive of obliteration and outcomes. De Oliveira et al. reported a modified SM criterion in which grade III lesions were subdivided into grade IIIA (due to size greater than 6 cm) and grade IIIB (due to deep venous drainage and/or eloquent location). Based on clinical outcomes, grade I/II lesions should be treated with microsurgical resection, grade III with microsurgery (grade IIIA) or radiosurgery (grade IIIB), and grade IV/V with a personalized, multidisciplinary approach (13). A second classification scheme, proposed by Spetzler and Ponce (28), shows a 3-tier system, in which grades I/II and grades IV/V are combined, resulting in predictive accuracies equivalent to the 5-tier surgical SM criteria (Table 7.2).

Although SM accurately predicts outcomes of surgery, it may not account for factors that predict radiosurgical obliteration. Karlsson and Schwartz individually developed indices to predict obliteration of AVMs based upon AVM size and marginal dose (29,30). However, as the radiobiological tolerance of the neural parenchyma at the AVM location is the dose-limiting factor, the following Pollock–Flickinger score can be applied to predict patient outcomes (31–33).

AVM score = (0.1) × (volume, mL) + (0.02) × (age, yr) + (0.5) × (location)

(Location: hemispheric/corpus callosum/cerebellar = 0; basal ganglia/thalamus/brainstem =1)

Pollock et al. (33) correlated the percentage of patients with AVM obliteration without new deficits with AVM scores in 220 patients. Deficit-free obliteration rates in patients with AVM scores of ≤1.00, 1 to 1.5, 1.5 to 2 and >2 were 89%, 70%, 64% and 46%, respectively ($r^2 = -0.98, p < .01$).

TABLE 7.1 SM Classification System

	Characteristic	Points
Size	Small (less than 3 cm)	0
	Medium (3 to 6 cm)	1
	Large (greater than 6 cm)	2
Location	Noneloquent	0
	Eloquent	1
Venous drainage	Superficial only	0
	Deep	1

Grade = Size + Location + Venous drainage.

TABLE 7.2 Simplified SM Classification System

Class	SM Grade	Management
A	I & II	Microsurgery
B	III	Multimodal treatment
C	IV & V	No treatment except for those with clinical symptoms or AVM-related aneurysm

INDICATIONS FOR RADIOSURGERY FOR OBLITERATION OF AVM

In patients presenting with brain hemorrhage in any compartment, seizures, or progressive neurological deficit, AVM should be considered in the differential diagnosis. Patients at particular risk for hemorrhage include those with AVMs whose venous drainage is through deep cerebral vessels and AVMs with high-pressure flow. Furthermore, although unruptured lesions generally only warrant observation until their eloquent location or large size cause neurologic symptoms, patients with a hemorrhagic presentation would require emergent evacuation of the hematoma.

Radiosurgery is optimal for grade III AVMs that are graded based on their deep venous drainage and/or eloquent location. Grade IIIB AVMs are particularly well suited for radiotherapy because of the risk of damage to eloquent regions if microsurgery is used. This also includes AVMs located in the posterior fossa due to the presence of critical neurovascular structures and brainstem regions.

The success of radiosurgery in ameliorating the nidus as well as clinical symptoms shows some heterogeneity among studies. However, positive predictors of obliteration include SM grade and size as well as location, smaller volume, the presence and location of draining veins, younger age, and larger marginal dose (34,35). Along with the positive predictors of obliteration, Sun et al. (35) report that prior embolization was a negative predictor of obliteration. Furthermore, stereotactic radiosurgery (SRS) was effective at reducing AVM-related headaches, but did not improve the performance status of patients.

IMAGING AND SELECTION OF RADIATION MODALITY

A complete neuroradiological evaluation of cerebral AVMs includes computed tomography, MRI, and digital subtraction magnetic resonance angiography (MRA). Although CT is the imaging modality of choice for evaluating a hemorrhage following a ruptured AVM, it may also reveal the tortuous veins and dilated arteries that characterize AVMs, as well as an AVM's location and size. MRI allows for a more exact determination of the AVM and, when combined with selective MRA on a single cerebral vessel, selective venous drainage may be assessed. Fluid-attenuated inversion recovery (FLAIR) MRI allows visualization of decreased flow and aneurysms associated with the AVM. The gold standard for diagnosis is 6-vessel cerebral angiography with all feeding arteries in order to assess size, shape, feeding arteries, draining veins, and AVM-associated aneurysms. Dosage analysis for treatment is classically completed using MRA or digital subtraction x-ray angiography. However, the newly available C-arm conebeam computerized tomography angiography should be considered as it has been shown to have better spatial resolution and contrast than MRA. Kang et al. (36) report that this imaging protocol significantly altered the region delineated for SRS planning, thus decreasing the risk of underdosing AVMs and treatment-induced injury to normal brain regions.

Accurate treatment planning is critical to ensure adequate dose delivery and to prevent adverse effects of radiation, which may undermine the benefit of treatment itself. Studies have revealed the most common reasons for partial obliteration are targeting errors, recanalization of previously embolized AVM, expansion of the nidus after recurrence of hemorrhage, and most important, inadequate dose (37,38). Treatment plans derived using a combination of MRI or CT with an angiogram ensure complete coverage of the AVM nidus and result in greater obliteration rates by allowing higher dose delivery and minimizing exposure to the neural bed harboring the AVM (39–41). Yu et al. (42) compared nidus coverage when MRI was used with and without an accompanying angiogram to delineate the target volume of AVM. The study recommended that MRI may be used alone when planning radiosurgery for small diffuse AVMs less than 2 cc with no embolization (42).

Dosing for patients with AVMs is planned using MRI, CT, and MRA at the time of treatment with the actual amount of radiation delivered ranging from 12 to 25 Gy in a single fraction. The dose delivered to the AVM margin is generally 50% to 70% of that delivered to the center of the AVM.

AVM RADIOSURGERY

Currently, the GK system is the most common platform for delivering focused radiation to the AVM nidus; however, its superiority as compared to other delivery platforms, such as linear accelerators (LINAC), has yet to be fully established.

GK differs from LINAC in that it delivers radiation in a single fraction and generally delivers a less homogenous dose to the lesion as compared to that of LINAC systems. Proton beam systems can deliver homogenous doses of radiation to irregularly shaped lesions, and because of their Bragg peak properties, further reduce delivery to surrounding tissue.

Although the mechanism of vessel damage remains uncertain, histology studies from vessels excised after GK therapy report that endothelial damage leads to intimal smooth muscle proliferation, collagen deposition, and sclerosis. A combination of later fibrin and platelet deposition as well as smooth muscle proliferation in the vessel walls narrows the vessel lumen and eventually completely occludes the lumen.

TREATMENT OF SMALL (LESS THAN 3 ML) LESIONS

The treatment of AVMs less than 3 mL have been shown to be safe and beneficial and should be considered in patients whose AVMs reside in eloquent brain regions. Prior to treatment, location of the AVM can be determined using MRI/MRA. Dose planning for the lesion can be determined using cerebral angiography in combination with contrast-enhanced CT for dosage calculations. Although many centers use embolization as a pretreatment for radiation therapy, embolization carries its own risks and is generally unnecessary for lesions less than 3 mL. The marginal dose for these lesions generally ranges between 12 and 22 Gy. Successful obliteration of AVMs is correlated with smaller AVM volume, larger marginal dose, prior hemorrhage, and male gender. Persistence of the AVM following radiosurgery for small lesions can be due to failure of visualizing the entire AVM, compression from a hematoma (resulting in not targeting the entire AVM due to image distortion from the hematoma), and recanalization after embolization procedures prior to radiosurgery treatment (35).

TREATMENT OF LARGE (GREATER THAN 3 ML) LESIONS

Radiotherapy has shown the most efficacy in treating AVMs that are less than 3 mL, as previous studies have shown poor efficacy (4,43–47) as well as high complication rates in the treatment of large lesions in a single fraction (23–26). Treatment of large AVMs poses risk of complication with either radiosurgical or surgical treatment. Although surgery would provide an immediate reduction in risk of hemorrhage, the risk of hemorrhage and deficits resulting from radiation injury are important concerns after treating large AVMs. The efficacy of the treatment plan for AVM is determined by the dose delivered at the periphery of the AVM (Dmin) (9). Furthermore, the risk of radiation injury correlates, both with dose and volume, because the dose gradient becomes less steep as the volume increases (48). In addition, increases in both the dose and volume of an AVM also increase the risk of hemorrhage during the latency period for obliteration (49,50). Emphasizing the role of size of AVM, Pollock et al. proposed an AVM score based on patients' age, volume of AVM, and location. In patients with an AVM score greater than 2, there was only a 46% probability of excellent outcomes (complete obliteration with no new deficits) with a 36% probability of a decline in function (as measured on Modified Rankin Score).

The radiosurgical treatment of large AVMs can be achieved by adjuvant embolization or by obliterating the nidus in a staged manner. In addition, hypofractionated SRS has also been found to be useful.

Salvage Therapy

To overcome the challenge of delivering radiation to a large volume while sparing normal brain parenchyma, suboptimal doses of radiation have been attempted with retreatment at a later time. By treating in multiple settings, it is possible a later treatment will be more efficacious due to a smaller nidus and a higher tolerable dose. Two groups report this method results in a general reduction of AVM volume (51,52).

Hypofractionated Stereotactic Radiosurgery

Hypofractionated stereotactic radiosurgery (HFSR) is used to deliver doses of approximately 25 Gy using four fractions to the AVM nidus using a linear accelerator with a stereotactic frame. Obliteration rates using HFSR are reported as 64% and 92% at 3 and 5 years, respectively, and are no different than single-fraction SRS (53). When using HFSR, the minimum dose necessary to achieve high occlusion rates is 7 Gy/fraction as doses less than 7 Gy result in occlusion in only 20% of patients. When greater than 7 Gy/fraction is delivered, occlusion rates are approximately 80%. Lindvall et al. (54) treated 29 patients with a mean AVM volume of 11.5 mL with hypofractionated regimens (6–7 Gy × 5 fractions) and attained 81% and 73% obliteration in AVMs that are 4 to 10 mL and greater than 10 mL, respectively, at 5 years. Chang et al. (55) compared single-dose SRS (15–25 Gy) to hypofractionated regimens 25 to 35 Gy over five fractions and found comparable 5-year obliteration rates (71% HFSR, 81%SRS). However, the rate of radiation necrosis was found to be lower in HFSR (1/33) than in SRS (4/42). Karlsson et al. (56) reported obliteration rates of 28 AVMs with a median volume of 78 mL treated with 42 Gy × 12 fractions. Obliteration of the nidus occurred in 2 (8%) patients at 4-year follow-up. However, results of this study suggest that patients with pretreatment hemorrhage should not undergo HFSR as the annual hemorrhage rate in this study was 6%, indicating a lack of protection against the risk of rupture in exceedingly large AVMs.

In conclusion, HFSR has not been shown to be effective in achieving complete obliteration of the AVM nidus of very large AVMs. This, along with an increased risk of rupture due to an AVM's large size, makes HFSR not particularly efficacious for the treatment of AVMs greater than 10 mL.

Staged Treatment

Large AVMs may also be treated by dividing the nidus into multiple smaller volumes, and then treating with multiple SRS sessions, or by repeatedly irradiating the entire nidus (52,57,58). When the AVM is divided into smaller volumes, the prescribed isodose volume is small and thus allows for treatment with marginal doses above 12 Gy. This strategy allows for a rapid falloff, limiting the exposure to normal parenchyma and is planned by analyzing the probability of radiation exposure above 12 Gy beyond the target volume (59,60). Although this procedure reduces the incidence of deficits arising from radiation injury, the partial obliteration of the nidus leads to an increase in flow through the untreated volume of the nidus, raising the transmural pressure and the predisposition to bleed (52,61,62). Although this strategy may be more efficacious, this property results in the possibility of posttreatment hemorrhage until the last segment is treated. Pollock et al. (52) compared the dosimetry of 10 patients who underwent staged-volume AVM radiosurgery with equivalent single-session procedures treating the entire volume of the nidus. As compared to patients receiving a single-session treatment, the staged-volume strategy significantly reduced the average exposure of AVM above 12 Gy by 11.1% (4.9%–21%), whereas the non AVM volume with exposure ≥12 Gy was reduced by 27.2% (12.5%–51.3%). Sirin et al. (57) reported 28 patients with an average AVM volume of 24.9 mL treated by staged-volume treatment at 3 to 8 months intervals. The obliteration rate was 33% (7/21 patients) among patients with at least 36 months follow-up. Four patients developed evidence of radiation injury on imaging and were successfully treated with steroids. One patient developed severe deficits due to radiation injury. Chung et al. (58) reported a series of six patients, with volumes ranging from 11.3 to 63.3 mL, all treated with marginal doses in excess of 16 Gy. Complete obliteration occurred in two patients, whereas the remaining four patients had partial obliteration. All patients had evidence of radiation injury and one patient had mild hemorrhage.

MULTIMODAL TREATMENT

AVMs are commonly approached using a combination of surgery, embolization, or radiosurgery. Radiosurgery may be used, if microsurgery is unable to resect the full AVM due to its location in eloquent brain territory. Radiosurgery may also be used following embolization to decrease flow through feeding arteries and draining veins and convert a large AVM to a mostly embolized lesion. In small AVMs, embolization may be curative; however, it is seldom performed considering that such lesions can be clearly treated surgically or radiosurgically. This combination is controversial as several groups have reported that preradiosurgery embolization results in increased nidus volume, persistent AV shunting, and recanalization of embolized vessels due to the time period required for radiosurgical obliteration of an AVM. To this effect, prior embolization was shown to be a negative predictor of AVM obliteration (35). Furthermore, embolization does not decrease the risk of post-radiation treatment hemorrhage. Although embolization is considered for patients with large AVMs, its success in small AVMs has been shown to be inferior to radiosurgery alone (63).

FOLLOW-UP

Successful treatment can be defined as obliteration of the AVM with no residual or new neurological deficits. Following treatment, patients should be followed with serial MR imaging until suggestive of obliteration. At this point, cerebral angiography should be used for confirmation (Figure 7.2). If CT and MR imaging are the only modalities used, high false-negative rates of a residual AVM nidus are possible. Following treatment, new areas of T2 signal occur in approximately 30% of patients, of whom two thirds are asymptomatic. Complete resolution of an AVM following radiosurgery generally requires 1 to 3 years, of which routine

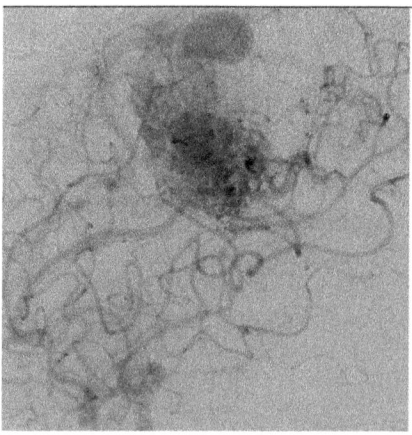
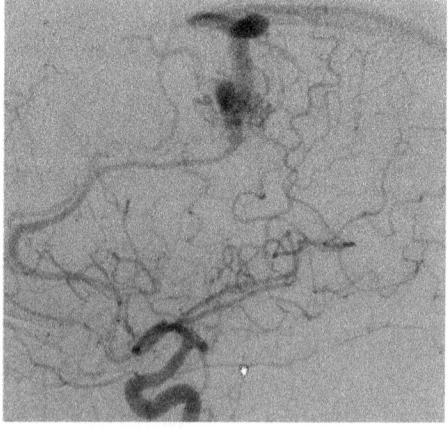

FIGURE 7.2 Pre- *(left)* and posttreatment *(right)* angiograms depicting obliteration of a right, frontal lobe AVM in a 37-year-old male following SRS. The AVM is fed by the right pericallosal and callosomarginal branches of the right anterior cerebral artery and distal branches of the right middle cerebral artery.

angiographic monitoring is imperative. Because of the time required for complete nidus closure, patients must be continually managed with antiepileptic drugs if clinically indicated. For patients with a residual nidus following the expected obliteration after 3 years, repeat radiosurgery is generally indicated.

COMPLICATIONS FOLLOWING TREATMENT

Morbidity following radiosurgery for AVMs has been estimated to be as high as 20% with the most common complications being headache, seizures, neurological deficits, and radiation-induced tissue injury. Two variables shown to be predictors of complications following treatment include AVM location and the volume of tissue receiving greater than 12 Gy of radiation (64). Complications occurring in a short period following treatment include cranial nerve deficits, seizures (especially in patients with lobar AVMs), and cyst formation. Regardless of the size of the original AVM, hemorrhage remains a potential catastrophic risk of radiosurgical treatment of AVMs both in the early and late recovery periods. Although radio surgery eliminates the risk of microsurgery, it is estimated that hemorrhage rates are 2% to 4% per year, similar to the natural history of AVM (65).

Subacute complications may also present within 1 year of treatment and are most often caused by posttreatment edema. Of note, in patients with prior history of AVM treatment, changes on MRI are often due to gliosis rather than edema.

CONCLUSION

Currently, radiation therapy is recommended for AVMs with a volume less than 3 mL or those in eloquent brain locations as published series have shown acceptable obliteration rates with minimal patient toxicities. Radiation therapy for larger AVMs (greater than 10 mL) is controversial as these lesions are best approached using fractionated radiation strategies to decrease the nidus volume between treatments. Following treatment for all AVMs, long-term imaging is required as the risk of hemorrhage remains the same as pretreatment during the 1 to 3 years that are required for radiation to induce its maximal treatment effect.

REFERENCES

1. Jessurun GA, Kamphuis DJ, van der Zande FH, Nossent JC. Cerebral arteriovenous malformations in The Netherlands Antilles. High prevalence of hereditary hemorrhagic telangiectasia-related single and multiple cerebral arteriovenous malformations. *Clin Neurol Neurosurg.* 1993;95(3):193–198.

2. Al-Shahi R, Bhattacharya JJ, Currie DG, et al. Prospective, population-based detection of intracranial vascular malformations in adults: the Scottish Intracranial Vascular Malformation Study (SIVMS). *Stroke.* 2003;34(5):1163–1169.
3. Al-Shahi R, Warlow C. A systematic review of the frequency and prognosis of arteriovenous malformations of the brain in adults. *Brain.* 2001;124(Pt 10):1900–1926.
4. Lunsford LD, Kondziolka D, Flickinger JC, et al. Stereotactic radiosurgery for arteriovenous malformations of the brain. *J Neurosurg.* 1991;75(4):512–524.
5. Arteriovenous malformations of the brain in adults. *N Engl J Med.* 1999;340(23): 1812–1818.
6. Brown RD Jr, Wiebers DO, Torner JC, O'Fallon WM. Frequency of intracranial hemorrhage as a presenting symptom and subtype analysis: a population-based study of intracranial vascular malformations in Olmsted Country, Minnesota. *J Neurosurg.* 1996;85(1):29–32.
7. Bollet MA, Anxionnat R, Buchheit I, et al. Efficacy and morbidity of arc-therapy radiosurgery for cerebral arteriovenous malformations: a comparison with the natural history. *Int J Radiat Oncol Biol Phys.* 2004;58(5):1353–1363.
8. Chang JH, Chang JW, Park YG, Chung SS. Factors related to complete occlusion of arteriovenous malformations after gamma knife radiosurgery. *J Neurosurg.* 2000;93(suppl 3): 96–101.
9. Flickinger JC, Pollock BE, Kondziolka D, Lunsford LD. A dose-response analysis of arteriovenous malformation obliteration after radiosurgery. *Int J Radiat Oncol Biol Phys.* 1996;36(4):873–879.
10. Inoue HK, Ohye C. Hemorrhage risks and obliteration rates of arteriovenous malformations after gamma knife radiosurgery. *J Neurosurg.* 2002;97(5 suppl):474–476.
11. Liscak R, Vladyka V, Simonova G, et al. Arteriovenous malformations after Leksell gamma knife radiosurgery: rate of obliteration and complications. *Neurosurgery.* 2007;60(6):1005–1014; discussion 1015–1006.
12. McInerney J, Gould DA, Birkmeyer JD, Harbaugh RE. Decision analysis for small, asymptomatic intracranial arteriovenous malformations. *Neurosurg Focus.* 2001;11(5):e7.
13. de Oliveira E, Tedeschi H, Raso J. Multidisciplinary approach to arteriovenous malformations. *Neurol Med Chir.* 1998;38 Suppl:177–85.
14. Ogilvy CS, Stieg PE, Awad I, et al. AHA Scientific Statement: Recommendations for the management of intracranial arteriovenous malformations: a statement for healthcare professionals from a special writing group of the Stroke Council, American Stroke Association. *Stroke.* 2001;32(6):1458–1471.
15. Pollock BE, Gorman DA, Coffey RJ. Patient outcomes after arteriovenous malformation radiosurgical management: results based on a 5- to 14-year follow-up study. *Neurosurgery.* 2003;52(6):1291–1296; discussion 1296–1297.
16. Pollock BE, Lunsford LD, Kondziolka D, Maitz A, Flickinger JC. Patient outcomes after stereotactic radiosurgery for "operable" arteriovenous malformations. *Neurosurgery.* 1994;35(1):1–7; discussion 7–8.
17. Schlienger M, Atlan D, Lefkopoulos D, et al. Linac radiosurgery for cerebral arteriovenous malformations: results in 169 patients. *Int J Radiat Oncol Biol Phys.* 2000; 46(5):1135–1142.
18. Shin M, Kawamoto S, Kurita H, et al. Retrospective analysis of a 10-year experience of stereotactic radio surgery for arteriovenous malformations in children and adolescents. *J Neurosurg.* 2002;97(4):779–784.

19. Shin M, Maruyama K, Kurita H, et al. Analysis of nidus obliteration rates after gamma knife surgery for arteriovenous malformations based on long-term follow-up data: the University of Tokyo experience. *J Neurosurg*. 2004;101(1):18–24.
20. Yen CP, Varady P, Sheehan J, Steiner M, Steiner L. Subtotal obliteration of cerebral arteriovenous malformations after gamma knife surgery. *J Neurosurg*. 2007;106(3):361–369.
21. Friedman WA, Blatt DL, Bova FJ, Buatti JM, Mendenhall WM, Kubilis PS. The risk of hemorrhage after radiosurgery for arteriovenous malformations. *J Neurosurg*. 1996;84(6):912–919.
22. Pan DH, Guo WY, Chung WY, Shiau CY, Chang YC, Wang LW. Gamma knife radiosurgery as a single treatment modality for large cerebral arteriovenous malformations. *J Neurosurg*. 2000;93(suppl 3):113–119.
23. Flickinger JC. An integrated logistic formula for prediction of complications from radiosurgery. *Int J Radiat Oncol Biol Phys*. 1989;17(4):879–885.
24. Flickinger JC, Kondziolka D, Lunsford LD, et al. Development of a model to predict permanent symptomatic postradiosurgery injury for arteriovenous malformation patients. Arteriovenous Malformation Radiosurgery Study Group. *Int J Radiat Oncol Biol Phys*. 2000;46(5):1143–1148.
25. Lax I, Karlsson B. Prediction of complications in gamma knife radiosurgery of arteriovenous malformation. *Acta Oncol*. 1996;35(1):49–55.
26. Voges J, Treuer H, Lehrke R, et al. Risk analysis of LINAC radiosurgery in patients with arteriovenous malformation (AVM). *Acta Neurochir Suppl*. 1997;68:118–123.
27. Spetzler RF, Martin NA. A proposed grading system for arteriovenous malformations. *J Neurosurg*. 1986;65(4):476–483.
28. Spetzler RF, Ponce FA. A 3-tier classification of cerebral arteriovenous malformations. Clinical article. *J Neurosurg*. 2011;114(3):842–849.
29. Karlsson B, Lindquist C, Steiner L. Prediction of obliteration after gamma knife surgery for cerebral arteriovenous malformations. *Neurosurgery*. 1997;40(3):425–430; discussion 430–421.
30. Schwartz M, Sixel K, Young C, et al. Prediction of obliteration of arteriovenous malformations after radiosurgery: the obliteration prediction index. *Can J Neurol Sci*. 1997;24(2):106–109.
31. Pollock BE, Flickinger JC, Lunsford LD, Maitz A, Kondziolka D. Factors associated with successful arteriovenous malformation radiosurgery. *Neurosurgery*. 1998;42(6):1239–1244; discussion 1244–1237.
32. Pollock BE, Flickinger JC. A proposed radiosurgery-based grading system for arteriovenous malformations. *J Neurosurg*. 2002;96(1):79–85.
33. Pollock BE, Flickinger JC. Modification of the radiosurgery-based arteriovenous malformation grading system. *Neurosurgery*. 2008;63(2):239–243; discussion 243.
34. Seifert V, Stolke D, Mehdorn HM, Hoffmann B. Clinical and radiological evaluation of long-term results of stereotactic proton beam radiosurgery in patients with cerebral arteriovenous malformations. *J Neurosurg*. 1994;81(5):683–689.
35. Sun DQ, Carson KA, Raza SM, et al. The radiosurgical treatment of arteriovenous malformations: obliteration, morbidities, and performance status. *Int J Radiat Oncol Biol Phys*. 2011;80(2):354–361.
36. Kang, J, Huang J, Gailloud P, Rigamonti D, Bernard V, Ehtiati T, Ford E. Planning evaluation of cone-beam CT angiography for target delineation in stereotactic radiosurgery of AVMs. San Diego, CA: ASTRO; 2010.
37. Gallina P, Merienne L, Meder JF, Schlienger M, Lefkopoulos D, Merland JJ. Failure in radiosurgery treatment of cerebral arteriovenous malformations. *Neurosurgery*. 1998;42(5):996–1002; discussion 1002–1004.

38. Kwon Y, Jeon SR, Kim JH, et al. Analysis of the causes of treatment failure in gamma knife radiosurgery for intracranial arteriovenous malformations. *J Neurosurg.* 2000;93(suppl 3):104–106.
39. Kondziolka D, Lunsford LD, Kanal E, Talagala L. Stereotactic magnetic resonance angiography for targeting in arteriovenous malformation radiosurgery. *Neurosurgery.* 1994;35(4):585–590; discussion 590–581.
40. Sanelli PC, Mifsud MJ, Stieg PE. Role of CT angiography in guiding management decisions of newly diagnosed and residual arteriovenous malformations. *AJR Am J Roentgenol.* 2004;183(4):1123–1126.
41. McGee KP, Ivanovic V, Felmlee JP, Meyer FB, Pollock BE, Huston J 3rd. MR angiography fusion technique for treatment planning of intracranial arteriovenous malformations. *J Magn Reson Imaging.* 2006;23(3):361–369.
42. Yu C, Petrovich Z, Apuzzo ML, Zelman V, Giannotta SL. Study of magnetic resonance imaging-based arteriovenous malformation delineation without conventional angiography. *Neurosurgery.* 2004;54(5):1104; discussion 1108–1110.
43. Coffey RJ, Nichols DA, Shaw EG. Stereotactic radiosurgical treatment of cerebral arteriovenous malformations. Gamma Unit Radiosurgery Study Group. *Mayo Clin Proc.* 1995;70(3):214–222.
44. Friedman WA, Bova FJ, Mendenhall WM. Linear accelerator radiosurgery for arteriovenous malformations: the relationship of size to outcome. *J Neurosurg.* 1995;82(2):180–189.
45. Kjellberg RN, Hanamura T, Davis KR, Lyons SL, Adams RD. Bragg-peak proton-beam therapy for arteriovenous malformations of the brain. *N Engl J Med.* 1983;309(5):269–274.
46. Miyawaki L, Dowd C, Wara W, et al. Five year results of LINAC radiosurgery for arteriovenous malformations: outcome for large AVMS. *Int J Radiat Oncol Biol Phys.* 1999;44(5):1089–1106.
47. Yamamoto M, Jimbo M, Hara M, Saito I, Mori K. Gamma knife radiosurgery for arteriovenous malformations: long-term follow-up results focusing on complications occurring more than 5 years after irradiation. *Neurosurgery.* 1996;38(5):906–914.
48. Flickinger JC, Kondziolka D, Pollock BE, Maitz AH, Lunsford LD. Complications from arteriovenous malformation radiosurgery: multivariate analysis and risk modeling. *Int J Radiat Oncol Biol Phys.* 1997;38(3):485–490.
49. Karlsson B, Lax I, Söderman M. Risk for hemorrhage during the 2-year latency period following gamma knife radiosurgery for arteriovenous malformations. *Int J Radiat Oncol Biol Phys.* 2001;49(4):1045–1051.
50. Karlsson B, Lindquist C, Steiner L. Effect of Gamma Knife surgery on the risk of rupture prior to AVM obliteration. *Minim Invasive Neurosurg.* 1996;39(1):21–27.
51. Karlsson B, Kihlstrom L, Lindquist C, Steiner L. Gamma knife surgery for previously irradiated arteriovenous malformations. *Neurosurgery.* 1998;42(1):1–5; discussion 5–6.
52. Pollock BE, Kline RW, Stafford SL, Foote RL, Schomberg PJ. The rationale and technique of staged-volume arteriovenous malformation radiosurgery. *Int J Radiat Oncol Biol Phys.* 2000;48(3):817–824.
53. Aoyama H, Shirato H, Nishioka T, et al. Treatment outcome of single or hypofractionated single-isocentric stereotactic irradiation (STI) using a linear accelerator for intracranial arteriovenous malformation. *Radiother Oncol.* 2001;59(3):323–328.
54. Lindvall P, Bergström P, Löfroth PO, et al. Hypofractionated conformal stereotactic radiotherapy for arteriovenous malformations. *Neurosurgery.* 2003;53(5):1036–42; discussion 1042.

55. Chang TC, Shirato H, Aoyama H, et al. Stereotactic irradiation for intracranial arteriovenous malformation using stereotactic radiosurgery or hypofractionated stereotactic radiotherapy. *Int J Radiat Oncol Biol Phys.* 2004;60(3):861–870.
56. Karlsson B, Lindqvist M, Blomgren H, et al. Long-term results after fractionated radiation therapy for large brain arteriovenous malformations. *Neurosurgery.* 2005;57(1):42–49; discussion 42.
57. Sirin S, Kondziolka D, Niranjan A, Flickinger JC, Maitz AH, Lunsford LD. Prospective staged volume radiosurgery for large arteriovenous malformations: indications and outcomes in otherwise untreatable patients. *Neurosurgery.* 2008;62(suppl 2):744–754.
58. Chung WY, Shiau CY, Wu HM, et al. Staged radiosurgery for extra-large cerebral arteriovenous malformations: method, implementation, and results. *J Neurosurg.* 2008;(109 suppl):65–72.
59. Raza SM, Jabbour S, Thai QA, et al. Repeat stereotactic radiosurgery for high-grade and large intracranial arteriovenous malformations. *Surgical Neurology.* 2007;68(1):24–34; discussion 34.
60. Kim HY, Chang WS, Kim DJ, et al. Gamma Knife surgery for large cerebral arteriovenous malformations. *J Neurosurg.* 2010;(113 suppl):2–8.
61. Colombo F, Pozza F, Chierego G, Casentini L, De Luca G, Francescon P. Linear accelerator radiosurgery of cerebral arteriovenous malformations: an update. *Neurosurgery.* 1994;34(1):14–20; discussion 20–11.
62. Spetzler RF, Hargraves RW, McCormick PW, Zabramski JM, Flom RA, Zimmerman RS. Relationship of perfusion pressure and size to risk of hemorrhage from arteriovenous malformations. *J Neurosurg.* 1992;76(6):918–923.
63. Andrade-Souza YM, Ramani M, Scora D, Tsao MN, Terbrugge K, Schwartz ML. Embolization before radiosurgery reduces the obliteration rate of arteriovenous malformations. *Neurosurgery.* 2007;60(3):443–451; discussion 451–442.
64. Flickinger JC, Kondziolka D, Maitz AH, Lunsford LD. An analysis of the dose-response for arteriovenous malformation radiosurgery and other factors affecting obliteration. *Radiother Oncol.* 2002;63(3):347–354.
65. Brown RD Jr, Wiebers DO, Forbes G, et al. The natural history of unruptured intracranial arteriovenous malformations. *J Neurosurg.* 1988;68(3):352–357.

Chapter 8

Role of Radiosurgery for Dural Arteriovenous Fistula

*Omar Choudhri &
Raphael Guzman*

BACKGROUND

Dural arteriovenous fistulae (dAVF) are insidious acquired lesions that comprise 10% to 15% of all intracranial arteriovenous malformations (1,2). Dural AVF is an abnormal connection between dural arteries and the leptomeningeal veins or venous sinuses located between leaves of the dura mater (3,4).

There are two main theories for pathogenesis of dural arteriovenous fistulae. The first implicates thrombosis of sinus or vein with resultant venous hypertension, which in turn causes angiogenesis leading to the abnormal shunting in response to hypoxia (5). The second theory suggests that preexisting arteriovenous shunts become active due to increase in venous pressure caused by obstruction of venous flow (6,7). dAVFs can be complex when arteries are recruited from branches of both the external and internal carotid artery before these arteries penetrate the dura (8).

dAVF most often present in adults in the fifth or sixth decade of life (17); the transverse, sigmoid, and cavernous sinuses are the most common locations (9,10).

CLINICAL PRESENTATION AND NATURAL HISTORY

The clinical presentation depends on the location of the dAVFs and the venous outflow pattern. Symptoms could include headaches, tinnitus, bruits, ocular

TABLE 8.1 Classification Schemes of Venous Drainage and the Clinical Application: Borden Classification

Type I	Drainage into the dural venous sinus
Type II	Drainage into the dural venous sinus with retrograde drainage into subarachnoid veins
Type III	Drainage into subarachnoid veins
Subtype a	Simple fistula
Subtype b	Multiple fistulas

Adapted from Borden JA, Wu JK, Shucart WA. A proposed classification for spinal and cranial dural arteriovenous fistulous mailformations and implications for treatment *J. Neurosurg* 1995;82(2): 166–179.

disturbances, seizures, focal neurologic deficits, and intracranial hemorrhage (11). Cavernous sinus fistulae most often present with ocular symptoms such as exophthalmos, retinal hemorrhages or cranial nerve palsies, whereas transverse sigmoid lesions present with bruits and tinnitus (12). Anterior fossa dAVF are more likely to present with hemorrhage as their only outflow is through pial venous channels.

A number of classification schemes have been proposed for risk stratification of patients. These include the classification systems by Djindijan et al. (13–15). Borden classification is the commonly used scheme that uses venous drainage patterns to determine prognosis (Table 8.1; 13). Generally an aggressive approach to treatment is employed in high-grade patients with features such as cortical venous drainage, venous ectasia, hemorrhage, or progressive neurological deficits (16).

Cerebral angiography is the gold standard for diagnosis of dAVF (3).

TREATMENT MODALITIES

Dural AVF can be targeted successfully with a multimodality treatment, including microsurgery, endovascular embolization, and radiosurgery (4,16,17). Patients may require one or a combination of the three modalities based on response, venous drainage pattern, and clinical presentation. Radiosurgery is the most recent treatment arm and its role in the array of treatments is still controversial even though its efficacy is clearly demonstrated by multiple studies.

Conservative

Dural AVF causing no symptoms (incidental discovery) or tinnitus only with a benign venous drainage pattern can be watched. Rarely dAVF undergoes spontaneous thrombosis on follow-up neuroimaging. For low-grade cavernous and transverse dAVF manual carotid compression over 4 to 6 weeks is reported to promote stasis and thrombosis with a 34% cure rate per Halbach et al. (18). We do not recommend this modality which has largely fallen out of favor.

Microsurgery

Surgical intervention includes feeding vessel ligation, venous sinus packing, and complete fistula excision (19). Surgery aims at permanent cure and can be straightforward in cases with a single feeding vessel. It is often used in combination with preoperative embolization and preferred for anterior fossa fistulae. In selected cases cure rates approach 100% with morbidity/mortality approaching 10% (20,21). This is mostly true for dAVF cases with a single feeder that can be approached safely surgically.

Endovascular Embolization

Endovascular treatment employs transvenous or transarterial access to selectively catheterize and embolize feeders. Various embolic agents such as onyx, cyanoacrylate glue, and coils may be employed to achieve 67% to 88% occlusion rates with a 3% complication rate (22,23). In most cases transvenous endovascular embolization is the first-line treatment (24).

Role of Radiosurgery: Historical Evidence and Current Data

Barcia-Salorio et al. (25) first used radiosurgery for dAVF in the 1980s on low-flow carotid-cavernous fistulae (CCF). Patients experience symptom resolution as early as 2 months after treatment with complete obliteration at 9 months (24). Since then radiosurgery in the form of Gamma Knife, CyberKnife, and linear accelerator has been used as a single therapy or in combination with embolization for treatment of dAVF (24,26). Its efficacy was described for both CCF and other dAVF (2,24).

Pathophysiology

Stereotactic radiation is targeted toward arterial feeders or fistulous points, where it causes radiation-induced changes and obliteration of the shunt. At the cellular level, radiation induces perivascular and subendothelial edema, endothelial injury, and resultant smooth muscle/fibroblast response. These changes contribute to small vessel occlusion of the arterial feeders over time (27).

Planning and Dose Calculation

A three-dimensional cerebral angiogram and stereotactic MRI are required for radiosurgical dose planning. MRI is particularly useful for contouring and limiting radiation to structures such as cranial nerves, cochlea, and brainstem. Doses ranging between 15 and 50 Gy have been employed in literature in dAVF radiosurgical plans (2). It is crucial to define the dAVF anatomy and understand the fistula hemodynamics by studying the cerebral angiogram (28).

Current Indications

Radiosurgery for dAVF can be used in three common settings: namely, (a) sole upfront therapy; (b) in combination with embolization; and (c) salvage therapy.

Sole Upfront Therapy

Radiosurgery is considered upfront for patients with dAVF who are not good candidates for surgery or embolization, such as patients who are medically unstable to undergo surgery or have a poor vascular access (29).

The obliteration rates differ between CCF and dAVF in other locations.

　i. CCF: CCF rarely presents with major hemorrhage. Instead these patients have prominent orbital symptoms such as proptosis and chemosis making these patients seek attention early (12). A cumulative complete obliteration rate of 77% with radiosurgery is reported by a recent meta-analysis (2,30). Given a high spontaneous regression rate in indirect CCF, this number may not be completely attributable to radiosurgery.

　ii. Other dAVF: Obliteration rates vary between 20% and 100% (2). The potential for hemorrhage during the latency period when the fistula is partially patent is a known risk with radiosurgery. It is thought, however, that the slow change in fistula hemodynamics seen with radiosurgery might be protective to some degree.

Radiosurgery Combined With Embolization

Endovascular embolization and radiosurgery are used synergistically in treating dAVF with multiple arterial feeders (16). Embolization offers a safe and effective means to immediately obliterate larger arterial feeders, whereas smaller feeders can be targeted with radiosurgery (31). Which procedure should be done first is still controversial. Performing embolization first shrinks the nidus requiring a smaller radiation dose. However, following embolization nidus identification becomes challenging and inadequate delineation can result in treatment failure. With combination therapy an obliteration rate of 62.5% is reported for CCF and 50% for non CCF (2).

Salvage Radiosurgery

Radiosurgery is often employed as a salvage modality when surgery and/or embolization fails to obliterate aggressive dAVF (6) as illustrated in Figure 8.1.

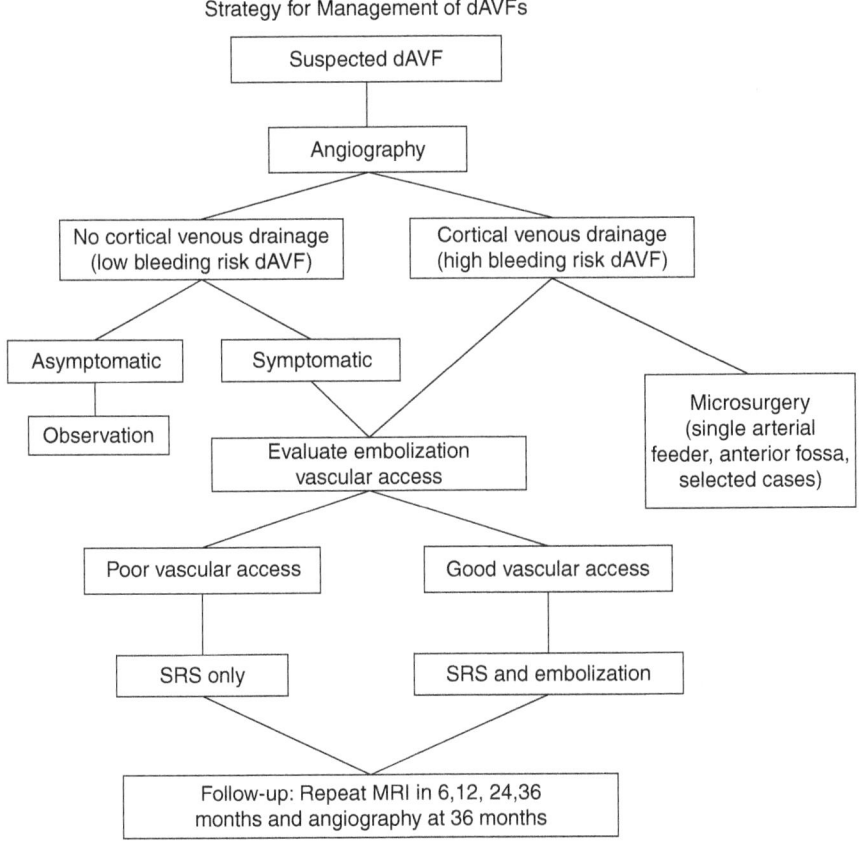

FIGURE 8.1 Treatment algorithm for dural AV fistulae.
Adapted from Yang HC, Kano H, Kondziolka D, et al. Stereotactic radiosurgery with or without embolization for intracranial dural arteriovenous fistulas. *Neurosurgery.* 2010;67(5):1276–1283; discussion 1284.

Complications

Complications after a radiosurgery treatment can include headache, nausea, vomiting, alopecia, fever, radiation-induced edema, seizures, neuropathy, and tumors (32). There have been isolated reports of unusual radiation-induced complications such as de novo cerebellar arteriovenous malformation (33). In most cases radiosurgery for dAVF is well tolerated.

CONCLUSIONS

Stereotactic radiosurgery has a definite role in the management of dAVF if surgery or embolization is not feasible or does not occlude all feeders to a fistula. Radiosurgery provides an added treatment arm for a gradual controlled obliteration of the fistula. All three treatment modalities may complement

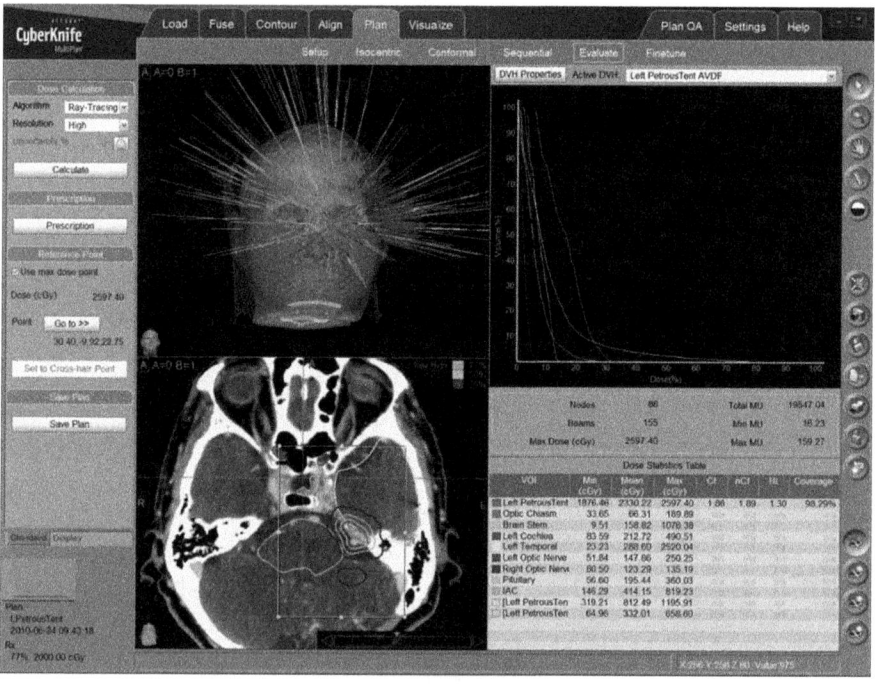

FIGURE 8.2 79-year-old female taken for CyberKnife stereotactic radiosurgery with 18 Gy to the fistula nidus along the left tentorium.
Borden JA, Wu JK, Shucart WA. A proposed classification for spinal and cranial dural arteriovenous fistulous malformations and implications for treatment. *J Neurosurg.* 1995;82:166–179.

each other. Combining embolization and radiosurgery can improve the obliteration rate for cavernous and noncavernous dAVF. Figure 8.1 illustrates an adapted algorithm from Yang et al. (16), which reflects our strategy for managing dAVF.

SUMMARY POINTS

- Radiosurgery can obliterate dAVFs by intimal injury, fibrosis, and smooth muscle hyperplasia.
- It can be used as a single modality or in combination with surgery and endovascular embolization.
- There is a latency period of at least 6 months after a radiosurgery treatment until the fistula is obliterated.
- Radiation doses between 20 and 30 Gy are usually employed in most cases.
- Follow-up is completed with diagnostic angiograms.

ILLUSTRATED CASE

A 79-year-old female presented to our hospital with sudden headache and CT showing a 4.5-cm left cerebellar hemorrhage; she had an external ventricular drain placed and the cerebral angiogram revealed a complex left dural, arteriovenous fistula fed by arterial supply from meningohypophyseal trunk as well as some from distal internal maxillary and distal middle meningeal branches. The fistula drained posteriorly and then cortically entered the cerebellar cortical veins with additional drainage into the junction of transverse and sigmoid sinuses. A venous aneurysm near the cerebellar hematoma was thought to be the source of hemorrhage. The hematoma was found to expand on repeat imaging and the patient deteriorated neurologically. She was hence taken to the operating room for a suboccipital craniectomy and hematoma evacuation. A portion of the dural fistula in the tentorium, extending from the tentorium to the superior cerebellar surface was resected. The venous aneurysm was coagulated and resected. Postoperative angiogram demonstrated that the dAVF was still present with patent feeders from the meningohypophyseal trunk. The patient was allowed to recover and brought back to the cath lab a few months later for definitive embolization. The embolization was unsuccessful, as the feeding vessel could not be catheterized. The patient was taken for CyberKnife stereotactic radiosurgery with 18 Gy to the fistula nidus along the left tentorium (Figure 8.2).

REFERENCES

1. Houser OW, Baker HL Jr, Rhoton AL Jr, Okazaki H. Intracranial dural arteriovenous malformations. *Radiology.* 1972;105(1):55–64.
2. Loumiotis I, Lanzino G, Daniels D, Sheehan J, Link M. Radiosurgery for intracranial dural arteriovenous fistulas (DAVFs): a review. *Neurosurg Rev.* 2011;34(3):305–315; discussion 315.
3. Katsaridis V. Treatment of dural arteriovenous fistulas. *Curr Treat Options Neurol.* 2009;11(1):35–40.
4. O'Leary S, Hodgson TJ, Coley SC, Kemeny AA, Radatz MW. Intracranial dural arteriovenous malformations: results of stereotactic radiosurgery in 17 patients. *Clin Oncol (R Coll Radiol).* 2002;14(2):97–102.
5. Lawton MT, Jacobowitz R, Spetzler RF. Redefined role of angiogenesis in the pathogenesis of dural arteriovenous malformations. *J Neurosurg.* 1997;87(2):267–274.
6. Cifarelli CP, Kaptain G, Yen CP, Schlesinger D, Sheehan JP. Gamma knife radiosurgery for dural arteriovenous fistulas. *Neurosurgery.* 2010;67(5):1230–1235; discussion 1235.
7. Kerber CW, Newton TH. The macro and microvasculature of the dura mater. *Neuroradiology.* 1973;6(4):175–179.
8. Uranishi R, Nakase H, Sakaki T. Expression of angiogenic growth factors in dural arteriovenous fistula. *J Neurosurg.* 1999;91(5):781–786.
9. Barrow DL, Spector RH, Braun IF, Landman JA, Tindall SC, Tindall GT. Classification and treatment of spontaneous carotid-cavernous sinus fistulas. *J Neurosurg.* 1985;62(2):248–256.
10. Malik GM, Pearce JE, Ausman JI, Mehta B. Dural arteriovenous malformations and intracranial hemorrhage. *Neurosurgery.* 1984;15(3):332–339.
11. See AP, Raza S, Tamargo RJ, Lim M. Stereotactic radiosurgery of cranial arteriovenous malformations and dural arteriovenous fistulas. *Neurosurg Clin N Am.* 2012;23(1):133–146.
12. Jung HH, Chang JH, Whang K, Pyen JS, Chang JW, Park YG. Gamma Knife surgery for low-flow cavernous sinus dural arteriovenous fistulas. *J Neurosurg.* 2010;(113 suppl):21–27.
13. Borden JA, Wu JK, Shucart WA. Correction: dural arteriovenous fistulous malformations. *J Neurosurg.* 1995;82(4):705–706.
14. Cognard C, Gobin YP, Pierot L, et al. Cerebral dural arteriovenous fistulas: clinical and angiographic correlation with a revised classification of venous drainage. *Radiology.* 1995;194(3):671–680.
15. Djindijan R MJ, Theron J: *Superselective Arteriography of the External Carotid Artery.* New York, NY: Springer, 1977.
16. Yang HC, Kano H, Kondziolka D, et al. Stereotactic radiosurgery with or without embolization for intracranial dural arteriovenous fistulas. *Neurosurgery.* 2010;67(5):1276–1283; discussion 1284.
17. Giller CA, Barnett DW, Thacker IC, Hise JH, Berger BD. Multidisciplinary treatment of a large cerebral dural arteriovenous fistula using embolization, surgery, and radiosurgery. *Proc (Bayl Univ Med Cent).* 2008;21(3):255–257.
18. Halbach VV HR, Hieshima GB, David FD. Endovascular therapy of dural fistulas. In: Vinuela F, Halbach VV, Dion JE, eds. *Interventional Neuroradiology: Endovascular Therapy of the Central Nervous System.* New York, NY: Raven; 1992:29–50.

19. Awad IA, Little JR, Akarawi WP, Ahl J. Intracranial dural arteriovenous malformations: factors predisposing to an aggressive neurological course. *J Neurosurg.* 1990;72(6):839–850.
20. Kakarla UK, Deshmukh VR, Zabramski JM, Albuquerque FC, McDougall CG, Spetzler RF. Surgical treatment of high-risk intracranial dural arteriovenous fistulae: clinical outcomes and avoidance of complications. *Neurosurgery.* 2007;61(3):447–57; discussion 457.
21. Sundt TM Jr, Piepgras DG. The surgical approach to arteriovenous malformations of the lateral and sigmoid dural sinuses. *J Neurosurg.* 1983;59(1):32–39.
22. Cognard C, Januel AC, Silva NA Jr, Tall P. Endovascular treatment of intracranial dural arteriovenous fistulas with cortical venous drainage: new management using Onyx. *AJNR Am J Neuroradiol.* 2008;29(2):235–241.
23. van Rooij WJ, Sluzewski M, Beute GN. Dural arteriovenous fistulas with cortical venous drainage: incidence, clinical presentation, and treatment. *AJNR Am J Neuroradiol.* 2007;28:651–655.
24. Pan HC, Sun MH, Sheehan J, et al. Radiosurgery for dural carotid-cavernous sinus fistulas: Gamma Knife compared with XKnife radiosurgery. *J Neurosurg.* 2010;(113 suppl):9–20.
25. Barcia-Salorio JL, Soler F, Barcia JA, Hernández G. Stereotactic radiosurgery for the treatment of low-flow carotid-cavernous fistulae: results in a series of 25 cases. *Stereotact Funct Neurosurg.* 1994;63(1–4):266–270.
26. Ratliff J, Voorhies RM. Arteriovenous fistula with associated aneurysms coexisting with dural arteriovenous malformation of the anterior inferior falx. Case report and review of the literature. *J Neurosurg.* 1999;91(2):303–307.
27. Hidaka H, Terashima H, Tsukamoto Y, Nakata H, Matsuoka S. Radiotherapy of dural arteriovenous malformation in the cavernous sinus. *Radiat Med.* 1989;7(3):160–164.
28. Kida Y. Radiosurgery for dural arteriovenous fistula. *Prog Neurol Surg.* 2009;22:38–44.
29. Heros RC. Gamma knife surgery for dural arteriovenous fistulas. *J Neurosurg.* 2006;104(6):861–3; discussion 865.
30. Wu HM, Pan DH, Chung WY, et al. Gamma Knife surgery for the management of intracranial dural arteriovenous fistulas. *J Neurosurg.* 2006;(105 suppl):43–51.
31. Koebbe CJ, Singhal D, Sheehan J, et al. Radiosurgery for dural arteriovenous fistulas. *Surg Neurol.* 2005;64(5):392–8; discussion 398.
32. Yamamoto M, Hara M, Ide M, Ono Y, Jimbo M, Saito I. Radiation-related adverse effects observed on neuro-imaging several years after radiosurgery for cerebral arteriovenous malformations. *Surg Neurol.* 1998;49:385–397; discussion 397–388.
33. Friedman JA, Pollock BE, Nichols DA, Gorman DA, Foote RL, Stafford SL. Results of combined stereotactic radiosurgery and transarterial embolization for dural arteriovenous fistulas of the transverse and sigmoid sinuses. *J Neurosurg.* 2001;94(6):886–891.

Chapter 9

The Role of Radiosurgery for the Treatment of Cerebral Cavernous Malformations

*Peter A. Gooderham &
Gary K. Steinberg*

Cerebral cavernous malformations (CMs) are the most common clinically relevant angiographically occult cerebral vascular malformations. With the widespread use of MRI, they are diagnosed with increasing frequency. Depending on the location, management can be very challenging. Although there has been a growing body of literature over the past two decades, radiosurgery remains a controversial treatment option in the management of CMs. The controversy stems from conflicting results reported for the treatment efficacy, lack of radiographic endpoint following radiosurgery, and incomplete understanding of the natural history of these lesions.

EPIDEMIOLOGY

Based on MRI and autopsy data, the prevalence of cerebral CMs is 0.4% to 0.8% of the general population (1). Multiple CMs are identified in 10% to 20% of patients. Familial cases, inherited in an autosomal dominant manner with incomplete penetrance, account for at least 20% of all CMs. Between 10% and 35% of CMs are located in the brainstem.

PRESENTATION AND NATURAL HISTORY

Superficial supratentorial CMs may present with seizure or less commonly with overt intracerebral hemorrhage. CMs located in the brainstem and deep supratentorial structures (thalamus and basal ganglia) tend to present with new or recurrent focal neurological deficits due intralesional or extralesional hemorrhage. Up to 40% of CMs are identified incidentally.

The annual risk of hemorrhage for a CM identified incidentally or due to seizure is 0.25% to 3%. The risk of hemorrhage seems higher in brainstem and deeply located CMs. It is unclear whether this is due to an actual difference in risk of bleeding, or a much higher risk of clinical deficit occurring with a small bleed. Following a hemorrhage, however, the risk of repeat hemorrhage from a CM is much higher, ranging from 4.5% to 40% per year. The risk of rebleeding appears to be highest in the first 1 to 2.5 years after the initial hemorrhage, with evidence of clustering of hemorrhages. In a retrospective natural history series looking at rehemorrhage risk in 141 patients, Barker found the monthly clinical rehemorrhage risk was 2% for the first 2.5 years with a subsequent decreased risk to less than 1% per month (2). As MRI findings suggest that many CMs have bled at some point, it is unclear whether and when the risk of rebleeding returns to prehemorrhage rates following a hemorrhage.

Up to 40% of patients with CMs present with seizures. Epilepsy associated with CMs can be controlled with antiepileptic medications in 60% of patients. The annual risk of new-onset seizures is 1.3% in patients with solitary CMs and 2.5% in patients with multiple CMs (1). As there is no neuropil within a CM proper, it is thought that the epileptogenic focus of CMs is the hemosiderin-stained, gliotic neuropil surrounding the lesion.

MANAGEMENT OF CEREBRAL CAVERNOUS MALFORMATIONS

The optimal management of CMs depends on balancing the natural history of the lesion with the risks of intervention. Treatment should be offered in cases when benefits of treatment outweigh the associated risks. This must be decided on an individual basis.

MICROSURGICAL RESECTION OF CAVERNOUS MALFORMATIONS

Recent reports have demonstrated that appropriately selected brainstem and deeply located CMs can be resected with acceptable morbidity and a low rate of incomplete resection. In Porter's series of 86 patients who underwent microsurgical resection of brainstem CMs, the overall morbidity rate was 35% with permanent or severe deficits occurring in 12% and perioperative mortality in 3.5% (3). A series of 56 patients with thalamic, basal ganglia, or brainstem CMs who underwent microsurgical resection was published by Steinberg. Immediate postoperative neurologic status was unchanged in 55%, worsened in 29%, and improved in 16%. Long-term outcomes (greater than 6 months) compared to status at presentation were unchanged in 45%, improved in 52%, and worsened in 5% (4). The goal of surgery must be complete resection, whenever feasible, as incomplete resection leaves the patient at significant risk of recurrence and rehemorrhage. Advances in microsurgical techniques, including accurate MRI-based frameless stereotaxy, have been instrumental in achieving these surgical results. Complete surgical resection of a CM remains the only treatment that results in cure of the lesion.

The surgical management of intractable epilepsy associated with CMs is well established. Seizure control rates up to 80% have been reported in the literature. The prognosis is worst for patients with a long preoperative history of epilepsy (1).

RADIOSURGERY FOR CAVERNOUS MALFORMATIONS

Radiosurgery for the treatment of CMs was introduced in the 1980s. It was initially used because of the success reported for the treatment of brain arteriovenous malformations. Because CMs are angiographically occult, purely radiographic endpoints for the treatment of these lesions with radiosurgery are not feasible. Determining the efficacy of this treatment has relied on changes of bleeding and rebleeding rates following radiosurgery. Because microsurgical resection is generally straightforward, safe, and effective for the management of symptomatic superficial supratentorial CMs, the majority of cases reported in radiosurgery series are deeply located supratentorial and brainstem lesions.

HISTOPATHOLOGICAL EFFECTS OF RADIOSURGERY

It has been proposed that the effect of radiosurgery on CMs would be analogous to the effects on the vessels of brain arteriovenous malformations; however, there appear to be differences. The vascular channels of brain arteriovenous malformations treated with radiosurgery have been shown to undergo early occlusion by coagulation of cytoplasmic debris and endothelial injury and ultimately permanent occlusion by fibrin thrombi (5). In contrast, cavernous malformations treated with radiosurgery have been found not to exhibit vascular obliteration when examined pathologically at a mean of 3.5 years posttreatment. There is evidence of fibrinoid necrosis and vessel fibrosis in some cases (6). The examined CMs after radiosurgery are all surgical specimens and may, therefore, underrepresent the effects of radiosurgery, as those lesions with the best response would not go on to further treatment.

EFFECT OF RADIOSURGERY ON RISK OF BLEEDING AND REBLEEDING

Promising results evaluating the role of radiosurgery in the management of CMs have been reported. Lunsford published a series of 103 patients with CMs treated with Gamma Knife radiosurgery (mean marginal dose 16 Gy). Of the 103 patients, 90% were located in deep structures or brainstem and 90% had presented with at least two clinical, imaging confirmed, hemorrhages prior to treatment. Prior to treatment, the mean annual hemorrhage rate was 32.5%. In the first 2 years after radiosurgery, the annual hemorrhage rate was 10.8% and after 2 years, the annual hemorrhage rate was 1.06% (7). Similar results were reported by Chang in a series of 56 patients treated with helium ion Bragg peak or linear accelerator radiosurgery (marginal doses 12–20 Gy). The annual hemorrhage rate following radiosurgery was 12.3% during the first 2 years and 1.9% thereafter (8). Amin-Hajani reported a series of 98 patients with CMs treated with proton beam radiosurgery. They reported a decrease in rehemorrhage risk from 17.4% per year before treatment to 4.5% per year following a 2-year latency after treatment (9). Although these results are promising, because of the tendency of hemorrhage events from CMs to cluster and because of the lack of control groups in the published series, it is difficult to determine the effect of radiosurgery. In a 2009 review of published series of radiosurgery for the treatment of CMs, Pham identified 23 retrospective studies. The included studies found variable efficacy of radiosurgery, with postradiosurgery hemorrhage rates of 7.3% to 22% per year in the first 2 years and 0.8% to 5.2% per year after the first 2 years. Although most included series demonstrated a reduction of hemorrhage rates after 2 years, several studies did not demonstrate any reduction (10).

COMPLICATIONS OF RADIOSURGERY FOR CAVERNOUS MALFORMATIONS

Although the Pittsburgh group has reported relatively low rates of complications when radiosurgery is used to treat deeply located CMs (13.5%; 7), other groups have reported rates as high as 59% (10). In the Harvard series, 26.5% of patients suffered a radiation-induced morbidity with 61.5% of these resulting in permanent neurological deficits (9). In a synthesis of published series, Steiner identified an overall neurological morbidity rate of 19% with half of these involving permanent deficits (11). Morbidity rates following radiosurgery are consistently highest when lesions are located in the brainstem, followed by the basal ganglia and thalamus. Morbidity rates appear to be highest in series where marginal doses greater than 16.5 Gy are employed (10).

RADIOGRAPHIC CHANGES FOLLOWING RADIOSURGERY

Up to 57% of CMs demonstrate regression in lesion volume after radiosurgery but none resolve on imaging following radiosurgery (7). Natural history studies have demonstrated that there is a great deal of spontaneous change in size of CMs. The dynamic nature of these lesions is highlighted in the prospective imaging assessment of 107 untreated CMs by Clatterbuck, in which they demonstrated a mean interval volume change of -991 mm^3 over 26 months. In this study, 35% of lesions demonstrated interval growth and 55% decreased in size (12). It is, therefore, difficult to ascribe meaning to the finding of radiographic change of these lesions following radiosurgery.

RADIOSURGERY FOR EPILEPSY ASSOCIATED WITH CAVERNOUS MALFORMATIONS

There are few reports of using radiosurgery for the management of epilepsy secondary to CMs. In 2000, Regis reported a series of 49 patients with drug-resistant epilepsy treated with Gamma Knife radiosurgery (mean marginal dose of 19 Gy). Of the 49 patients, 53% were seizure free at last follow-up with another 20% having a meaningful reduction in seizure rates (13). Although this suggests some degree of efficacy, these results are less successful than most modern surgical series for CM-associated epilepsy.

Radiosurgery Techniques

A high degree of conformality is paramount when targeting CMs located in the brainstem and deep cerebral structures. The optimal target is defined as being within the low-signal hemosiderin ring on T2-weighted MRI images. The low-signal hemosiderin margin itself is best avoided because the iron pigments within the neuropil can act as radiation sensitizers, potentially increasing morbidity. Associated developmental venous anomalies (DVAs) should not be included in the target volume (7). The ideal radiosurgery dose remains to be defined. Marginal doses of 15 to 16.2 Gy appear to be efficacious while minimizing associated morbidity (10). A single dose of corticosteroid is generally administered at the time of treatment.

CONCLUSIONS

As there is controversy regarding the efficacy and risk of radiosurgery for the management of CMs, it should be used very selectively. Most cerebrovascular centers recommend microsurgical resection for symptomatic CMs, including those in the deep supratentorial region or brainstem if they can be approached with low morbidity. Radiosurgery should be reserved for those patients with a CM that has proven to have an aggressive natural history, demonstrated by more than one clinical hemorrhage, for whom surgical resection carries an unacceptable risk due to either their location or the patient's poor surgical/anesthetic risk.

REFERENCES

1. Batra S, Lin D, Recinos PF, Zhang J, Rigamonti D. Cavernous malformations: natural history, diagnosis and treatment. *Nat Rev Neurol.* 2009;5(12):659–670.
2. Barker FG, 2nd, Amin-Hanjani S, Butler WE, et al. Temporal clustering of hemorrhages from untreated cavernous malformations of the central nervous system. *Neurosurgery.* 2001;49(1):15–24; discussion 24–15.
3. Porter RW, Detwiler PW, Spetzler RF, et al. Cavernous malformations of the brainstem: experience with 100 patients. *J Neurosurg.* 1999;90(1):50–58.
4. Steinberg GK, Chang SD, Gewirtz RJ, Lopez JR. Microsurgical resection of brainstem, thalamic, and basal ganglia angiographically occult vascular malformations. *Neurosurgery.* 2000;46(2):260–270; discussion 270–261.
5. Tu J, Stoodley MA, Morgan MK, Storer KP, Smee R. Different responses of cavernous malformations and arteriovenous malformations to radiosurgery. *J Clin Neurosci.* 2009;16(7):945–949.
6. Gewirtz RJ, Steinberg GK, Crowley R, Levy RP. Pathological changes in surgically resected angiographically occult vascular malformations after radiation. *Neurosurgery.* 1998;42(4):738–742; discussion 742–733.
7. Lunsford LD, Khan AA, Niranjan A, Kano H, Flickinger JC, Kondziolka D. Stereotactic radiosurgery for symptomatic solitary cerebral cavernous malformations considered high risk for resection. *J Neurosurg.* 2010;113(1):23–29.
8. Chang SD, Levy RP, Adler JR Jr, Martin DP, Krakovitz PR, Steinberg GK. Stereotactic radiosurgery of angiographically occult vascular malformations: 14-year experience. *Neurosurgery.* 1998;43(2):213–220; discussion 220–211.
9. Amin-Hanjani S, Ogilvy CS, Candia GJ, Lyons S, Chapman PH. Stereotactic radiosurgery for cavernous malformations: Kjellberg's experience with proton beam therapy in 98 cases at the Harvard Cyclotron. *Neurosurgery.* 1998;42(6):1229–1236; discussion 1236–1228.
10. Pham M, Gross BA, Bendok BR, Awad IA, Batjer HH. Radiosurgery for angiographically occult vascular malformations. *Neurosurg Focus.* 2009;26(5):E16.
11. Steiner L, Karlsson B, Yen CP, Torner JC, Lindquist C, Schlesinger D. Radiosurgery in cavernous malformations: anatomy of a controversy. *J Neurosurg.* 2010;113(1):16–21; discussion 21–12.
12. Clatterbuck RE, Moriarity JL, Elmaci I, Lee RR, Breiter SN, Rigamonti D. Dynamic nature of cavernous malformations: a prospective magnetic resonance imaging study with volumetric analysis. *J Neurosurg.* 2000;93(6):981–986.
13. Régis J, Bartolomei F, Kida Y, et al. Radiosurgery for epilepsy associated with cavernous malformation: retrospective study in 49 patients. *Neurosurgery.* 2000;47(5):1091–1097.

Section V

Radiosurgery for Functional Diseases

Section Editor

Lawrence R. Kleinberg

Chapter 10

Role of Radiosurgery for Trigeminal Neuralgia

*Alessandra Gorgulho &
Antonio A. F. De Salles*

Trigeminal neuralgia (TN) is the most common type of neuralgia with numerous therapeutic options. About a quarter of the patients diagnosed with TN will not respond to medication, whereas another quarter will develop intolerance to medication. Yet a common consensus regarding the optimal timing for a surgical intervention is still lacking. Studies evaluating quality of life in patients submitted to microvascular decompression (MVD) showed that an absolute majority of the patients would have had surgery earlier (1). For the sake of this chapter we will focus on the management of classical TN and secondary TN with typical features.

THERAPEUTIC OPTIONS FOR THE MANAGEMENT OF TRIGEMINAL NEURALGIA

Anticonvulsants are the first line of treatment. Carbamazepine is the most effective. The number needed to accomplish pain control is 1.7 to 1.8, whereas the number needed to harm equals 3.4 for minor side effects and 24 for severe effects (2). Side effects classified as minor significantly interfere with the quality of life of the patients. Oxcarbazepine has become preferable to carbamazepine due to reduced toxicity, while maintaining comparable levels of pain relief. Second-line options are baclofen and lamotrigine (class 2). Other antiepileptic drugs such as gabapentin, valproate, and phenytoin (including intravenous) seem to be effective (class 4).

Surgical modalities include: MVD, radiofrequency rhizotomy (RFR), balloon compression (BC), glycerol injection, and radiosurgery, which is the least invasive among all. MVD leads to the best long-term pain control (70% pain free at 10 years) with an incidence of facial numbness of only 1.7% (2–4). It is also the only surgical procedure that is not ablative. However, it does carry the highest short-term risk for complications among all the surgical options. Even though the perioperative complications are infrequent in experienced hands, the complications include death (incidence: 0.2%–0.5%), hemorrhage and stroke (incidence: 4%), hearing loss (incidence: 10%), meningitis, cerebrospinal fluid leak (incidence: 11%), and other complications of a craniotomy (4).

Radiosurgery can be delivered using a Gamma unit or a dedicated linear accelerator (LINAC) device. Clinical results observed with both devices are similar. Currently, the accuracy of some dedicated LINAC devices allow TN radiosurgery to be performed without invasive frame placement (5). Because of the noninvasive nature of radiosurgery, it is a very attractive option to patients who failed medical therapy.

TREATMENT ALGORITHM

Figure 10.1 describes the algorithm used at UCLA to recommend surgical procedures for TN (6). Briefly, patients under acute pain attack and after Hidantal

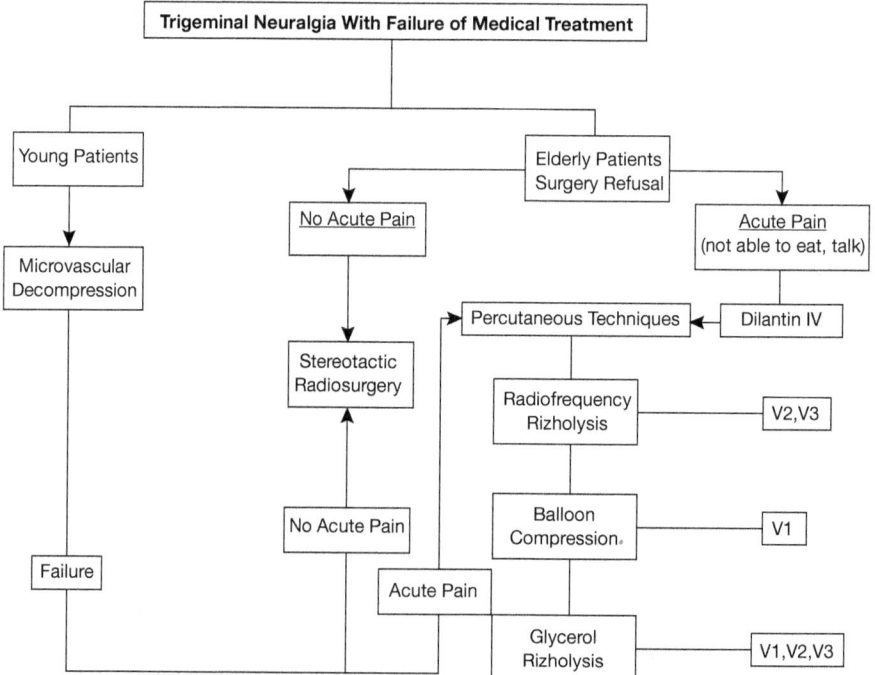

FIGURE 10.1 UCLA algorithm for TN surgical procedures.

intravenous infusion should undergo MVD or a percutaneous procedure. Usually we recommend BC for patients who are more fragile, who understand they may experience hypoesthesia in the entire hemiface after the procedure and are either unreliable or unwilling to undergo intraoperative stimulation for a precise location of the trigeminal nerve branch. It is also indicated for patients with V1 pain. RFR leads to selective branch numbness in the hemiface. The odds of the numbness subsiding over time are lower after RFR than BC. We tend to recommend RFR for TN secondary to multiple sclerosis (MS). It usually requires the procedure to be repeated during the course of the disease but does provide excellent long-lasting pain relief. We only recommend RFR for V2 and V3 pain because V1 numbness is associated with an unacceptably high level of corneal numbness, corneal ulcers, and dry eye complications. Paresthesias and anesthesia dolorosa after percutaneous procedures are reported in 12% and 4% of the patients, respectively. Young and healthy subjects showing a vascular conflict on thin cuts MRI evaluating the trigeminal pathway are candidates for MVD. The literature is controversial on the definition of elderly. Some authors observed more postoperative complications in the population 65 years and older, whereas others did not find increased morbidity in the elderly. Likely, age per se is not as important a risk factor as it is the cause for a rigorous preoperative evaluation of the patient's general health status. On the other hand, we observe in our clinic a trend of young and healthy patients who are candidates for MVD who elect radiosurgery as the first surgical treatment modality, seeking lack of invasiveness and comfort.

RADIOSURGERY FOR TRIGEMINAL NEURALGIA

Radiosurgery provides pain relief to 80% to 90% of the patients (6) after a mean time delay of 6 weeks after treatment delivery. Immediate pain relief after SRS is observed in only 20% of the cases. The time latency to triggering pain control is the main drawback of this technique, limiting its application to patients under acute pain attacks presenting with weight loss and the inability to eat or talk. The recurrence rate post SRS ranges from 25% to 53%, depending on the length of follow-up. In our series, 65% of the patients with classical TN are pain free and medication free at 3 years post SRS (7), whereas 80% are pain free with or without medication at 3 years. The literature reports similar rates (58%–69%) of pain control in the absence of medication at actuarial 3 years. At 5 years post SRS, 41% to 53% of the patients are pain free with or without medication (8–10). Other patients still experience improvement in the frequency and severity of pain attacks but do require the adjuvant use of medication. Prior surgical procedure is a negative predictor of successful pain outcome (7) in our series. This finding is echoed in other series. The results of SRS for secondary TN with typical features are not as good. For MS-triggered TN, we observe 66% of pain control with or without medication. The results are more modest for TN secondary to zoster. We achieve 50% success in the treatment of TN secondary to head and neck cancer infiltration, which is obviously a palliative procedure (7).

The most common complication after radiosurgery is facial numbness. The incidence varies considerably in the literature, ranging from 10% to 50%. It certainly reflects the scrutiny of followup and the treatment protocol, as it relates to radiation dose and positioning of the isocenter. Other complications such as bothersome dysesthesia are observed in a minority of the cases (incidence: 4%–10%). Anesthesia dolorosa is a rare complication and there have been few cases reported so far. Hearing decrease and foot weakness were described in two cases and one case, respectively, in a single-series cohort using nonisocentric radiosurgery technique (11). These complications were attributed to an inadvertent excess dose to the brainstem.

The dose of radiation prescribed varies from 80 to 90 Gy. A dose-searching trial showed that doses of 70 Gy or below do not lead to the same levels of pain control or to sustainability of pain relief. The three most common positionings of isocenters within the trigeminal pathway are: (a) at the root entry zone (Figure 10.2), which lies about 2 to 3 mm away from the brainstem surface; (b) at the midcisternal segment of the nerve; (c) at the *pars triangularis*, AKA far anterior

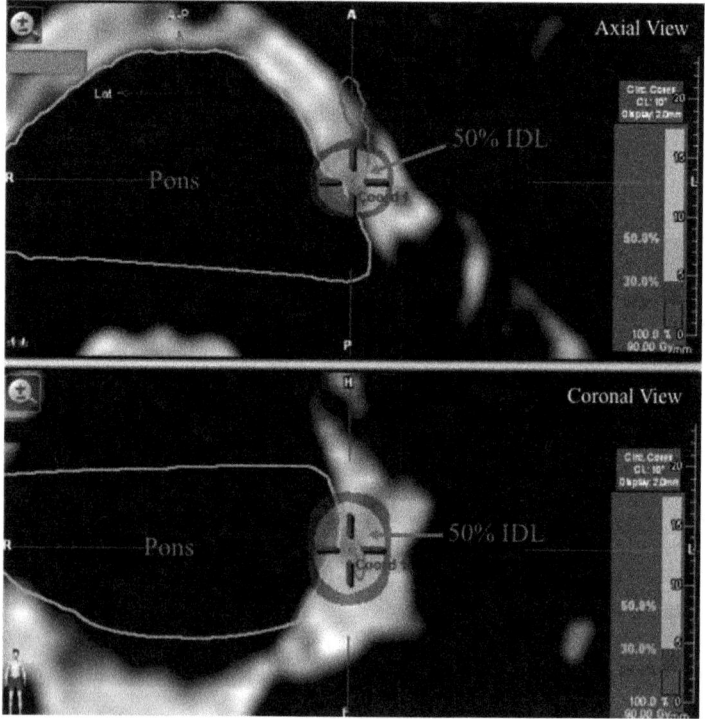

FIGURE 10.2 The root entry zone.

cisternal segment. Irradiation of an increased length of the nerve did not show improved pain relief rates but did show increased incidence of complications, mostly facial numbness (11,12).

Logistic regression analysis in our series showed a trend to better pain control as the dose of radiation to the nerve root entry zone (REZ) is increased (Figure 10.2; 7), and at the cost of higher incidence of facial numbness. These findings are corroborated by other reports (13,14). However, clinical outcomes from series using different protocols (i.e., targeting at the REZ or at the anterior far cisternal segment) are impossible to compare. Only a randomized controlled trial comparing the effects of different isocenter positioning will definitively establish where lies the "sweet spot" for radiation in regard to both pain outcomes. In our series, we also found a positive correlation between facial numbness occurrence, improved pain outcomes, and enhancement of the pons in the post-SRS MRI scans (15).

Radiosurgery as a retreatment option is feasible and yields to 80% pain control, but at the cost of a high incidence of facial numbness and an increase in facial numbness in patients who already experience it (16). Clinical results are similar among different treatment protocols (decreased dose, different target, same dose in the same target).

The radiosurgery treatment of TN should be performed by centers with excellence in radiosurgery. The treatment is targeted toward a 3-mm diameter nerve with a 4-mm (or 5-mm) collimator, delivering a high dose of radiation to the nerve. Absolute domain of the technology used, in-house accuracy tests, and stringent treatment protocols are an absolute prerequisite before consideration of performing radiosurgery for TN.

REFERENCES

1. Zakrzewska JL, Lopez BC, Kim SE, Coakham HB. Patient reports of satisfaction after microvascular decompression and partial sensory rhizotomy for trigeminal neuralgia. *Neurosurgery.* 2005; 56, 1304–1311.
2. Cruccu G, Gronseth G, Alksne J, et al. AAN-EFNS guidelines on trigeminal neuralgia management. *Eur J Neurol.* 2008;15:1013–1028.
3. Tatli M, Satici O, Kanpolat Y, Sindou M. Various surgical modalities for trigeminal neuralgia: literature study of respective long-term outcomes. *Acta Neurochir (Wien).* 2008;150:243–255.
4. Gronseth G, Cruccu G, Alksne J, et al. Practice parameter: the diagnostic evaluation and treatment of trigeminal neuralgia (an evidence-based review). *Neurology.* 2008;71:1183–1190.
5. Chen JC, Rahimian J, Rahimian R, et al. Frameless image-guided radiosurgery for initial treatment of typical trigeminal neuralgia. *World Neurosurg.* 2010;74(4–5):538–543.
6. Gorgulho AA, De Salles AA. Impact of radiosurgery on the surgical treatment of trigeminal neuralgia. *Surg Neurol.* 2006;66:350–356.
7. Smith Z, Gorgulho A, Bezrukiy N, et al. Dedicated linear accelerator radiosurgery for trigeminal neuralgia: a single-center experience in 179 patients with varied dose prescriptions and treatment plans. *IJROBP.* 2011;81(1):225–231.

8. Regis J, Arkha Y, Yomo S, et al. Radiosurgery in trigeminal neuralgia: long term results and influence of operative nuances. *Neurochirurgie.* 2009;55(2):213–222.
9. Han JH, Kim DG, Chung HT, et al. Long term outcome of gamma knife radiosurgery for treatment of typical trigeminal neuralgia. *IJROBP.* 2009;75(3):822–827.
10. Kondziolka D, Zorro O, Lobato-Polo J, et al. Gamma knife stereotactic radiosurgery for idiopathic trigeminal neuralgia. *JNS.* 2010;112:758–765.
11. Villavicencio AT, Lim M, Burneikiene S et al. CyberKnife radiosurgery for trigeminal neuralgia treatment: a preliminary multicenter experience. *Neurosurgery.* 2008;62:647–655.
12. Flickinger JC, Pollock BE, Kondziolka D, et al. Does increased nerve length within the treatment volume improve trigeminal neuralgia radiosurgery? A prospective double-blind, randomized study. *IJROBP.* 2001;51:449–454.
13. Brisman R, Mooij R. Gamma knife radiosurgery for trigeminal neuralgia: dose-volume histograms of the brainstem and trigeminal nerve. *J Neurosurg.* 2000;93(suppl 3):155–158.
14. Pollock BE. Radiosurgery for trigeminal neuralgia: is sensory disturbance required for pain relief? *J Neurosurg.* 2006;105:103–106.
15. Gorgulho A, De Salles AA, McArthur D, et al. Brainstem and trigeminal nerve changes after radiosurgery for trigeminal pain. *Surg Neurol.* 2006;66:127–135; discussion 135.
16. Park KJ, Kondziolka D, Berkowitz O, et al. Repeat gamma knife radiosurgery for trigeminal neuralgia. *Neurosurgery.* 2012; 70(2):295–305;discussion 305.

Chapter 11

Radiosurgery for Drug-Resistant Epilepsies: State of the Art, Results, and Perspectives

Jean Régis, Romain Caron, Fabrice Bartolomei, & Patrick Chauvel

Radiosurgery has been evaluated in our Epilepsy Surgery program since 1992. Nowadays, with 20 years of experience in this field, numerous experimental studies and clinical prospective trials are substantiating a reasonable worldwide experience which allows us to define seriously what can be expected from radiosurgery in this field. Our local clinical experience (217 patients), accumulated over the last 20 years, mainly includes treatment of temporal lobe epilepsy without space-occupying lesions (101 patients), 96 hypothalamic hamartomas, 7 callosotomies, and 13 other kinds of neocortical epilepsies. The analysis of our material, as well as other clinical and experimental data, suggests that the use of radiosurgery is beneficial only to those patients in whom strict preoperative definition of the extent of the epileptogenic zone (or network) has been achieved, and where strict rules of dose planning have been followed. As soon as these principles are not observed, the risk of treatment failure and/or side effects increases dramatically. Long-term outcome is now available for mesial temporal lobe epilepsy (MTLE) and hypothalamic hamartomas. Pure MTLE, especially in a patient with a high risk of verbal memory loss, or patients reluctant to undergo a microsurgical intervention, and patients with small type I, II, III hypothalamic hamartomas can be considered as current practice. The use of radiosurgery in more complex neocortical epilepsies with epileptogenic zone in a highly functional area (in first or second intention) is presently under evaluation. Although still in a preliminary stage, this field may be a very promising one for epilepsy radiosurgery.

RATIONALE

Radiosurgery is a neurosurgical technique during which high energy is delivered in a small, sharply limited target with stereotactic accuracy in a single session, with the aim either to create a lesion or to induce a desired biological effect (1,2). Since the first attempt by the pioneers in Stockholm, the practice of radiosurgery has substantially changed and in the vast majority of the indications, nondestructive low dosage inducing a subtle biological effect like apoptosis in tumors or endothelial proliferation in arteriovenous malformation (AVM) is used.

The Differential Effect Concept

There is a classical clinical observation that in 85% of the AVMs associated with resistant epilepsy, radiosurgery is followed by seizure cessation or dramatic improvement occurring much before the occlusion of the AVM itself. When the AVM is located in a highly functional area the seizure cessation is obtained without clinical deficit. This observation led us in 1992 to propose the concept of "clinical differential effect": radiosurgery can induce a functional effect, making the cortex surrounding the AVM no longer epileptic without destroying the underlying function of this cortical area thanks to its capacity to alter some systems specifically while sparing others! The first proof of this concept came from the demonstration of the existence of such an effect at the biochemical level in the striatum of rats (64). A group of rats received a single isocenter of 4 mm in the left striatum with a maximum dose of 50 Gy using the Gamma Knife (GK). Biochemical analyses demonstrated a stability of the level of the GABA acetyl decarboxylase in spite of the dramatic decrease of the level of the catecholemines (CAT), indicating an injury to the catecholaminergic system in spite of the sparing of the GABAergic system. Similarly, direct dosage of the GABA itself shows its stability in spite of the major decrease of the amino excitatory acids (glutamate and aspartate). This experimental demonstration led us to consider radiosurgery as a neuromulation therapy (1–3) and encouraged us to organize several prospective clinical trials (4–8). More recently the demonstration of the existence of a differential effect at the cellular level came from the Charlottesville group (9). In epileptic rats irradiated with 40 Gy in the temporal lobe using the GK immunohistochemical, the study suggested that at least one subtype of hippocampal interneurons is selectively vulnerable to Gamma Knife radiosurgery. Neuronal cells appear to have undergone a phenotypic shift with respect to calbindin and GAD-67 expression. There is a growing body of evidence in favor of a neuromodulatory effect (1,2,10).

A series of successive clinical trials has been organized in Marseille in order to evaluate GK surgery in epilepsy. In 1993 we organized a phase II prospective trial in four mesial temporal lobe epilepsy (MTLE) patients with a goal of dose ranging and toxicity evaluation (6,8). In 1995, the good safety and the impressive efficacy in the patient receiving the 24 Gy dosage led us to organize a Phase III prospective monocentric study in four MTLE patients (24 Gy, 7–8 mL) in order to evaluate the reproducibility of the efficacy (4). In 1996, we organized a prospective multicentric European study (21 MTLE patients) confirming the reproducibility of the safety and efficacy (7). In 1998, a dose de-escalation study (24, 20, and 18 Gy) showed that the efficacy decreased dramatically when the marginal doses were lower than 24 Gy (5). Finally, our neurologists performed a long-term evaluation (greater than 5 years follow-up) in the first 15 consecutive patients treated according to our standard protocol (11). This study confirmed the good safety efficacy of Gamma Knife surgery in this group of patients over the long term, with a rate of 60% of Engel I at a mean follow-up of 8 years (11–15). This compared well with the safety efficacy of open surgery in the long term. More recently, a multicentric prospective trial in the United States confirmed all our findings (16); as a result radiosurgery is the current practice for pure MTLE in our group (17).

There are convincing arguments for such an investigation of the potential role of radiosurgery in epilepsy surgery. We know that:

1. Radiosurgery (since its introduction in the 1950s) has been demonstrated to have advantages, in terms of safety and efficacy, for the treatment of numerous small deeply seated intracerebral lesions.
2. Radiosurgical treatment of small cortico-subcortical lesions associated with epilepsy has been demonstrated to lead to seizure cessation in a high percentage (58%–80% in AVM) of cases, long before the expected treatment of the lesion and sometimes even in spite of failing to cure the lesion itself.
3. Radiotherapeutic treatment of epilepsies with or without space-occupying lesions can lead to a reduction in seizure frequency and/or severity.
4. Experimental models of epilepsies treated with radiation therapy have demonstrated a dose-dependent positive effect of radiation on the frequency and severity of the seizures, and on the extent of discharge propagation.

Different kinds of radiation have been proposed for the treatment of epilepsies. Lars Leksell conceived GK radiosurgery as a tool for functional neurosurgery (18,19). Accordingly, he used GK in movement disorders, trigeminal neuralgia, and other pain syndromes, but not for epilepsy surgery (20). The first radiosurgical treatments for epilepsy surgery were performed by Talairach in the 1950s (21). Talairach was another pioneering expert in stereotaxis. Unlike Leksell, he had specific involvement in epilepsy surgery and led one of the first large comprehensive programs for epilepsy surgery. As early as 1974, he reported on the use of radioactive yttrium implants in patients with MTLE without space-occupying lesions, and showed a high rate of seizure control in patients with epilepsies confined to the mesial structures of the temporal lobe (21). Elomaa

(22), apparently ignoring the pioneering work of Talairach, promoted the idea of the use of focal irradiation for the treatment of temporal lobe epilepsy, based on the preliminary reports of Tracy and Von Wieser (23) and Baudouin et al. (15). Furthermore, clinical experience of the use of GK- and LINAC-based radiosurgery in AVMs and cortico-subcortical tumors (mostly metastases and low-grade glial tumors) revealed an antiepileptic effect of radiosurgery in the absence of a necrotizing effect (24–26). A series of experimental studies in small animals confirmed this effect (27,28) and has emphasized its relationship to the dose delivered (29–32). Barcia-Salorio et al. (33) and later Lindquist et al. (34–36) reported small and heterogeneous groups of patients treated with the aim of seizure cessation; results were, however, poor. Unfortunately, these data were never published in peer-reviewed articles and precise data are unavailable.

The department of Stereotactic and Functional Surgery in Marseille has two major fields of expertise, namely, epilepsy surgery and radiosurgery. This context has therefore facilitated the investigation and development of a potential role for GK radiosurgery in the treatment of intractable epilepsy. The first attempt to treat an MTLE occurred in Marseille in March 1993 (6). Since 1993, we have performed 217 cases of epilepsy surgery using GK radiosurgery.

Among 11,066 GK surgery procedures accomplished in our neurosurgical unit in a 20-year-period (between July 1992 and December 2012), only 217 were proposed in patients referred for epilepsy surgery (roughly 10 patients/year). During the same period, we have performed 759 nonradiosurgical, neurosurgical operations for epilepsy surgery. By the way, the philosophy of our team is to define the niche of patients in whom the safety–efficacy ratio makes it advantageous or at least compares favorably with open neurosurgery (37). Obviously, this represents a small subset of patients in our present experience (23%). However, a part of the patients we are actually operating on by GK are directly referred to us for this specific procedure. The real percentage of patients coming from our own clinical program of investigation for epilepsy and operated by GK is only 14.6%.

Hypothalamic Hamartomas

Hypothalamic hamartomas (HH) may be asymptomatic, associated with precocious puberty or with neurological disorders (including epilepsy, behavior disturbances, and cognitive impairment), or both. Usually the seizures begin early in life and are often particularly drug-resistant from the outset. The evolution is unfavorable in the majority of the patients because of behavioral symptoms (particularly aggressive behavior) and mental decline, which occur as a direct effect of the seizures (38), due to an epileptic encephalopathy. Interestingly, in our experience, the reversal of this encephalopathy after radiosurgery seems to start even before complete cessation of the seizures and seems to be correlated to the improvement in background electroencephalographic (EEG) activity. We may speculate that these continuous discharges are leading to the disorganization of several systems, including the limbic system, and that their disappearance accounts for the improvement seen in attention, memory, cognitive performance, impulsive behavior, and so on. Here, the goal of radiosurgery is the reversal of the epileptic encephalopathy rather than seizure cessation. Consequently, we consider that it is essential to operate on these young patients as early as possible, whatever the surgical approach considered (resection or radiosurgery).

The intrinsic epileptogenicity of hypothalamic hamartoma (HH) has been demonstrated (39,40) even though the mechanisms of the epilepsy associated with HH are still debatable. The boundary of the target zone of treatment is that of the lesion visualized on MRI. This contrasts greatly with cases of MTLE for which there is no such clear delineation of an epileptogenic zone on the images used for planning radiosurgical intervention.

We retrospectively analyzed radiosurgery in a series of 10 patients collected from centers around the world (41). The very good safety–efficacy ratio (all improved, 50% cured and no adverse effects except one case of poikilothermia) led us to organize a prospective multicenter trial. Our trial of 64 prospectively evaluated patients is unique by the number of patients and the strict methodology of this evaluation. We have published preliminary reports of this study (42–44) and the final evaluation is under publication. These 64 patients operated on between 1999 and 2007 have been all followed more than 3 years (36–107 months). According to our policy, the patient and the family are offered a second radiosurgery in case of partial benefit when the lesion is anatomically small and well defined. Due to significant but incomplete efficacy, 25 patients (62.5%) were treated twice. The preoperative cognitive deficits, behavioral disturbances, and investigated relationship of seizure severity and anatomical type to cognitive abilities were characterized (45,46). The goal of the preoperative work-up was to adequately select the candidates for inclusion and to evaluate the baseline neurological and endocrinological functions. All radiosurgical procedures were carried out using a GK model B, C, 4C, or Perfexion (Elekta Instrument, Stockholm). Consistently we elaborated multi-isocentric complex dose planning of high conformity and selectivity. We used low peripheral doses to take into account the close relationship with optic pathways and the hypothalamus (median 17 Gy; range 13–26 Gy). The lesions treated are generally small one (median 9.5 mm; range 5–26 mm). We pay special attention to the dose delivered to the mammillary body and to the fornix and we always try to tailor the dose plan for each patient, based on the use of a single run of shots with the 4-mm collimator. Patients were evaluated with respect to seizures, cognition, behavior, and endocrine status 6, 12, 18, 24, and 36 months after radiosurgery and then every year. Results are demonstrating that in 65% of these patients an Engel I+II is achieved. An Engel III is observed in 20% of the patients. The frequency of seizures(s) before radiosurgery was 92 s/month [mean, 427 ± 1009; min 3.3] and fell to 6 s/month [mean 34.6 ± 78; min = 0; max = 425] after the radiosurgery. In the majority of these patients a dramatic behavioral and cognitive improvement is observed. Psychiatric and cognitive comorbidity were cured in 28%, improved in 56%, and stable in 8% of the patients. Globally, very good results have been obtained in 60% of the patients. A microsurgical approach has been taken in the case of 6 patients (9.3%) with quite large HH and poor efficacy of radiosurgery: one patient was cured (Engel I), two had improved (Engel III), and 3 did not improve (Engel IV).

We are reporting no permanent or even transient neurological deficit. A transient increase in seizures was observed in 7 patients (17.5%). A transient nondisabling poikilothermia was observed in three cases. Due to the very critical location of these lesions, we always try to tailor the dose plan for each patient, based on the use of a single run of shots with a 4-mm collimator. We pay special attention to the dose delivered to the mammillary body and to the fornix.

Topological classification of the lesion based on a good high-resolution MRI is a key feature in the decision-making process (42). Previous classification based on anatomical (47–49) or surgical (50) consideration did not describe the large diversity of these lesions and their therapeutic consequences. As underlined by Palmini and coworkers, the exact location of the lesion in relation to the interpeduncular fossa and the walls of the third ventricle correlates with the extent of excision, seizure control, and complication rate (51). On this basis, we classify the HHs according to their topology based on our original classification (42,43). In our experience, this classification correlates with the clinical semiology and severity and is especially critical for surgical strategy selection. Type I (small HH located inside the hypothalamus extending more or less in the third ventricle) cases are certainly the best candidates for GKS. In this population, the risks for microsurgical removal are likely to be potentially high.

In type II (when the lesion is small and mainly in the third ventricle) radiosurgery is certainly the safer alternative. Even though the endoscopic and transcallosal interforniceal approaches have been proposed, the risks of short-term memory worsening, endocrinological disturbance (hyperphagia with obesity, low tyroxine, sodium metabolism disturbance), and thalamic or thalamocapsular infarcts have been reported also by the more enthusiastic and skillful neurosurgeons. However, in case of very severe repeated status epilepticus, we propose as a salvage surgery either a transcallosal interforniceal approach or an endoscopic approach (depending on the width of the third ventricle). In an emergency situation, if the lesion is small and the third ventricle large, the endoscopic approach is chosen.

In type III (lesion located essentially in the floor) the extremely close relationship among the mammillary body, the fornix, and the lesion is clearly leading us to prefer GKS. We speculate that sessile hypothalamic hamartomas have always more or less an "extension" in the hypothalamus close to the mammillary body. Thus, when a lesion is classified as a type II, it means that the lesion appears on the MRI to be mainly located in the third ventricle but is likely to have a "root" in the hypothalamus. The same assumption is made for type III.

In type IV (the lesion sessile in the cistern) a disconnection can be discussed (pterional approach with or without orbitozygomatic osteotomy). However, if the lesion is small, GKS can be recommended due to its safety and its capability to reach at the same time the small associated part of the lesion in the hypothalamus itself, frequently visible on high-resolution MR. In Delalande's experience, only two patients among 14 were seizure free after a single disconnection through a pterional approach (52). Consequently, we do use this approach in case of lesions too large for GKS as a first step of a staged approach. In most circumstances, the patient is improved but not seizure free after the first surgical step and GKS is performed at 3 months as a second step of the treatment.

Type V (pediculate) cases are rarely epileptic and can be easily cured by radiosurgery or disconnection through a pterional approach. In case of severe epilepsy the second therapeutic modality will allow certainly a faster seizure cessation. However, a distant extension of the HH in the hypothalamus close to the mammillary bodies must be cautiously searched for on high-resolution MR and its discovery will eventually lead to preference of GKS being treating both parts of the lesion, especially in cases where the cisternal component is small.

Type VI (giant) does not represent a good indication for first-line radiosurgery, as in nearly all the cases a combination of several therapeutic modalities should be considered. Even if GKS does not seem to be suitable when the lesion is large, "radiosurgical" disconnection has been envisaged (radiosurgery targeting only the superior part in the hypothalamus and/or the third ventricle leaving untreated all the lesion lower than the floor), but has been systematically disappointing. In our opinion, this strategy may cause loss of precious time for the child to be treated effectively. Consequently, we do not advocate for such a strategy. When microsurgical resection has left a small remnant in the third ventricle and a still active epilepsy, reoperation by GKS can be envisaged.

Two major questions remain. First, we know that complete treatment or resection of the lesion is not always mandatory (53–55), but we do not know how to predict in an individual patient the amount (and mapping) of the HH that must be treated in order to obtain a complete antiepileptic effect. Second, we know that these patients frequently present with an electroclinical semiology, suggesting involvement of the temporal or frontal lobe and which can mimic a secondary epileptogenesis phenomenon (40,52). In our experience, some of these patients can be completely cured by the isolated treatment of the HH, whereas in others, a partial result is obtained, with residual seizures despite a significant overall psychiatric and cognitive improvement. In this second group, it is tempting to propose that such a secondary epileptogenic area accounts for the partial failure.

Our initial results indicate that GKS is as effective as microsurgical resection and much safer (56). GKS also avoids the vascular risk related to radiofrequency lesioning or stimulation. With a transcallosal interforniceal approach both cognitive (long-term memory impairment) and severe endocrinological complications (23% long-term appetite stimulation and major weight gain) have been reported (57,58). Stabell et al. (59) have reported that with endoscopy a serious deterioration of memory and reading skills associated to a permanent oculomotor paresis takes place. In interstitial implants (iodine 125 seeds), Schulze-Bonhage (60) reported on a series of 24 patients, 5 patients developing a symptomatic edema, 4 patients with a weight gain of more than 5 kg, which was severe in 2, and a persistent decline of episodic memory in 2 patients. None of these complications have been observed after GKS. The disadvantage of radiosurgery is its delayed action. Longer follow-up is mandatory for proper evaluation of the role of GKS. Results are faster and more complete in patients with smaller lesions inside the third ventricle (Stage II). The early effect on subclinical EEG discharges appears to play a major role in the dramatic benefit to sleep quality, behavior, and cognitive-developmental improvement. GK surgery can safely lead to the reversal of the epileptic encephalopathy (41,43,44,61).

Due to the very poor clinical prognosis of the majority of these patients with HH and the invasiveness of microsurgical resection, GK can be now be considered the first-line intervention for small- and middle-size HH associated with epilepsy, as it can lead to dramatic improvements to the future of these young patients. The role of secondary epileptogenesis or of widespread cortical dysgenesis in these patients needs to be better evaluated and understood, in order to optimize patient selection and define the best treatment period.

Mesial Temporal Lobe Epilepsy

The first GK surgery operations for MTLE were performed in Marseille in March 1993. As no literature on similar experience was available then, we were obliged to base our technical choices on hypothesis and experience of radiosurgery for other pathological conditions. Four patients were treated with different technical strategies (dose, volume, target definition). The delayed huge radiological changes observed some months after radiosurgery (62) led us to stop such treatment and follow these first four patients. Due to the clinical safety of the procedure in these patients and the gradual disappearance of the acute MR changes after some months, we treated several new series of patients under strict prospective controlled trial conditions (with ethical committee approval). The treatment for the following 16 patients was based upon that of the first patient who had a successful outcome (as opposed to the three others who had partial or no effect). This "classic planning" was based on the use of two 18-mm shots, covering a volume of around 7 mL at the 50% isodose (24 Gy), and has turned out to produce a high rate of seizure cessation (63,64). For epileptological reasons, as well as for safety reasons, the targeting was very much centered on the parahippocampal cortex and spared a significant part of the amygdaloid complex and hippocampus. The refinement of the GK surgery technique, and the desire to find a dose that would create less transient acute MR changes, led us to reduce the dose from 24 to 20 Gy and 18 Gy at the margin. However, this brought about a significant decrease in the rate of seizure cessation. We have reviewed the long-term follow-up of our first 15 patients operated by GKS for MTLE at the state of the art (24 Gy). The mean follow-up was 8 years and at the last follow-up 73% were seizure free. These long-term results are comparing favorably to a microsurgical approach. No permanent neurological deficit was reported out of a visual field deficit in nine patients (11). After microsurgery for MTLE on the dominant side a verbal memory deficit is classically observed in 30% to 50% of the patients (65,66). It is very important to note that none of our patients have observed a neuropsychological worsening (using the evaluation published by Clusmann et al.) and especially no verbal memory decline (4,5,7,11). This finding of our four prospective trials has been confirmed by the U.S. prospective trial (67).

The timetable of events after radiosurgery and follow-up are quite standardized. Patients are informed that delayed efficacy of radiosurgery is its main drawback. Typically, the frequency of the seizures is not modified significantly for the first few months. Thereafter, there is a rapid and dramatic increase in auras for some days or weeks and then the seizures disappear. Usually the peak in seizure cessation is observed around the 8th to 18th month with a clear variability in the delay in onset. In one patient, this occurred 26 months after GK radiosurgery. We usually consider a delay of 2 years as a minimum for postradiosurgery follow-up. In the absence of initial radiological changes or clinical benefit, the recommendation is to wait for the onset of the MRI changes and their subsequent disappearance. All our patients had the same pattern of MR changes whichever marginal dose (18–24 Gy) and volume of treatment (5–8.5 cc) were used. However, the degree of these changes and their delay of onset varied according to the dose delivered to the margin, the volume treated, and the individual patient. In order to allow an optimal evaluation, we recommend that subsequent microsurgery not be considered before the third year after radiosurgery. Similarly, we believe that a patient who undergoes a cortectomy before the onset of the MR changes has occurred cannot be assumed to have failed radiosurgical treatment. Of course, before consideration of any further surgery, the question of the reason for the failure needs to be addressed. After reviewing files of patients treated for MTLE with radiosurgery, it was sometimes possible to identify likely causes of failure, such as:

1. Poor patient selection (e.g., patients with epilepsy involving more than the MTL structures)
2. Patients with the diagnosis of "treatment failure" (less than 3 years) who had been operated upon too early after radiosurgery (68)
3. Targeting of the amygdala and hippocampus (which is not in our opinion the optimal target in term of safety and efficacy) instead of parahippocampal cortex (69)
4. Insufficient dosage (68–70)

Our current strategy of treatment is based on our first series of MTLE patients who were strictly selected and treated systematically with a very simple but reproducible dose-planning strategy (4,6). The identification of putative improvements in the methodology requires a systematic analysis of the influence of the technical data from our experience and from the literature on the outcome of those patients.

The "Technical" Questions

The Dose Issue

The first targets used in functional GK radiosurgery (capsulotomy, thalamotomy of VIM or the centromedianum, pallidotomy) were treated using a high dose—(300–150 Gy) delivered in very small volumes (3–5 mm in diameter; 20). The goal was to destroy a predefined very small anatomical structure with stereotactic precision. Quite a significant variability in the delay and amplitude of the MR changes has been reported with fixed regimen of doses (31,71). Barcia-Salorio et al. (13) have presented several times a small and heterogeneous group of patients treated with different kinds of devices and dosage regimens. Apparently, some of those patients had no expanding lesion and were treated with very large volumes and very low dosage (around 10 Gy). Based on this experience, several teams have made the assumption that very low doses, as low as 10 to 20 Gy at the margin, should be as effective as the 24-Gy protocol (at the margin) that we used for our first series of patients with MTLE (4). A cautious examination of the last proceeding of Barcia-Salorio et al. (33) shows that the individual information concerning the dose at the margin, the volume, and the topography of the epileptogenic zone are not provided. Moreover, among the 11 patients reported, the real rate of seizure cessation is apparently only 36% (4/11), which is much lower than what we would expect with resection in MTLE. In a heterogeneous group of 176 patients, Yang et al. (70) confirmed that only a very low rate of seizure control is achieved when low doses (from 9 to 13 Gy at the margin) are used.

The experience of the radiosurgical treatment of HH indicates that 18 Gy at the margin appears to be a threshold in terms of probability of seizure cessation (41). In this group of patients (36 cases), only one showed MR changes. The majority of the AVM cases with worsening of the epilepsy were treated with a range of doses between 15 and 18 Gy. Similarly, poor results have been reported by Cmelak et al. (68) in one case of MTLE treated with LINAC-based radiosurgery, with 15 Gy at the 60% isodose line, who underwent surgical resection 1 year later. In this case, the authors first observed a slight improvement followed by an obvious worsening. A recent de-escalation study has allowed us to demonstrate poorer results in patients receiving doses of 18 or 20 Gy at the margin as compared to 24 Gy (62,72). Due to the rate of seizure cessation that is achievable by conventional resection, a radiosurgical strategy associated with a much lower rate of seizure cessation appears unacceptable. Fractionated stereotactically guided radiotherapy has been demonstrated to fail systematically in controlling seizures. Among 12 patients treated by Grabenbauer et al. none have achieved seizure cessation (73,74); only seizure reduction was obtained in this series.

Experimental studies on small animals have demonstrated the antiepileptic effect of radiosurgery (12,29,31), the dose dependence of this effect (29–31,75), and the possibility of obtaining a clear antiepileptic effect without macroscopic necrosis using certain doses (30). Of course, the rat models of epilepsy are far from being good models of human MTLE. However, taking into account the huge difference in volume of the target, it is intriguing to notice that according to our clinical experience in humans, a similar maximum dose range of 40 to 50 Gy is currently the range of dose providing the optimal safety–efficacy ratio.

The Target Definition

When the target is a lesion that is precisely defined radiologically, the question of the selection of the marginal dose can be quite easily addressed by correlating safety–efficacy and individual outcome to the marginal dose. This can be refined based upon stratification according to volume, location, age, and so on. However, in patients presenting with MTLE, this process is invalid for two reasons. First, there is no consensus regarding the requirement for extent of mesial temporal lobe resection. Second, the concept of MTLE syndrome with a stable extent of the epileptogenic zone and surgical target is increasingly the topic of debate (14,76).

The volume (in association with marginal dose) is well known to be a major determinant of the tissue effect, as shown in integrated risk/dose volume formulae (77). In the first series of patients that we treated, this marginal isodose volume (or prescription isodose volume) was approximately 7 mL (range 5–8.5).

An attempt to correlate dose/volume and the effect on seizures and on the MR changes (as evaluated by the volume of the contrast enhancement ring, extent of the high T2 signal, and the importance of the mass effect) has been published recently (72). In this study, we found, not surprisingly, that the higher the dose and the volume, the higher the risk of having more severe MR changes, but the chances of achieving seizure cessation also improved. However, these data have limited value. Hence, more precise identification of those structures of the mesial temporal lobe which need to be "covered" by the radiosurgical treatment may allow more selective, but just as efficacious, dose planning strategies, in spite of smaller prescription isodose volumes.

There is growing evidence to support the organization of the epileptogenic zone in networks, meaning that several different and possibly distant structures are discharging simultaneously at the onset of the electro-clinical seizure. This kind of organization explains why the risk of failure is so high when a simple topectomy (without preoperative investigations) is performed in severe drug-resistant epilepsies associated with a benign lesion (78). This has been also reported in MTLE (14,76). Certain nuclei of the amygdaloid complex; of the head, body, tail of the hippocampus; of the perirhinal, entorhinal (EC), and parahippocampal cortices may be associated with genesis of the seizures. The role of the EC cortex in epilepsy is supported by experimental studies on animals (79,80). The EC is considered to be the amplifier of the "amygdalohippocampal epileptic system." The pattern of the associated structures, including that of the structure playing the leader role, can vary significantly from one patient to another (14,76). There is a subgroup of patients who have clonic discharges and the involvement of the EC, amygdala, and head of the hippocampus, with a clear leader role of the EC. Wieser et al. (81) have analyzed the postoperative MR images of patients operated on by Yasargil (amygdalohippocampectomy) and were able to correlate the quality of the resection of each substructure of the mesial temporal lobe area and the outcome with respect to seizures. Only the quality of the removal of the anterior parahippocampal cortex was correlated strongly with a higher chance of seizure cessation (81). We tried to perform a similar study in patients treated with GK radiosurgery (72). We defined and manually drew the limits of subregions on the stereotactic images of all these patients. The amygdala, the head, the body, and the tail of the hippocampus were first delineated. The white matter, the parahippocampal cortex, and the cortex of the anterior wall of the collateral fissure were then separately drawn and divided into four sectors in the rostro-caudal axis, corresponding to the amygdala, the head, the body, and the tail of the hippocampus (72).

Patient Selection

Whang (without having first performed specific preoperative epileptological work-up; 82) treated patients with epilepsy associated with slowly growing lesions and observed seizure cessation in only 38% (12/31) of the patients. This kind of observation emphasizes the importance of preoperative definition of the extent of the epileptic zone and of its relationship with the lesion (78,83). In our institution, the philosophy is to adapt the investigations for each individual case. In some patients, the electroclinical data, the structural and functional imaging, and the neuropsychological examination are sufficiently concordant for surgery of the temporal lobe to be proposed without depth-electrode recording. In other cases, the level of evidence for MTLE is judged insufficient, and a stereoelectroencephalographic (SEEG) study is performed. The strategy of SEEG implantation is based on the primary hypothesis (mesial epileptogenic zone) and alternative hypotheses (early involvement of the temporal pole, lateral cortex, basal cortex, insular cortex, or other cortical areas). The goal of these studies is to record the patient's habitual seizures, in order to establish the temporospatial pattern of involvement of the cortical structures during these seizures. Clearly in these patients, the high resolution of depth-electrode recording allows fine tailoring of surgical resection, according to the precise temporospatial course of the seizures. The main limitation of radiosurgery is that of size of the target (prescription isodose volume). The radiosurgical treatment of MTLE is certainly the most selective surgical therapy for this group of patients. The requirement for precision and accuracy in the definition of the epileptogenic zone is consequently higher. Furthermore, if depth-electrode investigation enables demonstration of a particular subtype of MTLE, this can lead to tailoring of the treatment volume and frequently allows this to be reduced.

The Potential Concerns

The risk of long-term complications must always be cautiously scrutinized in functional neurosurgery. Radiotherapy is most frequently used in the brain for short-term life-threatening pathologies. The use of radiotherapy in young patients with benign diseases, such as pituitary adenomas or craniopharyngiomas, has been associated with a significant rate of cognitive decline (64,71) and tumor genesis (84), including some carcinogenesis (85). If the risk of radiation-induced tumor was similar with radiosurgery we should have by now already observed numerous cases. However, such reported cases (86–88) are extremely rare and frequently fail to meet the classical criteria by which tumors are deemed to be "radiation induced" (89). In fact it is considered that, if this risk exists, it is likely to be around 1/10,000, which is far lower than the mortality risk associated with temporal lobectomy (63,90–93).

Epilepsy is a life-threatening condition. The risk of sudden unexplained death in epileptic patients (SUDEP) is higher than in the general population (94,95). This risk is higher in patients treated with more than two antiepileptic drugs and IQ lower than 70 (as independent factors). Because seizure cessation after surgery reduces the mortality risk to that of the general population (95), microsurgical resection of the epileptogenic zone may confer a benefit in terms of the possibility of immediate seizure cessation and therefore reduced mortality risk, as compared to the more delayed benefits of radiosurgical treatment. Our patients are systematically informed about this disadvantage of radiosurgery.

What Are the Current Indications?

The demonstrated advantages of radiosurgery are the comfort of the procedure, the absence of general anesthesia, the absence of surgical complications and mortality, the very short hospital stay, and the immediate return to the previous level of functioning and employment. In MTLE the potential sparing of memory function is still a matter of debate and needs to be established using comparative studies. There is also a requirement for further demonstration of long-term efficacy and safety of radiosurgery. Worldwide, microsurgical cortectomies for MTLE are proving to be very satisfactory due to the rarity of surgical complications and a high rate of seizure freedom. In our experience, the most important selection parameters are the demonstration of the purely mesial location of the epileptogenic zone, as well as clear understanding by the patient of the advantages, disadvantages, and limitations. Another very good indication in our experience is that of patients with proven MTLE but previous failure of microsurgery, supposedly due to insufficient posterior extent of the resection. Best candidates are young patients, with middle severity epilepsy (working, or able to work), with a high level of functioning (able to understand well the limits and constraints of radiosurgery), a quite high risk of memory deficit with microsurgery (MTLE on the dominant side with little or no atrophy, some deficit of the verbal memory preoperatively), and potentially huge social and professional consequences in case of postoperative memory deficit (2,17,96).

CONCLUSIONS

The field of epilepsy surgery is a new and promising one for radiosurgery. However, determination of the extent of the epileptogenic zone requires specific expertise, which is crucial in order to achieve a reasonable rate of seizure cessation. In addition, the huge impact of fine technical detail on the efficacy and eventual toxicity of the procedure means that, at present, its use for these indications remains under evaluation, and further prospective work is absolutely required. It is difficult to know whether we really are at the dawn of a broader indication for the use of radiosurgery. In forthcoming years, our ability to identify the correct technical strategies should determine whether this is so!

REFERENCES

1. Régis J, Bartolomei F, Hayashi M, Chauvel P. Gamma Knife surgery, a neuromodulation therapy in epilepsy surgery! *Acta Neurochir Suppl.* 2002;84:37–47.
2. Régis J, Carron R, Park M. Is radiosurgery a neuromodulation therapy?: A 2009 Fabrikant award lecture. *J Neurooncol.* 2010;98:155–162.
3. Régis J, Kerkerian-Legoff L, Rey M, et al. First biochemical evidence of differential functional effects following Gamma Knife surgery. *Stereotact Funct Neurosurg.* 1996;66(suppl 1):29–38.
4. Régis J, Bartolomei F, Rey M, et al. Gamma knife surgery for mesial temporal lobe epilepsy. *Epilepsia.* 1999;40(11):1551–1556.
5. Régis J, Levivier M, Hayashi M. Radiosurgery for intractable epilepsy. *Tech Neurosurg.* 2003;9:191–203.
6. Régis J, Peragut JC, Rey M, Samson Y, Levrier O, Porcheron D, Regis H, Sedan R. First selective amygdalohippocampic radiosurgery for mesial temporal lobe epilepsy. *Stereotact Funct Neurosurg.* 64:191–201, 1994.
7. Régis J, Rey M, Bartolomei F, et al. Gamma knife surgery in mesial temporal lobe epilepsy: a prospective multicenter study. *Epilepsia.* 2004;45(5):504–515.
8. Régis J, Semah F, Bryan RN, et al. Early and delayed MR and PET changes after selective temporomesial radiosurgery in mesial temporal lobe epilepsy. *AJNR Am J Neuroradiol.* 1999;20(2):213–216.
9. Tsuchitani S, Drummond J, Kamiryo T, et al. Selective vulnerability of interneurons to low dosage radiosurgery. Presented at Society for Neuroscience Annual Meeting [abstract], New Orleans, LA. Nov 2003.

10. Quigg M, Rolston J, Barbaro NM. Radiosurgery for epilepsy: clinical experience and potential antiepileptic mechanisms. *Epilepsia.* 2012;53(1):7–15.
11. Bartolomei F, Hayashi M, Tamura M, et al. Long-term efficacy of gamma knife radiosurgery in mesial temporal lobe epilepsy. *Neurology.* 2008;70(19):1658–1663.
12. Barcia-Salorio JL, Vanaclocha V, Cerda M, Roldan P. Focus irradiation in epilepsy. Experimental study in the cat. *Appl Neurophysiol.* 1985;48:152.
13. Barcia-Salorio JL, Barcia JA, Hernández G, López-Gómez L. Radiosurgery of epilepsy. Long-term results. *Acta Neurochir Suppl.* 1994;62:111–113.
14. Bartolomei F, Wendling F, Bellanger JJ, Régis J, Chauvel P. Neural networks involving the medial temporal structures in temporal lobe epilepsy. *Clin Neurophysiol.* 2001;112(9):1746–1760.
15. Baudouin M, Stuhl L, Perrard A. Un cas d'épilepsie focale traité par la radiothérapie. *Rev Neurol.* 1951;84:60–63.
16. Barbaro NM, Quigg M, Broshek DK, et al. A multicenter, prospective pilot study of gamma knife radiosurgery for mesial temporal lobe epilepsy: seizure response, adverse events, and verbal memory. *Ann Neurol.* 2009;65(2):167–175.
17. Régis J, Bartolomei J, Chauvel P. Epilepsy. *Prog Neurol Surg.* 2007;20:267–278.
18. Leksell L. The stereotaxic method and radiosurgery of the brain. *Acta Chir Scand.* 1951;102(4):316–319.
19. Leksell L. Sterotaxic radiosurgery in trigeminal neuralgia. *Acta Chir Scand.* 1971;137(4):311–314.
20. Lindquist C, Kihlström L, Hellstrand E. Functional neurosurgery–a future for the gamma knife? *Stereotact Funct Neurosurg.* 1991;57(1–2):72–81.
21. Talairach J, Bancaud J, Szikla G, Bonis A, Geler S, Vedrenne C. Approche nouvelle de la neurochirurgie de l'epilepsie. Méthodologie stéréotaxique et résultats thérapeutiques. *Neurochirurgie.* 1974;20:92–98.
22. Elomaa E. Focal irradiation of the brain: an alternative to temporal lobe resection in intractable focal epilepsy? *Med Hypotheses.* 1980;6:501–503.
23. Von Wieser W. Die Roentgentherapie der traumatischen Epilepsie. *Mschr Psychiat Neurol.* 1939;101:422–424.
24. Heikkinen ER, Konnov B, Melnikov L, et al. Relief of epilepsy by radiosurgery of cerebral arteriovenous malformations. *Stereotact Funct Neurosurg.* 1989;53(3):157–166.
25. Rogers L, Morris H, Lupica K. Effect of cranial irradiation on seizure frequency in adults with low-grade astrocytoma and medically intractable epilepsy. *Neurology.* 1993;43:1599–1601.
26. Rossi G, Scerrati M, Roselli R. Epileptogenic cerebral low grade tumors: effect of interstital stereotactic irradiation on seizures. *Appl Neurophysiol.* 1985;48:127–132.
27. Barcia-Salorio JL, Roldan P, Hernandez G, Lopez Gomez L. Radiosurgical treatment of epilepsy. *Appl Neurophysiol.* 1985;48(1–6):400–403.
28. Gaffey C, Monotoya V, Lyman J, Howard J. Restriction of the spread of epileptic discharges in cats by mean of Bragg Peak intracranial irradiation. *Int J Appl Radiat Isotope.* 1981;32:779–787.
29. Chen ZF, Kamiryo T, Henson SL, et al. Anticonvulsant effects of gamma surgery in a model of chronic spontaneous limbic epilepsy in rats. *J Neurosurg.* 2001;94(2):270–280.
30. Maesawa S, Kondziolka D, Dixon CE, Balzer J, Fellows W, Lunsford LD. Subnecrotic stereotactic radiosurgery controlling epilepsy produced by kainic acid injection in rats. *J Neurosurg.* 2000;93(6):1033–1040.
31. Mori Y, Kondziolka D, Balzer J, et al. Effects of stereotactic radiosurgery on an animal model of hippocampal epilepsy. *Neurosurgery.* 2000;46(1):157–165; discussion 165.

32. Ronne-Engström E, Kihlström L, Flink R, et al. Gamma Knife surgery in epilepsy: an experimental model in the rat. Presented at European Society for Stereotactic and Functional Neurosurgery, 1993.
33. Barcia-Salorio JL, Garcia JA, Hernandez G, Lopez Gomez L. Radiosurgery of epilepsy: Long-term results. Presented at European Society for Stereotactic and Functional Neurosurgery, 1993.
34. Lindquist C. Gamma knife surgery in focal epilepsy. 1 year follow-up in 4 cases. Unpublished, 1992.
35. Lindquist C, Hellstrand E, Kilström L, Abraham-Fuchs K, Jernberg B, Wirth A. Stereotactic localisation of epileptic foci by magnetoencephalography and MRI followed by gamma surgery. Presented at International Stereotactic Radiosurgery Symposium, 1991.
36. Lindquist C, Kihlström L, Hellstrand E, Knutsson E. Stereotactic radiosurgery instead of conventional epilepsy surgery. Presented at European Society for Stereotactic and Functional Neurosurgery, 1993.
37. Régis J, Bartolomei F, Hayashi M, Roberts D, Chauvel P, Peragut JC. The role of gamma knife surgery in the treatment of severe epilepsies. *Epileptic Disord.* 2000;2(2):113–122.
38. Deonna T, Ziegler AL. Hypothalamic hamartoma, precocious puberty and gelastic seizures: a special model of "epileptic" developmental disorder. *Epileptic Disord.* 2000;2:33–37.
39. Kuzniecky R, Guthrie B, Mountz J, et al. Intrinsic epileptogenesis of hypothalamic hamartomas in gelastic epilepsy. *Ann Neurol.* 1997;42(1):60–67.
40. Munari C, Kahane P, Francione S, et al. Role of the hypothalamic hamartoma in the genesis of gelastic fits (a video-stereo-EEG study). *Electroencephalogr Clin Neurophysiol.* 1995;95(3):154–160.
41. Régis J, Bartolomei F, de Toffol B, et al. Gamma knife surgery for epilepsy related to hypothalamic hamartomas. *Neurosurgery.* 2000;47(6):1343–1351; discussion 1351.
42. Régis J, Hayashi M, Eupierre LP, et al. Gamma knife surgery for epilepsy related to hypothalamic hamartomas. *Acta Neurochir Suppl.* 2004;91:33–50.
43. Régis J, Scavarda D, Tamura M, et al. Epilepsy related to hypothalamic hamartomas: surgical management with special reference to gamma knife surgery. *Childs Nerv Syst.* 2006;22(8):881–895.
44. Régis J, Scavarda D, Tamura M, et al. Gamma knife surgery for epilepsy related to hypothalamic hamartomas. *Semin Pediatr Neurol.* 2007;14(2):73–79.
45. Frattali CM, Liow K, Craig GH, et al. Cognitive deficits in children with gelastic seizures and hypothalamic hamartoma. *Neurology.* 2001;57(1):43–46.
46. Weissenberger AA, Dell ML, Liow K, et al. Aggression and psychiatric comorbidity in children with hypothalamic hamartomas and their unaffected siblings. *J Am Acad Child Adolesc Psychiatry.* 2001;40(6):696–703.
47. Arita K, Ikawa F, Kurisu K, et al. The relationship between magnetic resonance imaging findings and clinical manifestations of hypothalamic hamartoma. *J Neurosurg.* 1999;91:212–220.
48. Debeneix C, Bourgeois M, Trivin C, Sainte-Rose C, Brauner R. Hypothalamic hamartoma: comparison of clinical presentation and magnetic resonance images. *Horm Res.* 2001;56(1–2):12–18.
49. Valdueza JM, Cristante L, Dammann O, et al. Hypothalamic hamartomas: with special reference to gelastic epilepsy and surgery. *Neurosurgery.* 1994;34(6):949–958; discussion 958.
50. Delalande O, Fohlen M. Disconnecting surgical treatment of hypothalamic hamartoma in children and adults with refractory epilepsy and proposal of a new classification. *Neurol Med Chir (Tokyo).* 2003;43(2):61–68.

51. Palmini A, Chandler C, Andermann F, et al. Resection of the lesion in patients with hypothalamic hamartomas and catastrophic epilepsy. *Neurology*. 2002;58(9):1338–1347.
52. Cascino GD, Andermann F, Berkovic SF, et al. Gelastic seizures and hypothalamic hamartomas: evaluation of patients undergoing chronic intracranial EEG monitoring and outcome of surgical treatment. *Neurology*. 1993;43:747–750.
53. Pascual-Castroviejo I, Moneo JH, Viano J, et al. Hypothalamic hamartomas: control of seizures after partial removal in one case. *Rev Neurol*. 2000;31:119–122.
54. Rosenfeld JV, Harvey AS, Wrennall J, Zacharin M, Berkovic SF. Transcallosal resection of hypothalamic hamartomas, with control of seizures, in children with gelastic epilepsy. *Neurosurgery*. 2001;48(1):108–118.
55. Watanabe T, Enomoto T, Uemura K, Tomono Y, Nose T. Gelastic seizures treated by partial resection of a hypothalamic hamartoma. *No Shinkei Geka*. 1998;26(10):923–928.
56. Wait SD, Abla AA, Killory BD, Nakaji P, Rekate HL. Surgical approaches to hypothalamic hamartomas. *Neurosurg Focus*. 2011;30(2):E2.
57. Anderson JF, Rosenfeld JV. Long-term cognitive outcome after transcallosal resection of hypothalamic hamartoma in older adolescents and adults with gelastic seizures. *Epilepsy Behav*. 2010;18(1–2):81–87.
58. Freeman JL, Zacharin M, Rosenfeld JV, Harvey AS. The endocrinology of hypothalamic hamartoma surgery for intractable epilepsy. *Epileptic Disord*. 2003;5(4):239–247.
59. Stabell KE, Bakke SJ, Egge A. Cognitive and neurological sequelae after stereoendoscopic disconnection of a hypothalamic hamartoma. A case study. *Epilepsy Behav*. 2012;24(2):274–278.
60. Schulze-Bonhage A, Trippel M, Wagner K, et al. Outcome and predictors of interstitial radiosurgery in the treatment of gelastic epilepsy. *Neurology*. 2008;71(4):277–282.
61. Mathieu D, Deacon C, Pinard CA, Kenny B, Duval J. Gamma Knife surgery for hypothalamic hamartomas causing refractory epilepsy: preliminary results from a prospective observational study. *J Neurosurg*. 2010;(113 suppl):215–221.
62. Hayashi M, Régis J, Hori T. Current treatment strategy with gamma knife surgery for mesial temporal lobe epilepsy. *No Shinkei Geka*. 2003;31(2):141–155.
63. Ganz JC. Gamma knife radiosurgery and its possible relationship to malignancy: a review. *J Neurosurg*. 2002;97(5 suppl):644–652.
64. Glosser G, McManus P, Munzenrider J, et al. Neuropsychological function in adults after high dose fractionated radiation therapy of skull base tumors. *Int J Radiat Oncol Biol Phys*. 1997;38(2):231–239.
65. Clusmann H, Schramm J, Kral T, et al. Prognostic factors and outcome after different types of resection for temporal lobe epilepsy. *J Neurosurg*. 2002;97(5):1131–1141.
66. Stroup E, Langfitt J, Berg M, McDermott M, Pilcher W, Como P. Predicting verbal memory decline following anterior temporal lobectomy (ATL). *Neurology*. 2003;60(8):1266–1273.
67. Quigg M, Broshek DK, Barbaro NM, et al.; Radiosurgery Epilepsy Study Group. Neuropsychological outcomes after Gamma Knife radiosurgery for mesial temporal lobe epilepsy: a prospective multicenter study. *Epilepsia*. 2011;52(5):909–916.
68. Cmelak AJ, Abou-Khalil B, Konrad PE, Duggan D, Maciunas RJ. Low-dose stereotactic radiosurgery is inadequate for medically intractable mesial temporal lobe epilepsy: a case report. *Seizure*. 2001;10(6):442–446.
69. Kawai K, Suzuki I, Kurita H, Shin M, Arai N, Kirino T. Failure of low-dose radiosurgery to control temporal lobe epilepsy. *J Neurosurg*. 2001;95(5):883–887.
70. Yang KJ, Wang KW, Wu HP, Qi ST. Radiosurgical treatment of intractable epilepsy with low radiation dose. *Di Yi Jun Yi Da Xue Xue Bao*. 2002;22(7):645–647.

71. McCord MW, Buatti JM, Fennell EM, et al. Radiotherapy for pituitary adenoma: long-term outcome and sequelae. *Int J Radiat Oncol Biol Phys.* 1997;39(2):437–444.
72. Hayashi M, Bartolomei F, Rey M, Farnarier P, Chauvel P, Regis J. MR changes after gamma knife radiosurgery for mesial temporal lobe epilepsy: an evidence for the efficacy of subnecrotic doses. In: Kondziolka D, ed. *Radiosurgery.* Basel, Karger; 2002:192–202.
73. Grabenbauer GG, Reinhold Ch, Kerling F, et al. Fractionated stereotactically guided radiotherapy of pharmacoresistant temporal lobe epilepsy. *Acta Neurochir Suppl.* 2002;84:65–70.
74. Stefan H, Hummel C, Grabenbauer GG, et al. Successful treatment of focal epilepsy by fractionated stereotactic radiotherapy. *Eur Neurol.* 1998;39(4):248–250.
75. Maesawa S, Kondziolka D, Balzer J, Fellows W, Dixon E, Lunsford LD. The behavioral and electroencephalographic effects of stereotactic radiosurgery for the treatment of epilepsy evaluated in the rat kainic acid model. *Stereotact Funct Neurosurg.* 1999;73(1–4):115.
76. Spencer SS, Spencer DD. Entorhinal-hippocampal interactions in medial temporal lobe epilepsy. *Epilepsia.* 1994;35(4):721–727.
77. Flickinger JC. An integrated logistic formula for prediction of complications from radiosurgery. *Int J Radiat Oncol Biol Phys.* 1989;17(4):879–885.
78. Régis j, Bartolomei F, Kida Y, et al. Radiosurgery of epilepsy associated with cavernous malformation: retrospective study in 49 patients. *Neurosurgery.* 2000;47:1091–1097.
79. Jones R, Heinemann U, Lambert J. The entorhinal cortex and generation of seizure activity: studies of normal synaptic transmission and epileptogenesis in vitro. In: Avanzini G, Engel J, Fariello R, Heinemann U, eds. *Neurotransmitters in Epilepsy.* New York, NY: Elsevier Science; 1992:173–180.
80. Wilson WA, Swartzwelder HS, Anderson WW, Lewis DV. Seizure activity *in vitro*: a dual focus model. *Epilepsy Res.* 1988;2(5):289–293.
81. Wieser HG, Siegel AM, Yasargil GM. The Zurich amygdalo-hippocampectomy series: a short up-date. *Acta Neurochir Suppl (Wien).* 1990;50:122–127.
82. Whang CJ, Kwon Y. Long-term follow-up of stereotactic Gamma Knife radiosurgery in epilepsy. *Stereotact Funct Neurosurg.* 1996;66(suppl 1):349–356.
83. Kitchen N. Experimental and clinical studies on the putative therapeutic efficacy of cerebral irradiation (radiotherapy) in epilepsy. *Epilepsy Res.* 1995;20(1):1–10.
84. Strasnick B, Glasscock ME 3rd, Haynes D, McMenomey SO, Minor LB. The natural history of untreated acoustic neuromas. *Laryngoscope.* 1994;104(9):1115–1119.
85. Simmons NE, Laws ER Jr. Glioma occurrence after sellar irradiation: case report and review. *Neurosurgery.* 1998;42(1):172–178.
86. Kaido T, Hoshida T, Uranishi R, et al. Radiosurgery-induced brain tumor. Case report. *J Neurosurg.* 2001;95(4):710–713.
87. Shamisa A, Bance M, Nag S, et al. Glioblastoma multiforme occurring in a patient treated with gamma knife surgery. Case report and review of the literature. *J Neurosurg.* 2001;94(5):816–821.
88. Yu JS, Yong WH, Wilson D, Black KL. Glioblastoma induction after radiosurgery for meningioma. *Lancet.* 2000;356(9241):1576–1577.
89. Cahan W, Woodard H, Highinbotham N, Stewart F, Coley B. Sarcoma arising in irradiated bone: report of eleven cases. *Cancer.* 1948;1:3–29.
90. Loeffler JS, Niemierko A, Chapman PH. Second tumors after radiosurgery: tip of the iceberg or a bump in the road? *Neurosurgery.* 2003;52(6):1436–1440; discussion 1440.
91. Lunsford LD, Niranjan A, Flickinger JC, Maitz A, Kondziolka D. Radiosurgery of vestibular schwannomas: summary of experience in 829 cases. *J Neurosurg.* 2005;(102 suppl):195–199.

92. Muracciole X, Cowen D, Régis J. Radiosurgery and brain radio-induced carcinogenesis: update. *Neurochirurgie.* 2004;50(2–3 Pt 2):414–420.
93. Rowe J, Grainger A, Walton L, Silcocks P, Radatz M, Kemeny A. Risk of malignancy after gamma knife stereotactic radiosurgery. *Neurosurgery.* 2007;60:60–65; discussion 65–66.
94. Ficker DM, So EL, Shen WK, et al. Population-based study of the incidence of sudden unexplained death in epilepsy. *Neurology.* 1998;51(5):1270–1274.
95. Sperling MR, Feldman H, Kinman J, Liporace JD, O'Connor MJ. Seizure control and mortality in epilepsy. *Ann Neurol.* 1999;46(1):45–50.
96. Régis J, Arkha Y, Yomo S, Bartolomei F, Peragut JC, Chauvel P. Radiosurgery for drug-resistant epilepsies: state of the art, results and perspectives. *Neurochirurgie.* 2008;54(3):320–331.

Section VI

Radiosurgery for Spine Lesions

Section Editor

Wesley Hsu

Chapter 12

Tumors of the Osseous Spine

A: Stereotactic Radiosurgery for Primary Osseous Spinal Tumors

Joseph A. Lin, Mohamad Bydon, Mohamed Macki, & Ali Bydon

Stereotactic radiosurgery is a technique for delivering ablative radiation to a lesion while minimizing damage to healthy tissue. Ionizing photons of x-ray or gamma-ray wavelength are focused on the lesion from multiple directions in three dimensions using CT, MRI, or angiography guidance, thereby maximizing the therapeutic dose delivered to the lesion. The Gamma Knife (Elekta), developed by Leksell, uses an array of 201 radioactive cobalt-60 sources to deliver gamma-ray photons in a head frame primarily oriented toward cranial lesions, limiting its use in the spine to lesions at the base of the skull (1). Linear-accelerator based devices, such as the CyberKnife (Accuray), Novalis (BrainLAB), and Synergy (Elekta) are more commonly used in the spine. These devices use a single linear accelerator to deliver x-ray photons; the linear accelerator robotically articulates around the patient (CyberKnife) or the patient table is mobile (Novalis and Synergy), allowing greater anatomical range to target lesions of the spine (2,3,4).

Stereotactic radiosurgery is becoming part of the standard treatment for both benign and malignant primary osseous spinal tumors, with demonstrated effectiveness in tumor control coupled with low morbidity. It is frequently used as an adjuvant therapy but is also emerging as a primary treatment option. Gwak et al. (5) found hypofractionated stereotactic radiation therapy to be effective as both adjuvant and sole primary therapy against chondromas and chordomas (traditionally radio-resistant tumors) at the base of the skull, with local control and minimal toxicity in nine patients through early follow-up periods. In patients with spinal metastases, stereotactic radiosurgery has provided timely and effective pain control (6). However, optimal dosing regimens, margins, and toxicity levels have not been well defined (5). Moreover, the toxicity to thoracic and abdominal organs as a result of stereotactic radiosurgery targeted to the spine requires consideration (6).

Well-circumscribed lesions with minimal or no spinal cord compression and stable biomechanics are acceptable pathologies for stereotactic radiosurgery. Tolerance to previous spinal radiotherapy, overt spinal instability, and cord compression are contraindications for stereotactic radiosurgery. As a frontline treatment, stereotactic radiosurgery may prevent future spinal instability and compression of the spinal cord and nerve roots, thus sparing the patient spinal surgery and instrumentation (7).

CHORDOMAS

Chordomas are rare cancers arising from remnants of the embryonic notochord. They are the most common primary malignant tumor of the spine, accounting for 1% to 4% of all bone malignancies, and typically affect older males but can be found in children. En bloc resection is the treatment of choice (8,9). Chordomas are considered resistant to conventional radiotherapy, with doses of at least 60 Gy required for efficacy (10). Despite the advent of modern image-guided radiotherapy, it is difficult to deliver such high doses without significant adverse effects, particularly because chordomas tend to develop near sensitive neural structures and grow in an irregular shape, complicating delivery (11).

Stereotactic radiotherapy can be used as an effective adjuvant for surgery in the management of chordomas, particularly if complete resection is not possible (11). En bloc resection followed by radiotherapy has been found to be better than either of them alone in providing long-term control of chordomas (12,13). For patients with relatively small residual tumors following surgical resection, treatment plans frequently call for adjuvant stereotactic radiotherapy or proton beam therapy. Proton beam therapy uses a particle accelerator such as a cyclotron to deliver ionizing protons (instead of photons as in radiotherapy). Protons rapidly lose energy within millimeters of reaching their maximal depth, so varying the energy of the proton beam allows precise delivery of radiation at a specific depth with minimal exit irradiation (14). However, given its high cost and the relatively small number of centers providing it, proton beam therapy is a more limited option.

En bloc resection remains the standard of care given the extensive body of evidence supporting it, with stereotactic radiosurgery serving mainly as an adjuvant for incomplete resection (8,9,15,16). However, recent studies have argued for a greater role in treatment plans for stereotactic radiosurgery. In a retrospective study of chordoma treatment methods by Eid et al. (17), the authors found that the local control rate, progression-free period, and overall survival of chordoma patients are comparable between en bloc resection and incomplete resection with adjuvant stereotactic radiosurgery (but not conventional radiotherapy). As noted above, Gwak et al. (5) successfully used hypofractionated stereotactic radiotherapy (21–43.6 Gy doses in three to five fractions) as both primary and adjuvant therapy against chordomas in nine patients. Pedroso et al. (18) reported using stereotactic radiosurgery as primary therapy for chordoma patients. They treated three patients using standard stereotactic radiosurgery (16–20 Gy in a single dose), one using hypofractionated stereotactic radiotherapy (42 Gy dose in three fractions), and four using fractionated stereotactic radiotherapy (45–75.6 Gy doses in 25–54 fractions). At follow-up ranging from 8 to 60 months (mean 23 months), all eight patients had local tumor control, and three of the patients who had received fractionated stereotactic radiotherapy had tumors decrease in volume or disappear on imaging. At longer follow-up, the control rate was 72% (19). Stereotactic radiosurgery is emerging as a useful complement to en bloc resection, the current standard of care for chordomas.

CHONDROMAS AND CHONDROSARCOMAS

Chondromas are rare and usually benign cartilage-forming tumors, comprising about 5% of primary bone tumors; less than 4% of chondromas are found in the spine, with males affected twice as often as females (20). Chondromas are radio-resistant, limiting the usefulness of radiation; primary treatment is complete surgical resection, as any residual tumor may lead to sarcomatous conversion (21,22). However, tumor recurrence is minimal if complete resection is accomplished (23). Nojima et al. (24) reported that after excision of periosteal chondromas not limited to the spine from 42 patients, none had recurrence after follow-up ranging from 10 months to 43 years.

Chondrosarcomas are extremely rare and highly malignant cartilaginous tumors that account for 7% to 12% of primary spine tumors and 25% of primary malignant spine neoplasms (20). They are distributed throughout the spine, with the majority appearing in the thoracic region (25). Tumor grading based on the WHO system (categorization by malignancy, growth rate, and risk of recurrence) is one of the most important factors in prognosis (25). Regardless of grade, en bloc resection with negative margins (as opposed to intralesional subtotal excision) gives the best chance of preventing long-term recurrence (21,26). These tumors are relatively resistant to both chemotherapy and radiotherapy (26). Although there is some evidence that stereotactic radiosurgery has an effect (5), its impact on chondrosarcoma outcomes remains unproven (20,25). A retrospective study by Boriani et al. (27) found that proton beam therapy may provide a benefit, but only as an adjuvant for en bloc resection. After it was first proposed by Suit et al. (28), combined proton beam therapy and radiotherapy for chondrosarcomas was successful in local control after surgical resection, as reported by Hug et al. (29). Four patients received the combined adjuvant radiation therapy after total resection (70.2–77.9 Gy equivalent doses of combined cobalt-60 and proton irradiation in 1.8–2.0 Gy equivalent fractions), whereas another two patients received the treatment after subtotal resection (75.1 and 75.6 Gy equivalent doses in 1.8–2.0 Gy equivalent fractions); all six were alive with locally controlled tumors after 10 years of follow-up.

OSTEOSARCOMAS

Osteosarcomas are rare, malignant bone-producing tumors that are often found in younger patients (median age of diagnosis, 15 years); however, spinal osteosarcomas, which make up 3% to 5% of osteosarcomas, tend to be found in patients over 40 years of age and have a poor prognosis (30,31). They account for 3% to 15% of primary spinal tumors and are usually found in the posterior elements of the sacral and thoracic spine (32). En bloc resection is the most common treatment option, although successfully achieving negative margins remains difficult (33). Chemotherapy is an important component of treatment for osteosarcomas of the extremities, but spinal osteosarcomas are less responsive to chemotherapy (30). Although the tumors are usually radio-resistant, adjuvant radiotherapy may be beneficial in improving survival and preventing recurrence, particularly if en bloc resection cannot be performed (34). The optimal treatment plan is unknown, but all three approaches—surgery, chemotherapy, and radiation—are supported by evidence, with surgical resection having the most impact (35).

Randomized clinical trials by Pisters et al. (36) and Yang et al. (37) showed that adjuvant radiation therapy after surgery (both complete and incomplete resection) is superior to surgery alone at preventing local recurrence of soft tissue sarcomas. In addition, the precision of modern techniques, such as proton beam and intensity-modulated radiotherapy, can avoid dose-limiting damage to normal tissue. Chemotherapy can increase radiation effectiveness by making these tumors more radiosensitive. Sundaresan et al. (38) found the combination of chemotherapy (T7 protocol, doxorubicin, cyclophosphamide, vincristine, cisplatin, and/or high-dose methotrexate) and radiation (30–45 Gy) as adjuvant therapy after surgical resection to be an improvement over narrower treatment plans for achieving local control of spinal osteosarcomas in 24 patients. Chang et al. (39) reported modest success in improving survival and local control using stereotactic radiosurgery as both adjuvant and sole primary therapy (34–93 Gy doses in one to three fractions) compared to conventional radiation therapy in 13 patients after median follow-up of 22 months (range 4–68 months). But for now, progress in improving outcomes for spinal osteosarcoma lags far behind the advances made in the treatment of osteosarcoma of the extremities (31). More research into the role of stereotactic radiosurgery in treatment of osteosarcomas is warranted.

EWING'S SARCOMA

Ewing's sarcoma accounts for about 10% of all primary bone tumors. It is typically seen in children and often metastasizes to the spine, although primary involvement of the spine is infrequent (40). Unlike other sarcomas, Ewing's sarcoma is fairly sensitive to radiotherapy. This makes radiation an important component in treatment regimens, playing a major role as an adjuvant to chemotherapy. Surgery can thus be avoided unless decompression is necessary (21,40). In addition, because complete resection with negative margins is challenging at times, radiation is often necessary for local tumor control. Schuck et al. (41) performed a retrospective analysis of 116 patients with primary Ewing's sarcoma of the spine and found no statistically significant difference in local recurrence rates among surgical resection, radiotherapy, and combined surgery and radiation. This data justifies the use of radiation therapy as a first-line treatment option in certain patients. Rock et al. (42) used stereotactic radiosurgery (50 Gy) and adjuvant chemotherapy (cisplatin, doxorubicin, methotrexate, and vincristine) to treat a 61-year-old woman whose Ewing's sarcoma recurred after surgical resection, chemotherapy, and conventional radiation. They reported a reduction in the size of the tumor maintained after 1 year of follow-up. Chang et al. (39) also effectively used stereotactic radiosurgery as both adjuvant and sole primary therapy in the treatment of Ewing's sarcoma in two patients (39). The radiosensitivity of Ewing's sarcoma and the precision of modern techniques make stereotactic radiosurgery an important tool in the treatment of this disease.

MULTIPLE MYELOMA (PLASMACYTOMAS)

Multiple myeloma is a plasma cell cancer that commonly spreads to bone, forming plasmacytomas. Median survival is approximately 3.5 years with standard chemotherapy, and about 4.5 years with high-dose chemotherapy followed by autologous stem cell transplantation. Standard chemotherapy is the treatment of choice for patients 65 years of age and older, whereas autologous stem cell transplantation is the treatment of choice for patients younger than 65 (43). Plasmacytomas are malignant plasma cells growing in soft or bony tissue and can involve the spine, infiltrating the vertebrae, inhibiting osteoblasts, and activating osteoclasts, thereby undermining bone integrity. Approximately 11% to 24% of multiple myeloma patients experience spinal cord compression (44,45).

Radiation therapy is the treatment of choice for plasmacytomas, with chemotherapy also an efficacious part of treatment plans, allowing effective treatment options for pain and spinal cord compression (46,47). Commonly, diffuse involvement of the spine limits surgical resection and reconstruction (21). Jin et al. (48) treated 31 lesions in 24 patients with multiple myeloma experiencing epidural spinal cord compression. Using stereotactic radiosurgery alone (10–18 Gy), the authors controlled pain in 86% of patients, improved symptoms in five of seven patients presenting with neurological deficits, and observed radiographic response in 81% of patients, with median follow-up of 11.2 months (range 1 to 55 months). Neither radiation nor chemotherapy are curative, but they provide important tools to increase survival time and maintain quality of life for patients.

ANEURYSMAL BONE CYSTS

Aneurysmal bone cysts are characterized as vascular, expanding lesions filled with cavities, and they are typically seen in patients younger than 20. They account for about 1% of bone tumors, and 10% to 30% of aneurysmal bone cysts are found in the spine (49). Although usually benign, they can grow aggressively, making aneurysmal bone cysts of the spine a distinct concern (50). Relatively little is known about their etiology, and the optimal treatment is undetermined (51). En bloc resection provides the least chance of recurrence, but is not always possible. Other treatment options have been shown to have limited efficacy, including arterial embolization, implantation of demineralized bone particles, and injection of a solution of alcohol and zein, a corn protein (51).

Radiotherapy may serve as an important primary therapy or adjuvant to surgery when complete resection cannot be achieved. Feigenberg et al. (52) reported using radiotherapy (20–60 Gy doses in fractions of 1.5–2.0 Gy) to treat nine patients with aneurysmal bone cysts; six of the patients were treated primarily with radiotherapy alone, whereas the other three had undergone subtotal resection. After median follow-up of 17 years (range 20 months to 20 years), none had experienced local recurrence, secondary malignancies, or significant side effects. These developments underscore the potential utility of stereotactic radiosurgery in treating aneurysmal bone cysts.

GIANT CELL TUMORS

Giant cell tumors are rare bone tumors believed to originate from macrophage lineages; they are thought to be usually benign despite being locally aggressive and prone to recurrence, accounting for 5% of primary bone tumors (53). About 1% to 9% of giant cell tumors are found in the spine, more often in the vertebral body than the posterior element (54). Surgery is the treatment of choice (53): Boriani et al. (54) reported that en bloc resection provided the best prevention of local recurrence in higher grade tumors, whereas intralesional resection was adequate for lower grade tumors.

Radiation therapy has been found to be a useful component of treatment plans. Caudell et al. (53) retrospectively reviewed 25 patients with giant cell tumors, 17 of whom had spinal tumors; 13 patients were treated primarily with radiotherapy, with the other 12 experiencing recurrences despite resection or previous radiotherapy. After median follow-up of 8.8 years (range 8 months to 34 years), radiotherapy delivered acceptable local control as primary therapy or as adjuvant to surgery. However, radiotherapy was not found to be efficacious in patients who had undergone previous radiotherapy. Malone et al. (55) retrospectively reviewed 21 patients with giant cell tumors treated with radiotherapy either primarily or after recurrence, finding a control rate of 100% after mean follow-up of 15.4 years (range 2–35 years). Kim et al. (56) effectively treated a patient with giant cell tumors in both petrous bones using stereotactic radiosurgery (15.0 Gy dose on the right, 8.0 Gy dose in two fractions on the left) after previous surgery and conventional radiation therapy had failed. After 28 months of follow-up, the authors found consistently decreased tumor volumes.

OSTEOID OSTEOMAS AND OSTEOBLASTOMAS

Osteoid osteomas and osteoblastomas are rare bone-forming tumors found in relatively young males and accounting for less than 1% of bone tumors (57,58). Twenty percent of osteoid osteomas and 40% of osteoblastomas are found in the spine, usually in the posterior elements (59,60). Osteoblastomas are larger (greater than 2 cm), more aggressive, and may become malignant, whereas osteoid osteomas are smaller and typically benign. Surgery is the primary treatment for osteoid osteoma and osteoblastoma as complete resection is often curative (21). Berberoglu et al. (61) used a combination of conventional radiotherapy (50 Gy) and chemotherapy (cisplatin and doxorubicin) to treat a pediatric patient with recurrent osteoblastoma after surgery. The authors observed local control and tumor reduction after 6 years of follow-up. Singer and Deutsch (62) also used conventional radiotherapy (50 Gy dose in 25 fractions) to treat a pediatric patient with osteoblastoma after failure of surgical excision. The patient was recurrence- and symptom-free after 10 years of follow-up. However, these rare examples limit radiotherapy to cases in which complete resection is impossible.

HEMANGIOMAS

Hemangiomas are benign vascular proliferations. Spinal vertebral body hemangiomas are incidentally found in about 11% of autopsies and are often asymptomatic. Symptomatic and aggressive hemangiomas, particularly those causing spinal cord compression, require intervention, which is commonly primary radiotherapy or surgical decompression with or without adjuvant radiotherapy. Effective alternatives include transarterial embolization, ethanol injection, and percutaneous vertebroplasty (63). Faria et al. (64) treated nine patients with symptomatic hemangiomas using conventional radiotherapy (30–40 Gy doses in fractions of 2 Gy) as primary treatment, with seven out of the nine asymptomatic after median follow-up of 28 months (range 6–62 months). Yang et al. (65) treated 23 patients with symptomatic hemangiomas using conventional radiotherapy (20–43 Gy doses in fractions of 1.2–2.5 Gy) as both primary treatment and adjuvant to surgical decompression, with symptom relief in nearly all patients after 5 to 20 years of follow-up. Less frequently, stereotactic radiosurgery has been used in the treatment of hemangiomas. Gerszten et al. (66) retrospectively studied 15 patients with benign spinal tumors who received stereotactic radiosurgery as primary treatment (16 Gy mean dose) and mean follow-up of 12 months; one patient had a spinal hemangioma, which improved with remarkable reduction of tumor size. Current evidence supporting stereotactic radiosurgery as treatment for spinal hemangiomas is limited and its role is likely to prove minor, especially given the extent of existing treatment options.

CONCLUSION

Primary osseous spinal tumors have various treatments depending on pathology and extent of disease. Spinal stereotactic radiosurgery is emerging as a safe and effective option for the treatment of a variety of spinal lesions, offering an alternative for both primary and adjuvant therapy.

REFERENCES

1. Leksell L. Stereotactic radiosurgery. *J Neurol Neurosurg Psychiatr*. 1983;46(9):797–803.
2. Lutz W, Winston KR, Maleki N. A system for stereotactic radiosurgery with a linear accelerator. *Int J Radiat Oncol Biol Phys*. 1988;14(2):373–381.
3. Adler JR Jr, Chang SD, Murphy MJ, Doty J, Geis P, Hancock SL. The CyberKnife: a frameless robotic system for radiosurgery. *Stereotact Funct Neurosurg*. 1997;69(1–4 Pt 2):124–128.
4. Cosgrove VP, Jahn U, Pfaender M, Bauer S, Budach V, Wurm RE. Commissioning of a micro multi-leaf collimator and planning system for stereotactic radiosurgery. *Radiother Oncol*. 1999;50(3):325–336.
5. Gwak HS, Yoo HJ, Youn SM, et al. Hypofractionated stereotactic radiation therapy for skull base and upper cervical chordoma and chondrosarcoma: preliminary results. *Stereotact Funct Neurosurg*. 2005;83(5–6):233–243.
6. Benzil DL, Saboori M, Mogilner AY, Rocchio R, Moorthy CR. Safety and efficacy of stereotactic radiosurgery for tumors of the spine. *J Neurosurg*. 2004;101(suppl 3):413–418.
7. Peter G. Radiosurgery for benign spine tumors and vascular malformations. Winn HR, ed. *Youman's Neurological Surgery*. Vol. 3. Philadelphia: Saunders and Elsevier; 2011.
8. Healey JH, Lane JM. Chordoma: a critical review of diagnosis and treatment. *Orthop Clin North Am*. 1989;20(3):417–426.
9. Boriani S, Chevalley F, Weinstein JN, et al. Chordoma of the spine above the sacrum. Treatment and outcome in 21 cases. *Spine*. 1996;21(13):1569–1577.
10. Chugh R, Tawbi H, Lucas DR, Biermann JS, Schuetze SM, Baker LH. Chordoma: the nonsarcoma primary bone tumor. *Oncologist*. 2007;12(11):1344–1350.
11. Kano H, Iqbal FO, Sheehan J, et al. Stereotactic radiosurgery for chordoma: a report from the North American Gamma Knife Consortium. *Neurosurgery*. 2011;68(2):379–389.
12. al-Mefty O, Borba LA. Skull base chordomas: a management challenge. *J Neurosurg*. 1997;86(2):182–189.

13. Ammirati M, Bernardo A. Management of skull base chordoma. *Crit Rev Neurosurg.* 1999;9(2):63–69.
14. Levin WP, Kooy H, Loeffler JS, DeLaney TF. Proton beam therapy. *Br J Cancer.* 2005;93(8):849–854.
15. Boriani S, Bandiera S, Biagini R, et al. Chordoma of the mobile spine: fifty years of experience. *Spine.* 2006;31(4):493–503.
16. Baratti D, Gronchi A, Pennacchioli E, et al. Chordoma: natural history and results in 28 patients treated at a single institution. *Ann Surgical Oncology.* 2005;10(3):291–296.
17. Eid AS, Chang UK, Lee SY, Jeon DG. The treatment outcome depending on the extent of resection in skull base and spinal chordomas. *Acta Neurochir (Wien).* 2011;153(3):509–516.
18. Pedroso AG, De Salles AAF, Frighetto L, et al. Preliminary Novalis experience in the treatment of skull base chordomas with stereotactic radiosurgery and stereotactic radiotherapy. Kondziolka D, ed. *Radiosurgery.* Vol. 5. Karger, 2004.
19. De Salles AA, Gorgulho AA, Selch M, De Marco J, Agazaryan N. Radiosurgery from the brain to the spine: 20 years experience. *Acta Neurochir Suppl.* 2008;101:163–168.
20. McLoughlin GS, Sciubba DM, Wolinsky JP. Chondroma/Chondrosarcoma of the spine. *Neurosurg Clin N Am.* 2008;19(1):57–63.
21. Hsu W, Kosztowski TA, Zaidi HA, Dorsi M, Gokaslan ZL, Wolinsky JP. Multidisciplinary management of primary tumors of the vertebral column. *Curr Treat Options Oncol.* 2009;10(1–2):107–125.
22. Palaoglu S, Akkas O, Sav A. Chondroma of the cervical spine. *Clin Neurol Neurosurg.* 1988;90(3):253–255.
23. Morard M, De Tribolet N, Janzer RC. Chondromas of the spine: report of two cases and review of the literature. *Br J Neurosurg.* 1993;7(5):551–556.
24. Nojima T, Unni KK, McLeod RA, Pritchard DJ. Periosteal chondroma and periosteal chondrosarcoma. *Am J Surg Pathol.* 1985;9(9):666–677.
25. Chow WA. Update on chondrosarcomas. *Curr Opin Oncol.* 2007;19(4):371–376.
26. Katonis P, Alpantaki K, Michail K, et al. Spinal chondrosarcoma: a review. *Sarcoma.* 2011;2011:378957.
27. Boriani S, De Iure F, Bandiera S, et al. Chondrosarcoma of the mobile spine: report on 22 cases. *Spine.* 2000;25(7):804–812.
28. Suit HD, Goitein M, Munzenrider J, et al. Definitive radiation therapy for chordoma and chondrosarcoma of base of skull and cervical spine. *J Neurosurg.* 1982;56(3):377–385.
29. Hug EB, Fitzek MM, Liebsch NJ, Munzenrider JE. Locally challenging osteo- and chondrogenic tumors of the axial skeleton: results of combined proton and photon radiation therapy using three-dimensional treatment planning. *Int J Radiat Oncol Biol Phys.* 1995;31(3):467–476.
30. Bielack SS, Kempf-Bielack B, Delling G, et al. Prognostic factors in high-grade osteosarcoma of the extremities or trunk: analysis of 1,702 patients treated on neoadjuvant Cooperative Osteosarcoma Study Group protocols. *J Clinical Oncology.* 2002;20(3):776–790.
31. Schoenfeld AJ, Hornicek FJ, Pedlow FX, et al. Osteosarcoma of the spine: experience in 26 patients treated at the Massachusetts General Hospital. *Spine J.* 2010;10(8):708–714.
32. Ozaki T, Flege S, Liljenqvist U, et al. Osteosarcoma of the spine: experience of the Cooperative Osteosarcoma Study Group. *Cancer.* 2002;94(4):1069–1077.
33. Rao G, Suki D, Chakrabarti I, et al. Surgical management of primary and metastatic sarcoma of the mobile spine. *J Neurosurg Spine.* 2008;9(2):120–128.

34. Hsu W, Nguyen T, Kleinberg L, et al. Stereotactic radiosurgery for spine tumors: review of current literature. *Stereotact Funct Neurosurg.* 2010;88(5):315–321.
35. Ozaki T, Flege S, Liljenqvist U, et al. Osteosarcoma of the spine: experience of the Cooperative Osteosarcoma Study Group. *Cancer.* 2002;94(4):1069–1077.
36. Pisters PW, Harrison LB, Leung DH, Woodruff JM, Casper ES, Brennan MF. Long-term results of a prospective randomized trial of adjuvant brachytherapy in soft tissue sarcoma. *J Clin Oncol.* 1996;14(3):859–868.
37. Yang JC, Chang AE, Baker AR, et al. Randomized prospective study of the benefit of adjuvant radiation therapy in the treatment of soft tissue sarcomas of the extremity. *J Clin Oncol.* 1998;16(1):197–203.
38. Sundaresan N, Rosen G, Huvos AG, Krol G. Combined treatment of osteosarcoma of the spine. *Neurosurgery.* 1988;23(6):714–719.
39. Chang UK, Cho WI, Lee DH, et al. Stereotactic radiosurgery for primary and metastatic sarcomas involving the spine. *J Neurooncol.* 2012;107(3):551–557.
40. Grubb MR, Currier BL, Pritchard DJ, Ebersold MJ. Primary Ewing's sarcoma of the spine. *Spine.* 1994;19(3):309–313.
41. Schuck A, Ahrens S, von Schorlemer I, et al. Radiotherapy in Ewing tumors of the vertebrae: treatment results and local relapse analysis of the CESS 81/86 and EICESS 92 trials. *Int J Radiat Oncol Biol Phys.* 2005;63(5):1562–1567.
42. Rock J, Kole M, Yin FF, Ryu S, Guttierez J, Rosenblum M. Radiosurgical treatment for Ewing's sarcoma of the lumbar spine: case report. *Spine.* 2002;27(21):E471–E475.
43. Barlogie B, Shaughnessy J, Tricot G, et al. Treatment of multiple myeloma. *Blood.* 2004;103(1):20–32.
44. Wallington M, Mendis S, Premawardhana U, Sanders P, Shahsavar-Haghighi K. Local control and survival in spinal cord compression from lymphoma and myeloma. *Radiother Oncol.* 1997;42(1):43–47.
45. Woo E, Yu YL, Ng M, Huang CY, Todd D. Spinal cord compression in multiple myeloma: who gets it? *Aust N Z J Med.* 1986;16(5):671–675.
46. Mill WB, Griffith R. The role of radiation therapy in the management of plasma cell tumors. *Cancer.* 1980;45(4):647–652.
47. Soutar R, Lucraft H, Jackson G, et al. Guidelines on the diagnosis and management of solitary plasmacytoma of bone and solitary extramedullary plasmacytoma. *Br J Haematol.* 2004;124(6):717–726.
48. Jin R, Rock J, Jin JY, et al. Single fraction spine radiosurgery for myeloma epidural spinal cord compression. *J Exp Ther Oncol.* 2009;8(1):35–41.
49. Boriani S, De Iure F, Campanacci L, et al. Aneurysmal bone cyst of the mobile spine: report on 41 cases. *Spine.* 2001;26(1):27–35.
50. Cottalorda J, Bourelle S. Modern concepts of primary aneurysmal bone cyst. *Arch Orthop Trauma Surg.* 2007;127(2):105–114.
51. Zenonos G, Jamil O, Governale LS, Jernigan S, Hedequist D, Proctor MR. Surgical treatment for primary spinal aneurysmal bone cysts: experience from Children's Hospital Boston. *J Neurosurg Pediatr.* 2012;9(3):305–315.
52. Feigenberg SJ, Marcus RB Jr, Zlotecki RA, Scarborough MT, Berrey BH, Enneking WF. Megavoltage radiotherapy for aneurysmal bone cysts. *Int J Radiat Oncol Biol Phys.* 2001;49(5):1243–1247.
53. Caudell JJ, Ballo MT, Zagars GK, et al. Radiotherapy in the management of giant cell tumor of bone. *Int J Radiat Oncol Biol Phys.* 2003;57(1):158–165.
54. Boriani S, Bandiera S, Casadei R, et al. Giant cell tumor of the mobile spine: a review of 49 cases. *Spine.* 2012;37(1):E37–E45.

55. Malone S, O'Sullivan B, Catton C, Bell R, Fornasier V, Davis A. Long-term follow-up of efficacy and safety of megavoltage radiotherapy in high-risk giant cell tumors of bone. *Int J Radiat Oncol Biol Phys.* 1995;33(3):689–694.
56. Kim IY, Jung S, Jung TY, et al. Gamma knife radiosurgery for giant cell tumor of the petrous bone. *Clin Neurol Neurosurg.* 2012;114(2):185–189.
57. Canale ST, Beaty JH: Osteoblastoma. In: Daugherty K, Jones L, eds. *Campbell's Operative Orthopaedics.* 11th ed. St Louis, MO: Mosby and Elsevier, 2007.
58. Canale ST, Beaty JH. Bone-forming tumors. In: Daugherty K, Jones L, eds. *Campbell's Operative Orthopaedics.* 11th ed. St Louis, MO: Mosby and Elsevier, 2007.
59. Fountain EM, Burge CH. Osteoid osteoma of the cervical spine. A review and case report. *J Neurosurg.* 1961;18:380–383.
60. Jackson RP, Reckling FW, Mants FA. Osteoid osteoma and osteoblastoma. Similar histologic lesions with different natural histories. *Clin Orthop Relat Res.* 1977;(128):303–313.
61. Berberoglu S, Oguz A, Aribal E, Ataoglu O. Osteoblastoma response to radiotherapy and chemotherapy. *Med Pediatr Oncol.* 1997;28(4):305–309.
62. Singer JM, Deutsch GP. The successful use of radiotherapy for osteoblastoma. *Clin Oncol (R Coll Radiol).* 1993;5(2):124–125.
63. Acosta FL Jr, Dowd CF, Chin C, Tihan T, Ames CP, Weinstein PR. Current treatment strategies and outcomes in the management of symptomatic vertebral hemangiomas. *Neurosurgery.* 2006;58(2):287–95; discussion 287.
64. Faria SL, Schlupp WR, Chiminazzo H Jr. Radiotherapy in the treatment of vertebral hemangiomas. *Int J Radiat Oncol Biol Phys.* 1985;11(2):387–390.
65. Yang ZY, Zhang LJ, Chen ZX, Hu HY. Hemangioma of the vertebral column. A report on twenty-three patients with special reference to functional recovery after radiation therapy. *Acta Radiol Oncol.* 1985;24(2):129–132.
66. Gerszten PC, Ozhasoglu C, Burton SA, et al. CyberKnife frameless single-fraction stereotactic radiosurgery for benign tumors of the spine. *Neurosurgical Focus.* 2003;14(5):e16.

Chapter 12

Tumors of the Osseous Spine

B. Stereotactic Radiosurgery for Metastatic Spinal Tumors

Wesley Hsu

Metastatic spinal disease is the source of significant morbidity, as 40% of all cancer patients develop spinal metastases (1). Stereotactic radiosurgery (SR) is currently well established as having a role in the treatment of intracranial metastatic disease (2,3). The experience gained using SR for intracranial metastatic disease is now being translated to metastatic spine tumors (Figure 12B.1). There are currently several large institutional series documenting the efficacy of SR for spinal metastatic disease (Table 12B.1; 3-12).

When considering radiation therapy for spine tumors, it is important that each patient be evaluated using a multidisciplinary approach involving an oncologist, radiation oncologist, and surgeon. An oncologist can help prognosticate a particular patient's life expectancy and overall ability to tolerate an invasive surgical procedure. A neurosurgeon or orthopedic surgeon who specializes in spine oncology can lend insight into whether a patient could potentially benefit from a surgery as it relates to palliation of symptoms (i.e., pain control) or even local recurrence-free survival. A surgeon's input with respect to the overall stability of the spine may influence whether or not a patient undergoes surgical stabilization with or without tumor debulking/resection. In many instances, surgery in combination with radiation therapy may be the best treatment plan for a given patient. A team approach to metastatic spine disease is critical to promote optimal patient outcomes.

TABLE 12B.1 Stereotactic Radiosurgery for Metastatic Spine Disease

Author and Year	No. of Patients/ Lesions	Age (Mean/Med)	Intra/Extra/Metastatic Lesions	Method	Mean Follow-Up (Mo)	Prior Treatment Surgery	Prior Treatment Radiation	(Gy)/Isodose/Fractions	Target Dose Spinal Cord Dose Limit	LC	OS	PI	New Neuro Deficit	Improved Deficit	Toxicity	Major Non-neuro
Amdur et al. (2009)	21/25	>18	0/3/22	Elekta Synergy	2–27 (med 8)	0	57%	15/100% (95% to PTV)	No prior RT: 12 Gy to 0.1 mL Prior RT: 5 Gy to 0.5 mL	95%	25%	43%	0	NR		0
Benzil et al. (2004)	31/35	40–82 (mean 61)	4/5/2026	Novalis	NR	NR	NR	5–50.4/85 % –90%/1–28	2.4–42.8 Gy total dose	NR	97%	94%	3%	NR		6%
Chang et al. (2007)	63/74	21–82 (med 59)	0/0/74	ExaCT Varian	0.9–49.6 (med 21.3)	38%	55.60%	30 Gy/5 fractions or 27 Gy/3 fractions	<10 Gy	84%	70% * at 1 year		NR	0%		5%
De Salles et al. (2004)	14/22	48–82 (mean 60.2)	3/0/19	Novalis	1–16 (med 6.1)	50%	93%	8–21/91%	NR	56%	71%	50%	NR	NR		0
Degen et al. (2005)	51/72	mean 53	0/14/58	Cyber-Knife	mean 12	0	53%	10–37.5/50–100%/1–5	2.2–27.1 Gy	100%	59%	97%	21%	NR		0

Study	Intra/Extra/Total	Age	?/?/?	System	Follow-up (med)	?	?	Dose constraint	LC	PI	?	?	OS
Gerszten et al. (2007)	393/500	18–85 (mean 56)	0/0/500	Cyber-Knife	3–53 (med 21)	2%	69%	12.5–25/80%	<8 Gy to mean 0.6 cm	88%	NR	86%	0	0
Jin et al. (2007)	196/270	NR	0/0/270	Novalis	NR	NR	NR	10–18/90%	<10 Gy to 10% volume	NR	NR	85%	NR	0
Milker-Zabel et al. (2003)	18/19	16–76 (med 55.2)	0/0/19	NR	3.5–33.1 (med 12.3)	0	100%	24–45/90%	<20 Gy point dose	95%	65% at 1 year	81%	5.50%	42%
Nelson et al. 2009	32/33	45–82 (med 60)	0/1/32	NR	3–21 (med 7)	NR	69%	5.1–16/ NR/1–4	varied	87%	66% at 1 year	97%	0	0
Ryu et al. (2007)	177/230	14–85	0/0/230 (med 61)	Novalis	0.5–49	0 (med 6.4)	0	8–18/90%	<10 Gy to 10% volume	NR	49% at 1 year	NR	1	NR
Yamada et al. (2008)	93/103	38–91 (med 62)	0/0/103	NR	2–45	0	0	18–24/100%	12–14 Gy	90% point dose	36% at 3 years	NR	0	1%

Intra—intradural primary tumor; Extra—extradural primary tumor; med—median; NR—not recorded; PTV—planning target volume; LC—local control; OS—overall survival; PI—pain improvement; RT—radiotherapy. *Narcotic usage fell from 60% to 36% in 6 months.

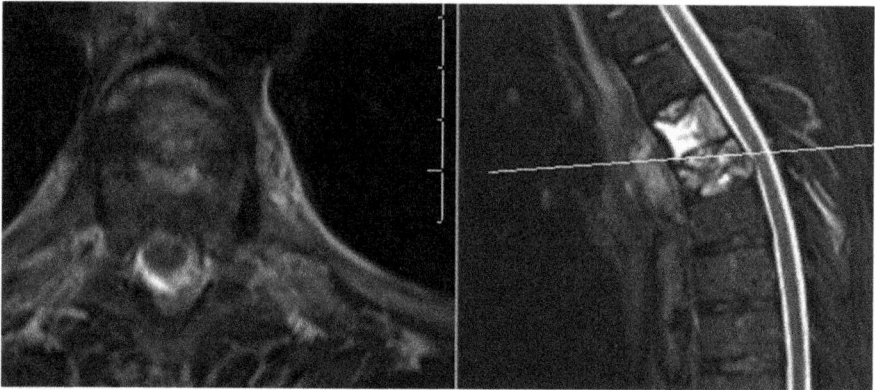

FIGURE 12B.1 57-year-old man with stage 4 esophageal cancer and metastatic spinal cancer to the T5 and T6 vertebral bodies. The patient had significant mechanical back pain. The axial view demonstrates that the tumor was abutting the spinal cord, making it difficult to properly dose the radiation to the epidural space.

EFFICACY OF STEREOTACTIC RADIOSURGERY FOR METASTATIC SPINE DISEASE

A growing body of literature supports the use of SR in the context of metastatic spinal disease. Gerstzen et al. (13) reported the largest series of spine tumors treated with SR. Three hundred ninety-three patients were treated for 500 lesions involving the vertebral body, and the vast majority were metastatic lesions. Of the 336 patients with pain as the primary indication for SR, 86% of these patients experienced long-term improvement in pain control; it was more likely with certain tumor histologies (breast, melanoma, renal, and lung cancer). Eighty-eight percent of patients had radiographic evidence of local control. Interestingly, no patient had evidence of tumor progression at adjacent vertebral body levels. Nelson et al. (10) also did not find adjacent level treatment failures in their series of 32 patients. In contrast, Ryu et al. reported that 4% of patients developed progression at adjacent vertebral levels in their series (14). When tumors do recur, it appears that that they tend to do so near the spinal cord. Chang et al. (15) found that the most common location of recurrence was the epidural space (47%), followed by the pedicles and posterior elements (18%). This is not surprising, as these areas are the most likely to receive lower doses of radiation in an effort to prevent radiation toxicity to the adjacent spinal cord and nerve roots. This suggests that the recurrence was along the portion of the tumor receiving the smallest dose or, perhaps, could have been a marginal miss (15).

Overall, the studies suggest that SR appears to provide excellent local control for metastatic spine cancer. All but one study report a greater than 80%

local control rate. Desalles et al. (7) report the lowest rate of local control (56%). However, in closely examining their series, 93% of patients in their series were previously radiated, and 50% had prior surgical intervention for these lesions. In contrast, studies such as Degen et al. reported 100% local control in patients who had no prior radiation treatment (6). Also, Amdur et al. (4), in a study of a prospective series of 21 patients with metastatic spine cancer, reported that 95% of treated lesions were locally controlled after SR therapy. The high rate of local control may be partially explained by the short survival time of this cohort, as the median survival was only 8 months.

In terms of pain control, SR appears to have excellent efficacy in improving pain attributable to metastatic disease. After SR, 43% to 97% of patients experienced improvement in back pain. This data is comparable to those reported for patients receiving standard fractionated radiotherapy for spine metastases (16).

STEREOTACTIC RADIOSURGERY CAN IMPROVE NEUROLOGIC OUTCOMES

There is a role for SR alone or in combination with surgery in the context of metastatic spine cancer causing neurologic deficits. SR has been shown to improve neurologic deficits secondary to tumor-induced radiculopathy. However, the role of SR in reversing preexisting neurological decline from cord compression is unclear. Many studies have excluded patients with metastatic spine tumors that lead to significant spinal cord compression. Milker-Zabel et al. (8) report that 42% of patients obtained improvement in neurologic symptoms after SR. In contrast, Nelson et al. (10) reports that none of the seven patients with neurologic deficits from cord compression improved after SR. However, it is unclear whether the neurologic deficits were acute or chronic in these patient populations.

The role of SR in spinal cord compression causing an acute decline in neurologic function is unclear. The pivotal 2005 study by Patchell et al. (17) demonstrates that surgical decompression of metastatic tumors causing epidural compression was clearly superior to fractionated radiation therapy (30 Gy over 10 fractions) with respect to long-term clinical outcomes, including the ability to ambulate after treatment. Excluded from this study were patients with radiosensitive tumors (multiple myeloma/plasmacytoma, germ cell tumors) who were likely to respond favorably to standard radiation. However, it is unclear whether SR would provide any improvement in outcomes compared to standard fractionated radiation in this patient population. Based on current evidence, SR alone is not recommended for the treatment of this patient population unless clinical comorbidities preclude safe surgical intervention.

STEREOTACTIC RADIOSURGERY IN COMBINATION WITH SURGERY

The epidural space between the vertebral body and the spinal cord is the most common area of treatment failure after SR for metastatic spinal tumors. As mentioned previously, this observation is most likely secondary to underdosing the epidural space for fear of causing radiation-induced myelopathy. In situations in which the spinal cord is abutting the vertebral body containing a metastatic tumor, one reasonable treatment algorithm is to have a surgical oncologist perform a partial corpectomy of the vertebral body adjacent to the spinal cord (Figure 12B.2). This algorithm is often employed in situations in which a patient has back pain that is at least partially attributable to spinal instability and has a clinical picture that does not warrant an en bloc resection of the vertebral body to prevent local recurrence. In such an instance, the goal of surgery is to stabilize the spine with internal fixation (pedicle screws/rods) and resect enough of the vertebral body to allow for a full dose of radiation to all of the remaining tumor. Such an approach eliminates the potential morbidity of removing the entire vertebral body and allows for optimal dosing of radiation to the remaining tumor burden. The timing of radiation after surgical intervention to prevent radiation-induced wound breakdown is unclear, although it is common practice to wait 3 to 4 weeks after surgery.

SIDE EFFECTS

Overall morbidity that is directly attributable to SR is quite low. Decline in neurologic function after SR is usually a manifestation of tumor progression rather

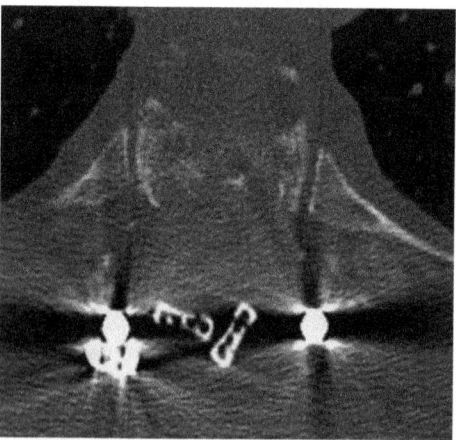

FIGURE 12B.2 The patient underwent a partial corpectomy of the C6 vertebral body to remove the portion of the vertebral body adjacent to the spinal cord. The patient also underwent spinal stabilization and had significant improvement of his mechanical back pain postoperatively.

than radiation toxicity. In Benzil et al.'s (5) review of 31 patients with SR, two patients developed radiculitis after SR. Both patients had biologically effective dose (BED) values greater than 60 Gy. Ryu et al. (11,14) recently updated their institutional series of patients with metastatic spine cancer treated with SR. One hundred seventy-seven patients were treated for 230 lesions using single-dose SR (8–18 Gy). Of the 86 patients who were alive after 1 year, only one patient experienced radiation-induced myelopathy.

Vertebral compression fracture is another phenomenon that has occurred after SR (12,14,15). Although they are thought to occur secondary to tumor progression, compression fractures have been documented after SR in patients without evidence of tumor progression (12). Although some believe that the treated vertebral body is structurally weaker, thereby predisposing the individual to a lower threshold of axial stress to cause a compression fracture, the mechanism of fracture has yet to be fully defined. In some instances, the tumor itself provides significant structural stability to the spinal column, and a rapid destruction of tumor by SR treatment could paradoxically lead to a decrease in spinal stability and predispose a patient to fractures. Therefore, it is important for physicians to instruct patients to seek immediate medical attention if their back pain worsens acutely and/or they develop neurologic deficits. Furthermore, patients should be followed closely with serial radiographs/CT scans to monitor for early signs of spinal instability.

CONCLUSION

The role of stereotactic radiosurgery for tumors of the spine continues to be refined. Issues such as proper treatment dosage, spinal cord radiation tolerance, single-dose versus multidose SR continue to be investigated. However, despite the amazing accuracy and precision of our tools, we also have to acknowledge that the side effects can be devastating. Further refinements in hardware, software, and techniques are still required.

The current literature provides support for SR as a primary treatment option for metastatic spine disease without evidence of spinal cord compression. Evidence suggests that SR provides excellent local control and pain relief. Continued follow-up of these patients will help to elucidate the long-term outcomes of these patients.

REFERENCES

1. Klimo P Jr, Schmidt MH. Surgical management of spinal metastases. *Oncologist.* 2004;9(2):188–196.

2. Muacevic A, Wowra B, Siefert A, Tonn JC, Steiger HJ, Kreth FW. Microsurgery plus whole brain irradiation versus Gamma Knife surgery alone for treatment of single metastases to the brain: a randomized controlled multicentre phase III trial. *J Neurooncol.* 2008;87(3):299–307.
3. Smith ML, Lee JY. Stereotactic radiosurgery in the management of brain metastasis. *Neurosurg Focus.* 2007;22(3):E5.
4. Amdur RJ, Bennett J, Olivier K, et al. A prospective, phase II study demonstrating the potential value and limitation of radiosurgery for spine metastases. *Am J Clin Oncol.* 2009;32(5):515–520.
5. Benzil DL, Saboori M, Mogilner AY, Rocchio R, Moorthy CR. Safety and efficacy of stereotactic radiosurgery for tumors of the spine. *J Neurosurg.* 2004;101(suppl 3):413–418.
6. Degen JW, Gagnon GJ, Voyadzis JM, et al. CyberKnife stereotactic radiosurgical treatment of spinal tumors for pain control and quality of life. *J Neurosurg Spine.* 2005;2(5):540–549.
7. De Salles AA, Pedroso AG, Medin P, et al. Spinal lesions treated with Novalis shaped beam intensity-modulated radiosurgery and stereotactic radiotherapy. *J Neurosurg.* 2004;101(suppl 3):435–440.
8. Milker-Zabel S, Zabel A, Thilmann C, Schlegel W, Wannenmacher M, Debus J. Clinical results of retreatment of vertebral bone metastases by stereotactic conformal radiotherapy and intensity-modulated radiotherapy. *Int J Radiat Oncol Biol Phys.* 2003;55(1):162–167.
9. Jin JY, Chen Q, Jin R, et al. Technical and clinical experience with spine radiosurgery: a new technology for management of localized spine metastases. *Technol Cancer Res Treat.* 2007;6(2):127–133.
10. Nelson JW, Yoo DS, Sampson JH, et al. Stereotactic body radiotherapy for lesions of the spine and paraspinal regions. *Int J Radiat Oncol Biol Phys.* 2009;73(5):1369–1375.
11. Ryu S, Jin JY, Jin R, et al. Partial volume tolerance of the spinal cord and complications of single-dose radiosurgery. *Cancer.* 2007;109(3):628–636.
12. Yamada Y, Bilsky MH, Lovelock DM, et al. High-dose, single-fraction image-guided intensity-modulated radiotherapy for metastatic spinal lesions. *Int J Radiat Oncol Biol Phys.* 2008;71(2):484–490.
13. Gerszten PC, Burton SA, Ozhasoglu C, Welch WC. Radiosurgery for spinal metastases: clinical experience in 500 cases from a single institution. *Spine (Phila Pa 1976).* 2007;32:193–199.
14. Ryu S, Rock J, Rosenblum M, Kim JH. Patterns of failure after single-dose radiosurgery for spinal metastasis. *J Neurosurg.* 2004;101(suppl 3):402–405.
15. Chang EL, Shiu AS, Mendel E, et al. Phase I/II study of stereotactic body radiotherapy for spinal metastasis and its pattern of failure. *J Neurosurg Spine.* 2007;7(2):151–160.
16. Rose CM, Kagan AR. The final report of the expert panel for the radiation oncology bone metastasis work group of the American College of Radiology. *Int J Radiat Oncol Biol Phys.* 1998;40(5):1117–1124.
17. Patchell RA, Tibbs PA, Regine WF, et al. Direct decompressive surgical resection in the treatment of spinal cord compression caused by metastatic cancer: a randomised trial. *Lancet.* 2005;366(9486):643–648.

Chapter 13

Radiotherapy and Radiosurgery in the Management of Intramedullary Spinal Cord Tumors

Mari Groves & George Jallo

OBJECTIVES

This chapter will review radiation treatment of intramedullary spinal cord tumors (IMSCTs) as an adjuvant to surgery. The differences in the treatment approach depending on histology will be discussed as well as consideration for stereotactic radiosurgery (SRS).

INTRODUCTION

Primary spinal cord tumors account for approximately 2% to 6% of all central nervous system neoplasms (1–3). Over 90% of IMSCTs are primary glial tumors, which include astrocytomas and ependymomas. Medical therapy, including radiotherapy, is typically not the primary form of treatment, as some tumors can achieve long-term survival with complete surgical excision (3–7). However, for recurrent and more aggressive neoplasms, as well as in cases of subtotal resection (STR), radiotherapy can be used as an adjunct to additional surgery or as a palliative measure (8).

Treatment measures have been well established for primary intracranial tumors. However, emerging literature shows inherent genetic differences and natural history of spinal lesions compared to their intracranial counterparts that may influence responses to radiation and chemotherapy (9,10). Since radiation relies on rapidly dividing cells to have a maximum effect, its effect on the slow-growing lesions in the spinal cord may be limited. However, several studies at multiple institutions suggest an improved survival and/or local control with adjuvant radiotherapy (11–15).

Tumor etiology plays a significant role in whether radiation therapy is considered following a partial resection. Compared to benign tumors, malignant tumors often progress more rapidly, and radiation can potentially provide a more significant upfront effect (4,12,13,16). Radiation injury is also a consideration, especially in the younger population, as negative side effects can sometimes take decades to manifest (17). Some clinicians may favor delaying radiation treatment as long as possible until there is local recurrence and surgical means have been exhausted. Intramedullary lesions are typically contiguous with normal spinal cord; therefore, concern for spinal cord toxicity and preservation of neurological function is of highest importance (17).

RADIOTHERAPY FOR ASTROCYTOMAS

Astrocytomas are more infiltrative and poorly defined; therefore, treatment with perioperative radiation is less controversial (4,13,16). Five-year survival rates climb as high as 60% to 90% for postoperative radiation (Table 13.1). Local failure typically occurs within 2 to 3 years and is more common in patients with an STR of less than 80% of tumor successfully resected at the time of surgery (4,6). However, given the insidious natural history of these lesions it is unclear whether they would have a similar course even without radiation treatment. There does not appear to be a dose-response relationship that improves local control or survival.

Patients who show progression of a low-grade lesion on routine MRI imaging should have a second attempt at resection at that time. Following resection, radiation can be considered. At routine dosage of 4500 cGy there is retention of motor function and improved survival. A retrospective study of 136 consecutive patients showed that postoperative radiotherapy improved survival for patients with World Health Organization (WHO grade 2 to 4 gliomas, but not WHO grade 1 (pilocytic) tumors (18). In cases of pilocytic astrocytomas, radiotherapy should be initiated only when there is definite clinical or radiographic progression. In another study of 52 patients with low-grade astrocytoma, postoperative radiation improved progression-free survival but not overall survival (14).

High-grade or malignant astrocytomas have an extremely poor prognosis despite resection and improvements in delivery of radiation. There are case reports of survival at 4 years in patients who have undergone aggressive radiation in doses that cause "radiocordectomy" (12,19). However, most cases proceed to local failure and cerebrospinal fluid (CSF) dissemination with metastatic lesions despite radiation at the primary site. It is not clear whether radiation benefits survival or impacts neurological decline. Aggressive radiation treatment may be an option in patients with poor motor function (Table 13.2; 4,12,13,16,19–21).

TABLE 13.1 Radiotherapy for Low-Grade Intramedullary Spinal Cord Astrocytomas

Authors	Number of Patients Irradiated (Total No of Pts)	PFS at 5y (%)	PFS at 10y (%)
Schwade et al. (1978) (22)	7 (34)	59	—
Kopelson and Linggood (1982) (13)	9 (23)	89	89
Garcia et al. (1985) (23)	14 (14)	60	50
Lindstadt et al. (1989) (20)	12 (12)	91	91
Chun et al. (1990) (24)	15 (16)	60	40
Whitaker et al. (1991) (25)	43 (58)	50	—
Huddart et al. (1993) (26)	27 (27)	59	—
Hulshof et al. (1993) (27)	12 (13)	43	—
Shirato et al. (1995) (12)	6 (7)	50	50 (8 y)
Jyothirmayi et al. (1997) (28)	23 (23)	55	—
McLaughlin et al. (1998) (19)	8 (8)	86	57
Abdel-Wahab (1999) (29)	24 (24)	54	46
Rodrigues et al. (2000) (14)	37 (37)	54	43
Nowak and Glinski (2002) (30)	13 (13)	—	46
Quigley et al. (2007) (15)	10 (26)	79	—
TOTAL	260 (335)	50–91	40–91

PFS, progression-free survival.

TABLE 13.2 Radiotherapy for High-Grade Intramedullary Spinal Cord Astrocytomas

Authors	Number of Patients	Survival Rate at 5y
Kopelson and Linggood (1982) (13)	5	0 (median ~ 2y)
Cooper and Epstein (1985) (4)	3	0 (median ~ 2y)
Cohen et al. (1989) (16)	19	0 at 2y; 21 median at 6m
Lindstadt et al. (1989) (20)	3	0 (median ~ 2y)
Ciapetta et al. (1991) (21)	4	22.7m average (2pt >24m)
Shirato et al. (1995) (12)	6	4 at 3y (2pt >24m)
McLauglin et al. (1998) (19)	4	0 (median ~ 2y)
Rodrigues et al. (2000) (14)	15	20% PFS at 5y
Tseng et al. (2010) (31)	1	0 (death at 33m)

PFS, progression-free survival; m, months; y, years.

RADIOTHERAPY FOR EPENDYMOMAS

Ependymomas arise from the ependymal lining of the ventricles and central canal and are generally well encapsulated with distinct borders. They are the most common lesions found in adults between the ages of 30 to 50 years of age. Ependymomas have a low rate of recurrence when a gross total resection (GTR) has been successfully performed (6,19,32–37). However, these patients still have survival rates at 5 and 10 years of 50% to 100% with recurrence reported between 5% and 10% (Table 13.3). Patients with STRs have a much higher recurrence rate. Most studies are limited by a small patient population, short-term follow-up, and inadequate controls. Treatment includes surgical resection with a goal of GTR. If there is residual tissue or regrowth, a second operation is done to try to remove any tissue that is easily removed. Any residual tumor can then be treated with radiation. Traditionally, a total dosing of 5000 cGy in 180 to 200 cGy fractions

TABLE 13.3 Radiotherapy for Intramedullary Spinal Cord Ependymomas

Author	Number of Patients Irradiated (Total Number of Pts)	PFS at 5y (%)	PFS at 10y (%)	15y (%)
Kopelson and Linggood (1982) (13)	8	100	72	
Garrett (1983) (38)	41	83		
Garcia (1985) (23)	8 (8)	60	60	
Shaw (1986) (39)	22 (22)	95	95	
Lindstadt (1989) (20)	18(18)	93	93	
Chun (1990) (24)	16 (17)	87	67	
Whitaker (1991) (25)	43 (58)	69	62	
Wen (1991) (34)	13	95	86	
Hulshof (1993) (27)	11 (34)	91	91	
Clover (1993) (40)	8 (11)	100	80	
Shirato (1995) (12)	8 (22)	100	100	
McLauglin (1998) (19)	10 (10)	100	100	
Schild (1998) (41)	35 (35)	97	94	75
Abdel-Wahab (1999) (29)	25 (25)	64.2	45.9	
Nowak and Glinski (2002) (30)	27 (27)		84	
Wahab (2007) (42)	22 (22)			80
Total	316 (363)	60–100	46–100	78

PFS, progression-free survival.

using external beam radiation is used in order to limit the potential for spinal cord toxicity (11).

RADIOTHERAPY IN THE PEDIATRIC POPULATION

Radiotherapy in children can be associated with significant adverse effects, and oncologists will attempt to avoid or delay radiation therapy as long as possible (43–46). Adults have a higher tolerance for radiation than children, and in children, the radiation dose should be reduced by 10% (11). Children are more likely to have low-grade lesions that are amenable to total resection. Their course is indolent and often does not require radiation.

STEREOTACTIC RADIOTHERAPY

SRS is quickly becoming an accepted form of treatment in intracranial as well as certain extradural spinal lesions. This form of radiation delivers a highly conformal, high-dose radiation to a defined area while mitigating radiation exposure to other portions of the normal spinal cord. There is limited data on whether intramedullary lesions that are presumed to be infiltrative can benefit from such a contained area of radiation. There is no direct comparison between conventional delivery methods of radiation with stereotactic treatment.

One recent retrospective study examined 10 patients from 1998 to 2003 of whom seven patients had hemangioblastomas and three had ependymomas (47). These patients underwent a prescribed dose of 1,800 to 2,500 cGy (mean 2100 cGy) in 1 to 3 stages. There were no significant complications, but the mean follow-up was only 1 year. Three lesions were smaller on follow-up imaging and the remaining tumors were stable.

Although SRS has some promise for improvement in local control, there is concern that the highly conformal treatment will limit treatment in the margins of these IMSCT. Tumors that have large volumes and/or are highly elongated may also not be appropriate candidates for SRS. Extramedullary tumors that result in compression of the spinal cord may also pose a technical challenge for SRS planning.

COMPLICATIONS

Spinal cord lesions are unique in that the area most at risk for radiation toxicity and the area radiated are typically the same. The normal cord and cauda equina are dose limiting; however, tumor recurrence is more likely in these areas

(11). Peripheral nerves and exiting nerve roots are at risk for late effects as well. Areas outside of the spinal canal are influenced by the location of the tumor and include the laryngeal airway, pharyngeal mucosa, great vessels, lungs, heart, esophagus, kidneys, liver, bowel, and reproductive organs. Long-term complications depend on the dose per daily fraction as well as the location and length of cord irradiated (48).

Multiple radiation techniques used throughout the past several decades have served as the basis for determining spinal cord tolerance. Traditional dosing for spinal cord tolerance includes conventional fractionation of 180 to 200 cGy with total doses as high as 4500 to 5000 cGy. Multiple studies have quoted a 5% risk of damage at 5 years, although there is no prospective study to elucidate a specific dose (11). Several studies have irradiated the spinal cord incidentally when treating other lesions and there has been no significant myelopathy with dosing of 4500 to 5000 cGy. There is increasing clinical support that treating higher than 5500 cGy does not have a significantly increased risk of myelitis. Patients had a 6% incidence of myelitis if treated with 5500 cGy, and many of these patients exceeded 6000 cGy (49,50).

SUMMARY

Patients with newly diagnosed primary IMSCT should first undergo surgical resection with the goal of GTR. Radiation should be used in cases of high-grade lesions or as an adjuvant when GTR cannot be achieved in low-grade lesions. Some low-grade lesions can be observed and radiated with demonstration of tumor progression. The role of SRS for IMSCTs, particularly infiltrative lesions, remains unclear at this time.

KEY POINTS

- Primary therapy for IMSCTs is surgical resection.
- In cases in which GTR is not possible or surgery is not an option, radiotherapy should be considered.
- High-grade lesions often have poor prognosis despite radiation; however, these lesions are not amenable to surgical resection and radiation is considered first-line therapy.
- SRS should be considered for small lesions, but studies showing efficacy are limited.
- Pediatric patients can often defer radiation treatment until tumor progression is noted.

REFERENCES

1. Kane PJ, el-Mahdy W, Singh A, Powell MP, Crockard HA. Spinal intradural tumours: part II–intramedullary. *Br J Neurosurg.* 1999;13(6):558–563.
2. Hanbali F, Fourney DR, Marmor E, et al. Spinal cord ependymoma: radical surgical resection and outcome. *Neurosurgery.* 2002;51(5):1162–72; discussion 1172.
3. Constantini S, Miller DC, Allen JC, Rorke LB, Freed D, Epstein FJ. Radical excision of intramedullary spinal cord tumors: surgical morbidity and long-term follow-up evaluation in 164 children and young adults. *J Neurosurg.* 2000;93(2 suppl):183–193.
4. Cooper PR, Epstein F. Radical resection of intramedullary spinal cord tumors in adults. Recent experience in 29 patients. *J Neurosurg.* 1985;63(4):492–499.
5. Epstein F. Spinal cord astrocytomas of childhood. *Adv Tech Stand Neurosurg.* 1986;13:135–169.
6. Epstein FJ, Farmer JP, Freed D. Adult intramedullary spinal cord ependymomas: the result of surgery in 38 patients. *J Neurosurg.* 1993;79(2):204–209.
7. Jallo GI, Kothbauer KF, Epstein FJ. Intrinsic spinal cord tumor resection. *Neurosurgery.* 2001;49(5):1124–1128.
8. Sgouros S, Malluci CL, Jackowski A. Spinal ependymomas—the value of postoperative radiotherapy for residual disease control. *Br J Neurosurg.* 1996;10(6):559–566.
9. Parsa AT, Fiore AJ, McCormick PC, Bruce JN. Genetic basis of intramedullary spinal cord tumors and therapeutic implications. *J Neurooncol.* 2000;47(3):239–251.
10. Johnson R, Wright KD, Gilbertson RJ. Molecular profiling of pediatric brain tumors: insight into biology and treatment. *Curr Oncol Rep.* 2009;11(1):68–72.
11. Isaacson SR. Radiation therapy and the management of intramedullary spinal cord tumors. *J Neurooncol.* 2000;47(3):231–238.
12. Shirato H, Kamada T, Hida K, et al. The role of radiotherapy in the management of spinal cord glioma. *Int J Radiat Oncol Biol Phys.* 1995;33(2):323–328.
13. Kopelson G, Linggood RM. Intramedullary spinal cord astrocytoma versus glioblastoma: the prognostic importance of histologic grade. *Cancer.* 1982;50(4):732–735.
14. Rodrigues GB, Waldron JN, Wong CS, Laperriere NJ. A retrospective analysis of 52 cases of spinal cord glioma managed with radiation therapy. *Int J Radiat Oncol Biol Phys.* 2000;48(3):837–842.
15. Gavin Quigley D, Farooqi N, Pigott TJ, et al. Outcome predictors in the management of spinal cord ependymoma. *Eur Spine J.* 2007;16(3):399–404.
16. Cohen AR, Wisoff JH, Allen JC, Epstein F. Malignant astrocytomas of the spinal cord. *J Neurosurg.* 1989;70(1):50–54.
17. Schultheiss TE, Kun LE, Ang KK, Stephens LC. Radiation response of the central nervous system. *Int J Radiat Oncol Biol Phys.* 1995;31(5):1093–1112.
18. Minehan KJ, Brown PD, Scheithauer BW, Krauss WE, Wright MP. Prognosis and treatment of spinal cord astrocytoma. *Int J Radiat Oncol Biol Phys.* 2009;73(3):727–733.
19. McLaughlin MP, Buatti JM, Marcus RB Jr, Maria BL, Mickle PJ, Kedar A. Outcome after radiotherapy of primary spinal cord glial tumors. *Radiat Oncol Investig.* 1998;6(6):276–280.
20. Linstadt DE, Wara WM, Leibel SA, Gutin PH, Wilson CB, Sheline GE. Postoperative radiotherapy of primary spinal cord tumors. *Int J Radiat Oncol Biol Phys.* 1989;16(6):1397–1403.
21. Ciappetta P, Salvati M, Capoccia G, Artico M, Raco A, Fortuna A. Spinal glioblastomas: report of seven cases and review of the literature. *Neurosurgery.* 1991;28(2):302–306.

22. Schwade JG, Wara WM, Sheline GE, Sorgen S, Wilson CB. Management of primary spinal cord tumors. *Int J Radiat Oncol Biol Phys*. 1978;4(5–6):389–393.
23. Garcia DM. Primary spinal cord tumors treated with surgery and postoperative irradiation. *Int J Radiat Oncol Biol Phys*. 1985;11(11):1933–1939.
24. Chun HC, Schmidt-Ullrich RK, Wolfson A, Tercilla OF, Sagerman RH, King GA. External beam radiotherapy for primary spinal cord tumors. *J Neurooncol*. 1990;9(3):211–217.
25. Whitaker SJ, Bessell EM, Ashley SE, Bloom HJ, Bell BA, Brada M. Postoperative radiotherapy in the management of spinal cord ependymoma. *J Neurosurg*. 1991;74(5):720–728.
26. Huddart R, Traish D, Ashley S, Moore A, Brada M. Management of spinal astrocytoma with conservative surgery and radiotherapy. *Br J Neurosurg*. 1993;7(5):473–481.
27. Hulshof MC, Menten J, Dito JJ, Dreissen JJ, van den Bergh R, González González D. Treatment results in primary intraspinal gliomas. *Radiother Oncol*. 1993;29(3):294–300.
28. Jyothirmayi R, Madhavan J, Nair MK, Rajan B. Conservative surgery and radiotherapy in the treatment of spinal cord astrocytoma. *J Neurooncol*. 1997;33(3):205–211.
29. Abdel-Wahab M, Corn B, Wolfson A, et al. Prognostic factors and survival in patients with spinal cord gliomas after radiation therapy. *Am J Clin Oncol*. 1999;22(4):344–351.
30. Nowak-Sadzikowska J, Gliński B. The value of postoperative radiotherapy of primary spinal cord glioma. *Rep Pract Oncol Radiother*. 2002; 7(4):139–147.
31. Tseng HM, Kuo LT, Lien HC, Liu KL, Liu MT, Huang CY. Prolonged survival of a patient with cervical intramedullary glioblastoma multiforme treated with total resection, radiation therapy, and temozolomide. *Anticancer Drugs*. 2010;21(10):963–967.
32. Rawlings CE 3rd, Giangaspero F, Burger PC, Bullard DE. Ependymomas: a clinicopathologic study. *Surg Neurol*. 1988;29(4):271–281.
33. Sonneland PR, Scheithauer BW, Onofrio BM. Myxopapillary ependymoma. A clinicopathologic and immunocytochemical study of 77 cases. *Cancer*. 1985;56(4):883–893.
34. Wen BC, Hussey DH, Hitchon PW, et al. The role of radiation therapy in the management of ependymomas of the spinal cord. *Int J Radiat Oncol Biol Phys*. 1991;20(4):781–786.
35. Taricco MA, Guirado VM, Fontes RB, Plese JP. Surgical treatment of primary intramedullary spinal cord tumors in adult patients. *Arq Neuropsiquiatr*. 2008;66(1):59–63.
36. Kucia EJ, Maughan PH, Kakarla UK, Bambakidis NC, Spetzler RF. Surgical technique and outcomes in the treatment of spinal cord ependymomas: part II: myxopapillary ependymoma. *Neurosurgery*. 2011;68(1 suppl Operative):90–4; discussion 94.
37. Chang UK, Choe WJ, Chung SK, Chung CK, Kim HJ. Surgical outcome and prognostic factors of spinal intramedullary ependymomas in adults. *J Neurooncol*. 2002;57(2):133–139.
38. Garrett PG, Simpson WJ. Ependymomas: results of radiation treatment. *Int J Radiat Oncol Biol Phys*. 1983;9(8):1121–1124.
39. Shaw EG, Evans RG, Scheithauer BW, Ilstrup DM, Earle JD. Radiotherapeutic management of adult intraspinal ependymomas. *Int J Radiat Oncol Biol Phys*. 1986;12(3):323–327.
40. Clover LL, Hazuka MB, Kinzie JJ. Spinal cord ependymomas treated with surgery and radiation therapy. A review of 11 cases. *Am J Clin Oncol*. 1993;16(4):350–353.
41. Schild SE, Nisi K, Scheithauer BW, et al. The results of radiotherapy for ependymomas: the Mayo Clinic experience. *Int J Radiat Oncol Biol Phys*. 1998;42(5):953–958.
42. Wahab SH, Simpson JR, Michalski JM, Mansur DB. Long term outcome with postoperative radiation therapy for spinal canal ependymoma. *J Neurooncol*. 2007;83(1):85–89.
43. Rousseau P, Habrand JL, Sarrazin D, et al. Treatment of intracranial ependymomas of children: review of a 15-year experience. *Int J Radiat Oncol Biol Phys*. 1994;28(2):381–386.

44. Perilongo G, Massimino M, Sotti G, et al. Analyses of prognostic factors in a retrospective review of 92 children with ependymoma: Italian Pediatric Neuro-oncology Group. *Med Pediatr Oncol.* 1997;29(2):79–85.
45. Grill J, Le Deley MC, Gambarelli D, et al.; French Society of Pediatric Oncology. Postoperative chemotherapy without irradiation for ependymoma in children under 5 years of age: a multicenter trial of the French Society of Pediatric Oncology. *J Clin Oncol.* 2001;19(5):1288–1296.
46. Valera ET, Serafini LN, Machado HR, Tone LG. Complete surgical resection in children with low-grade astrocytomas after neoadjuvant chemotherapy. *Childs Nerv Syst.* 2003;19(2):86–90.
47. Ryu SI, Kim DH, Chang SD. Stereotactic radiosurgery for hemangiomas and ependymomas of the spinal cord. *Neurosurg Focus.* 2003;15(5):E10.
48. Wara WM, Phillips TL, Sheline GE, Schwade JG. Radiation tolerance of the spinal cord. *Cancer.* 1975;35(6):1558–1562.
49. Marcus RB Jr, Million RR. The incidence of myelitis after irradiation of the cervical spinal cord. *Int J Radiat Oncol Biol Phys.* 1990;19(1):3–8.
50. van der Kogel AJ. Retreatment tolerance of the spinal cord. *Int J Radiat Oncol Biol Phys.* 1993;26(4):715–717.

Chapter 14

Radiotherapy and Radiosurgery in the Management of Sacral Tumors

Mari Groves, Patricia Zadnik, & Daniel Sciubba

OBJECTIVES

This chapter will review external-beam radiotherapy (EBRT) in the treatment of sacral tumors as an adjuvant to surgery as well as intensity-modulated radiotherapy (IMRT), stereotactic radiosurgery (SRS), proton beam and carbon ion radiotherapy. The differences in the treatment approach for metastases versus primary malignant tumors versus benign tumors will be described.

INTRODUCTION

Sacral tumors are relatively rare but can cause significant patient morbidity and mortality (1). The treatment of sacral tumors is dependent upon the cell of tumor origin, with primary malignant bone lesions, benign bone tumors, and metastatic lesions comprising the majority of tumors. Radiotherapy can be used as a curative, palliative, or adjunct therapy for sacral tumors and has been shown to reduce bone pain in metastatic tumors (2–4) and reduce local recurrence rates in subtotal chordoma resections (4–10).

Historically, radiotherapy to the sacrum has been limited by the relative inaccuracy of treatment planning. Relatively low doses of radiation have been administered in multiple fractions, often well below the known curative dose. Further, the inability to place a patient in a fixed stereotactic device and the concerns for exposure of surrounding tissue to high doses of radiation have limited radiosurgical approaches. Recent advances such as CyberKnife, proton beam therapy (PBRT), and intensity-modulated radiation therapy have afforded higher doses and steeper dose gradients, maximizing tumor damage and reducing patient morbidity.

RADIOTHERAPY FOR GIANT CELL TUMORS

Benign giant cell tumors are the most common sacral tumor, accounting for about 70% of all sacral neoplasms (11). Although benign, these tumors can grow very large and cause pain and neurologic impairment. Treatment for giant cell tumors involves excision, curettage, and local chemoablation with phenol. Arterial embolization may also be used prior to operative excision to decrease the blood supply to this highly vascular tumor. Adjuvant radiotherapy has been reported in several small case series (Table 14.1), with the average dose between 34 and 56 Gy (12).

COMPLICATIONS

Radiotherapy for giant cell tumors is controversial, as there is a reported 11% risk of malignant transformation following radiation (12). Ruggieri et al. (12) reported in a retrospective study of patients with sacral giant cell tumors treated with intralesional excision and radiotherapy that there was a significantly increased risk of complications with radiation although there was no difference in the time to local recurrence. As such, it is necessary to discuss the high risk of sarcomatous transformation following radiation for giant cell tumors of the sacrum.

RADIOTHERAPY FOR CHORDOMAS

Chordomas are the most common primary malignant tumors of the sacrum, resulting from abnormal growth of notochordal remnants and typically arise from the midline at the level of S4-S5 (13). Chordomas are classically slow-growing, and at the time of presentation, most patients have a large tumor with significant extralesional extension into nearby pelvic structures. Patients typically present with pain, bowel and bladder dysfunction, and impaired sexual function. Surgery is considered necessary if a patient presents with neurologic compromise in the setting of epidural compression (14). Radiotherapy as an adjunct, including EBRT, SRS, PBRT, and carbon ion radiotherapy have been reported with varying success. However, these studies are significantly limited by small patient sample size (Table 14.2).

TABLE 14.1 Radiotherapy for Giant Cell Tumors

Adjuvant Radiotherapy Following Surgical Excision

Study	Year	Patient Sample Size	Outcome Measure	Results
Ruggieri	2010	21	Survival to local recurrence	90% at 60 and 120 months
Leggon	2004	10	Survival to local recurrence	80% at 36 months, no difference in surgery alone; 11% rate of sarcoma
Turcotte	1993	26	Survival to local recurrence	67% at 84 months

This table describes the primary outcome measure and results for selected studies of adjuvant radiotherapy following surgical excision of giant cell tumors of the sacrum.

EBRT is typically recommended following intralesional resection as an adjuvant therapy. However, new studies are emerging that demonstrate durable symptom improvement and improved overall survival, decreased rate of local recurrence, and durable symptom improvement when radiotherapy follows extralesional resection (8). Proton beam therapy has also been used to treat patients with chordoma, with the most benefit seen in primary versus recurrent tumor (7). From these studies, a dose of 40 to 60 Gy or 70 CGE has shown benefit in reducing recurrence (1,3,5–10,15–19; Table 14.2).

SRS has been reported as an adjuvant treatment following surgery, although the number of patients with sacral chordomas was small ($n = 3$) (20). The authors report an improvement in patient pain scores and no new neurological deficits following radiosurgery. Carbon ion therapy alone has been used to treat sacral chordomas and when compared to surgery, carbon ion therapy alone results in higher patient emotional acceptance scores, better urinary–anorectal control, and lower local recurrence rates (21).

COMPLICATIONS

Many patients undergoing radiation therapy have persistent deficits following surgery, and their tumors are likely to recur. Sacral surgery is complex and often results in significant patient morbidity, including impaired or absent bowel and bladder continence, impaired sexual function, perianal pain, and pelvic instability. Adjuvant radiotherapy is associated with lumbosacral plexopathy when given at high doses (22). Further, damage to the bowel and spinal cord must be avoided by minimizing the volume of cauda equina and spinal cord within the treatment area.

TABLE 14.2 Radiotherapy for Sacral Chordomas

Study	Year	Patient Sample Size	Dose	Outcome Measure	Results
Radiotherapy as Adjuvant Treatment					
Sundaresan	1979	36	60–70 Gy (treatment), 40–50 Gy (palliation)	10 years OS%	40%
Amendola	1986	3	50–60 Gy	Symptom control	Durable symptom improvement 1–6 years
Samson	1993	53	NA	10 years OS%	NA
Catton	1996	23	40–50 Gy	Symptoms, OS	61% with improved symptoms, 62 month mean OS
Cheng	1999	23	54 Gy	10 years OS%	49%
York	1999	13		Disease-free interval (DFI)	2.12 years versus 8 months DFI
Fuchs	2005	52	42 Gy	10 years OS%	52%
Moojen	2011	15	>50 Gy	10 years OS%	42%
Stereotactic Radiosurgery					
Henderson	2009	3	40 Gy	Local control rates, OS	Sacral patient sample size too small
Proton Beam Radiotherapy					
Park	2006	27	71 CGE (primary) 77 CGE (recurrent)	Local control in primary versus recurrent tumor	Local control in 86% primary, 14.3% recurrent tumors
Rutz	2007	26	72 CGE	3 years PFS, OS	PFS 77%, OS 84%
Carbon Ion Radiotherapy					
Schultz-Ertner	2004	8	50.4 Gy photon with 18CGE	Local recurrence	88% local control in sacral chordomas at 3 years
Imai	2004	30	70.4 CGE	5 years local control rate	96% local control at 5 years
Nishida	2011	7	70.4 CGE	Local recurrence rate	NSS decreased local control rates

This table describes the primary outcome measure and results for selected studies of adjuvant radiotherapy following surgical excision, stereotactic radiosurgery, carbon ion radiosurgery, and proton beam radiotherapy. OS, overall survival; PFS, progression-free survival; CGE, cobalt Gray equivalents; NSS, not statistically significant.

RADIOTHERAPY FOR SACRAL METASTASES

Radiotherapy for spinal metastatic lesions serves an important role in palliative care for this patient population, which often has a poor prognosis. Radiotherapy can lead to a reduction in pain in 50% to 80% of these patients (23). Radiotherapy may be given when the primary tumor is radiosensitive, with doses reported between 18 and 24 Gy (Tables 14.2 and 14.3) and SRS

TABLE 14.3 Radiosensitivity of Metastatic Tumors

Radiosensitive	Lymphoma, myeloma
Intermediate radiosensitivity	Breast cancer, prostate cancer
Radioresistant	Renal cell carcinoma, NSCLC, melanoma

This table describes the degree of sensitivity of each tumor type to radiation. NSCLC: non-small cell lung cancer.

TABLE 14.4 Radiotherapy for Sacral Metastases

Study	Year	Patient Sample Size	Dose	Outcome Measure	Results
Stereotactic Radiosurgery					
Gibbs	2003	3	18 Gy	SRS related side effects	None
Gerszten	2007	103	19 Gy	Long-term pain improvement, radiographic control	Pain improvement in 86%, radiographic control in 88%
Saghal	2009	25	24 Gy (3 fractions)	PFP	96% PFP in radiosurgery versus 85%
IMRT					
Rose	2009	18	18–24 Gy	Vertebral body fracture	Lumbosacral spine metastases are 4.6 to 6.8 times more likely to fracture with IMRT

This table reviews several studies of SRS and IMRT in patients with sacral metastases.

may be considered for radioresistant lesions. Radiosurgery is recommended for patients with solitary or oligometastatic lesions, a 5-mm margin between spinal cord and lesion to be irradiated, an acceptable Karnofsky Performance Status, no spinal cord compression, and a minimum of 6 months life expectancy (24). Previous radiation to the spinal cord is another consideration when choosing EBRT versus SRS, as spinal cord radiation sensitivity limits cumulative dosing.

A review of the literature reveals that SRS is a safe and efficacious approach to treating spinal metastases, preventing radiographic progression of tumor and improving pain control (3,9,25,26; Table 14.4). A large study of 500 patients with spinal metastases, 103 in the sacral region, demonstrated that spinal radiosurgery can be safely conducted using the principles of intracranial radiosurgery (3). In this series, the area within the spinal canal exposed to radiation greater than 8 Gy was less than 0.6 cm^3. Gerszten and colleagues further reported no clinically or radiographically evident spinal cord damage after treatment with a mean dose of 20 Gy (range 15–25 Gy). Sahgal et al. (26) further demonstrated that radiosurgery confers an improved progression-free probability (PFP) when

TABLE 14.5 Summary of Treatment Recommendations

Type of Tumor	Considerations	Radiation Dose (Gy)
Metastasis	Radiosensitivity of the primary cancer, patient life expectancy, and quality of life	18–24
Benign tumors (e.g., osteoid osteoma, osteblastoma, aneurysmal bone cyst, giant cell tumor)	Risk of radiation-induced malignancy	30–50
Primary malignant tumors (e.g., chordoma)	Possible radical surgical resection, protecting existing bowel/bladder function, and neurologic status	40–60

used on previously irradiated patients. In that series, the authors do not report any new cases of radiation-induced damage to the spinal cord.

COMPLICATIONS

Metastatic lesions between T10 and the sacrum are 4.6 to 6.8 times more likely to fracture following radiation with IMRT (25). If surgical intervention is planned concurrently, radiation to the area of instrumentation may contribute to failed fusion. Further, for a patient with a significantly limited life expectancy, daily radiation treatments may be burdensome, and patient preference should be incorporated into the treatment plan.

SUMMARY

For a review of the treatment recommendations for various tumor types see Table 14.5 above.

KEY POINTS

- Radiotherapy should be tailored to patient need and tumor type.
- Preexisting neurologic impairment and local recurrence are important predictors of patient outcome.
- Radiotherapy for metastatic lesions is guided by radiosensitivity of the lesion and patient prognosis.
- Evidence is emerging that immediate adjuvant radiotherapy following en bloc and subtotal resection results in lower rates of local recurrence in sacral chordomas.
- Radiotherapy for benign sacral tumors is complicated by a very real risk of malignant transformation.

REFERENCES

1. Catton C, O'Sullivan B, Bell R, et al. Chordoma: long-term follow-up after radical photon irradiation. *Radiother Oncol.* 1996;41(1):67–72.
2. Chawla S, Abu-Aita R, Philip A, Lundquist T, Okunieff P, Milano MT. Stereotactic radiosurgery for spinal metastases: case report and review of treatment options. *Bone.* 2009;45(4):817–821.
3. Gerszten PC, Burton SA, Ozhasoglu C, Welch WC. Radiosurgery for spinal metastases: clinical experience in 500 cases from a single institution. *Spine.* 2007;32(2):193–199.
4. Sciubba DM, Chi JH, Rhines LD, Gokaslan ZL. Chordoma of the spinal column. *Neurosurg Clin N Am.* 2008;19(1):5–15.
5. York JE, Kaczaraj A, Abi-Said D, et al. Sacral chordoma: 40-year experience at a major cancer center. *Neurosurgery.* 1999;44(1):74–9; discussion 79.
6. Samson IR, Springfield DS, Suit HD, Mankin HJ. Operative treatment of sacrococcygeal chordoma. A review of twenty-one cases. *J Bone Joint Surg Am.* 1993;75(10):1476–1484.
7. Park L, Delaney TF, Liebsch NJ, et al. Sacral chordomas: impact of high-dose proton/photon-beam radiation therapy combined with or without surgery for primary versus recurrent tumor. *Int J Radiat Oncol Biol Phys.* 2006;65(5):1514–1521.
8. Moojen WA, Vleggeert-Lankamp CL, Krol AD, Dijkstra SP. Long-term results: adjuvant radiotherapy in en bloc resection of sacrococcygeal chordoma is advisable. *Spine.* 2011;36(10):E656–E661.
9. Gibbs IC, Chang SD. Radiosurgery and radiotherapy for sacral tumors. *Neurosurg Focus.* 2003;15(2):E8.
10. Amendola BE, Amendola MA, Oliver E, McClatchey KD. Chordoma: role of radiation therapy. *Radiology.* 1986;158(3):839–843.
11. Kollender Y, Meller I, Bickels J, et al. Role of adjuvant cryosurgery in intralesional treatment of sacral tumors. *Cancer.* 2003;97(11):2830–2838.
12. Leggon RE, Zlotecki R, Reith J, Scarborough MT. Giant cell tumor of the pelvis and sacrum: 17 cases and analysis of the literature. *Clin Orthop Relat Res.* 2004;(423):196–207.
13. Muro K, Das S, Raizer JJ. Chordomas of the craniospinal axis: multimodality surgical, radiation and medical management strategies. *Expert Rev Neurother.* 2007;7(10):1295–1312.
14. Fourney DR, Gokaslan ZL. Current management of sacral chordoma. *Neurosurg Focus.* 2003;15(2):E9.
15. Sundaresan N, Galicich JH, Chu FC, Huvos AG. Spinal chordomas. *J Neurosurg.* 1979;50(3):312–319.
16. Rutz HP, Weber DC, Sugahara S, et al. Extracranial chordoma: Outcome in patients treated with function-preserving surgery followed by spot-scanning proton beam irradiation. *Int J Radiat Oncol Biol Phys.* 2007;67(2):512–520.
17. Schulz-Ertner D, Nikoghosyan A, Thilmann C, et al. Results of carbon ion radiotherapy in 152 patients. *Int J Radiat Oncol Biol Phys.* 2004;58(2):631–640.
18. Fuchs B, Dickey ID, Yaszemski MJ, Inwards CY, Sim FH. Operative management of sacral chordoma. *J Bone Joint Surg Am.* 2005;87(10):2211–2216.
19. Imai R, Kamada T, Tsuji H, et al.; Working Group for Bone, Soft Tissue Sarcomas. Carbon ion radiotherapy for unresectable sacral chordomas. *Clin Cancer Res.* 2004;10(17):5741–5746.

20. Henderson FC, McCool K, Seigle J, Jean W, Harter W, Gagnon GJ. Treatment of chordomas with CyberKnife: Georgetown university experience and treatment recommendations. *Neurosurgery.* 2009;64(2 suppl):A44–A53.
21. Nishida Y, Kamada T, Imai R, et al. Clinical outcome of sacral chordoma with carbon ion radiotherapy compared with surgery. *Int J Radiat Oncol Biol Phys.* 2011;79(1):110–116.
22. Ashenhurst EM, Quartey GR, Starreveld A. Lumbo-sacral radiculopathy induced by radiation. *Can J Neurol Sci.* 1977;4(4):259–263.
23. Helissey C, Levy A, Jacob J, et al. External beam radiotherapy in the management of spinal metastases: review of current strategies and perspectives for highly conformal irradiation modalities. *Discov Med.* 2011;11(61):505–511.
24. Swift PS. Radiation for spinal metastatic tumors. *Orthop Clin North Am.* 2009;40(1):133–44, vii.
25. Rose PS, Laufer I, Boland PJ, et al. Risk of fracture after single fraction image-guided intensity-modulated radiation therapy to spinal metastases. *J Clin Oncol.* 2009;27(30):5075–5079.
26. Sahgal A, Ames C, Chou D, et al. Stereotactic body radiotherapy is effective salvage therapy for patients with prior radiation of spinal metastases. *Int J Radiat Oncol Biol Phys.* 2009;74(3):723–731.

Chapter 15

Radiosurgery of Vascular Disorders

Samuel Ryu

SPINAL ARTERIOVEINOUS MALFORMATION

Spinal vascular malformations represent rare and insufficiently studied pathological entities characterized by considerable variation. Insufficient study of this disease is connected with the rarity and complexity of its diagnosis and treatment.

Clinical Presentation

Spinal arteriovenous malformations (AVMs) are rare, comprising about 4% of primary intraspinal masses. Spinal AVMs are classified into four pathological groups based on the location of the anomalous vascular connection. Type I is a dural arteriovenous fistula, and type IV is a perimedullary arteriovenous fistula. Type I is the most common type in adults. These types can be treated with endovascular and/or microsurgical resection. Type II and III AVMs are located within the parenchyma of the spinal cord. Type II is sometimes called a glomus lesion. It consists of a compact intramedullary nidus. Type III, or juvenile AVM is characterized by a large and diffuse intramedullary nidus. This is often associated with a significant extramedullary and, occasionally, a paraspinal component.

Spinal AVMs cause progressive neurological deficit over months to years. Common symptoms are back pain, transient neurological deficit, progressive sensory loss, and lower extremity weakness. Sudden onset of myelopathy can develop secondary to hemorrhage to intramedullary or subarachnoid space and venous congestion, rarely by steal effects.

Evaluation

The imaging studies are complimentary to each other in accurately identifying the AVM nidus.

1. Selective spinal angiography is difficult and has a significant complication rate. Three-dimensional rotational spinal angiography (1) can be fused with the standard thin-section CT scan.
2. CT: Thin-section (1.25–2.5 mm slice thickness) contrast enhanced axial and sagittal computer tomography can be used to image the relevant region of the spine.
3. MRI may detect the lesion with safety and good sensitivity.
4. Myelography shows serpiginous intradural filling defect. It should be done prone and supine to avoid missing a dorsal AVM.

Treatment

1. Microsurgical resection
2. Endovascular technique (e.g., embolization)
3. Radiosurgery

Intramedullary AVMs are high-risk lesions because of their location. If feasible, endovascular embolization and/or microsurgical resection can be used. However, many of type II and type III spinal cord AVMs are not amenable to surgical approach. It may be even riskier at the thoracic level, where collateral blood supply may be reduced.

Radiosurgery may allow spinal lesions to be irradiated with an accuracy and high degree of conformity that is comparable to the experience with radiosurgery for intracranial lesions. The experience of radiosurgery for spinal AVM is limited. It is recommended one borrow and exercise the results of radiosurgery for brain AVM. The AVM nidus should be visualized by angiogram with or without image fusion of other diagnostic tests. Accurate target definition is important as well as delineation of the adjacent topographic spinal cord structures.

The optimum radiosurgery target volume and dose are not defined for spinal AVM at this time. A single high-radiation dose can be used based on the experience of brain AVM when it is feasible, considering the tolerability of the spinal cord to such a high dose of radiation. Stanford group used a fractionated or staged radiosurgery in two to five sessions with an average marginal dose of 20.5 Gy (2). The results are encouraging. A reduction in the AVM volume was seen in six of seven patients on an interim MRI scan after a median follow-up of 27 months. Four of these patients had postoperative angiography that demonstrated residual nidus that was reduced in size. One patient demonstrated complete angiographic obliteration 26 months after radiosurgery.

Supportive care should be provided as needed. Dexamethasone is usually used to prevent exacerbating adjacent spinal cord edema, typically with 8 to 12 mg per day initially followed by a slow taper. Antinausea medications should be considered, particularly when treating lesions in the upper cervical or medullary levels. This can lead to radiation exposure to the area postrema within the medulla.

CAVERNOUS HEMANGIOMA

Spinal cavernomas are usually a soft circumscribed formation of small cavernous, dilated, blood-filled cavities. These cavities are lined by endothelium and contain no smooth muscle. Spinal cavernomas are rare. They are usually without symptoms, but may become symptomatic in the later decades of life. The majority of cavernomas of the spinal cord are intramedullary. Cavernomas can also involve the vertebral body.

Surgery is the primary mode of treatment. Radiosurgery is generally not a consideration unless the patient has significant comorbidities that may preclude surgical intervention. Experience of radiosurgery for intramedullary cavernomas is limited, and it may be prudent to use the experience of radiosurgery for intracranial lesions (3). Radiosurgery may be a good treatment for alleviation of neurological symptoms or pain. An experience of radiosurgery for thoracic epidural cavernous hemangioma has been reported (4). A fractionated radiosurgical regimen 32 Gy in four fractions resulted in good symptom control and radiographic reduction of the lesion at 1 and 3 years MRI follow-up. Experience of fractionated radiation suggests that radiation doses 30 to 40 Gy in 1.6–2.5 Gy were also useful in various sites, including three cases of vertebral body hemangiomas (5). In our experience, single-dose 16 Gy to the vertebral body was well tolerated and was able to control the symptoms.

REFERENCES

1. Prestigiacomo CJ, Niimi Y, Setton A, Berenstein A. Three-dimensional rotational spinal angiography in the evaluation and treatment of vascular malformations. *AJNR Am J Neuroradiol*. 2003;24(7):1429–1435.
2. Sinclair J, Chang SD, Gibbs IC, Adler JR Jr. Multisession CyberKnife radiosurgery for intramedullary spinal cord arteriovenous malformations. *Neurosurgery*. 2006;58(6):1081–1089; discussion 1081.
3. Monaco EA, Khan AA, Niranjan A, et al. Stereotactic radiosurgery for the treatment of symptomatic brainstem cavernous malformations. *Neurosurg Focus*. 2010;29(3):E11.
4. Sohn MJ, Lee DJ, Jeon SR, Khang SK. Spinal radiosurgical treatment for thoracic epidural cavernous hemangioma presenting as radiculomyelopathy: technical case report. *Neurosurgery*. 2009;64(6):E1202–E1203; discussion E1203.
5. Schild SE, Buskirk SJ, Frick LM, Cupps RE. Radiotherapy for large symptomatic hemangiomas. *Int J Radiat Oncol Biol Phys*. 1991;21(3):729–735.

Chapter 16

Complications and Dose Selection of Radiosurgery for Spine Lesions

Edward A. Monaco III & Peter C. Gerszten

Stereotactic radiosurgery (SRS) for spinal lesions evolved from the success of intracranial radiosurgery first devised by Lars Leksell (1). Its principles are identical: the administration of conformal high-dose radiation to a target with rapid dose falloff, limiting toxicity to adjacent structures. The first clinical application of linear accelerator-based (LINAC) SRS for spinal lesions was published by Hamilton et al. (2). Since then, there has been a burgeoning interest in spinal SRS. Although spinal SRS has several advantages over conventional radiation therapy (e.g., single session/hypofractionated regimens, repeatability, utility after failure, conventional radiation failure, limited toxicity to surrounding structures) it is not without potential complications. Complications of spinal SRS are related to dose, conformality, and radiation tolerance of tissues. Because of fundamental differences in the administration of conventional radiation therapy and SRS, conventional tolerance doses do not apply to SRS. A balance must be struck between the administration of a lesion-controlling dose and radiation toxicity to adjacent tissues, in particular, the spinal cord and cauda equina. Herein, we discuss the current understanding of complications in spinal SRS and appropriate dose selection for the treatment of various lesions.

COMPLICATIONS

SRS Treatment Planning

Creating a conformal SRS treatment that yields tumor control but limits radiation toxicity begins with treatment planning. The first task is to delineate the radiosurgical target volume. The gross tumor volume (GTV) or the volume that represents all visible tumors on imaging is contoured. For malignant tumors, a margin of one to two millimeters is added for the clinical target volume (CTV), which includes an area likely to contain microscopic disease. The planning target volume (PTV), or the volume that is being dosed, is often the CTV. With benign tumors, a margin is not necessary and the PTV is the GTV. After identifying the target, normal structures are delineated. The most critical structures at risk for radiation injury are the spinal cord and cauda equina. The volumes of the spinal cord and the cauda equina (for which the entire spinal canal is contoured) are outlined. This volume is defined by some groups to include spinal cord 6 mm above and below the target (3). Depending on the spinal levels of the target, other "at risk" structures are defined, including pharynx, esophagus, bowel, kidney, and lung. Dose to these structures can be minimized via inverse planning algorithms.

Nonneurological Toxicity

Nonneurological toxicity can involve any nearby organ. In the cervicothoracic region, esophageal injury can result rarely in conditions ranging from acute transient esophagitis to tracheoesophageal fistula. The rates of esophageal injury vary. In the largest retrospective spine SRS series, which included 285 cervicothoracic levels treated, no esophageal toxicity was reported (4). Yamada et al. (5) reported two cases of mild esophagitis and one delayed tracheoesophageal fistula formation in 93 patients. In 19 postsurgical patients treated with SRS to the cervical or thoracic spine, Moulding et al. (6) reported three patients with mild esophagitis and one with tracheoesophageal fistula. Sheehan et al. (7) did not observe esophageal toxicity after SRS treatment of 91 metastatic tumors in the cervical and thoracic spine. Only one report has specifically examined esophageal injury following spine SRS. Cox et al. (8) retrospectively evaluated 182 patients for esophageal injury following SRS from C5 to T10. The overall rate of any toxicity was 27%, with 75% of the toxicity low grade. The rate of high-grade toxicity was 6.8% and included esophagitis, esophageal ulcer, stenosis, and tracheoesophageal fistulae. On this basis, Cox et al. recommend that the dose to the esophagus from a single fraction to be limited to 14 Gy to 2.5 cm^3 and a point dose of less than 22 Gy.

Skin toxicity can also rarely occur, typically in the setting of SRS involving the posterior spinal elements. However, it is usually mild and self-limiting. Moulding et al. (6) reported one mild skin reaction in 21 patients, whereas Yamada et al. (5) noted three instances in 93 consecutive patients.

Following spine SRS, some authors have noted radiation-related fractures or progressive kyphosis. In one series, 2 of 93 patients suffered vertebral fractures without evidence of tumor progression (5). Rose et al. (9) evaluated 62 consecutive patients treated by single-fraction SRS for metastatic tumors and noted a nearly 40% rate of fracture progression. Fractures were more common with lytic disease, when tumors involved most of the vertebral body, and when occurring below T10. Damast et al. (10) reported on a population of patients all previously treated with conventional radiation therapy and observed nine vertebral body fractures in 94 patients (9.6%; 10). Finally, 73% of 1-year survivors of spine metastases treated with SRS developed segmental kyphosis, which was associated with decreased symptomatic improvement (7).

Other rare reported complications include pharyngitis, laryngitis, gastrointestinal ulcer, and tissue fibrosis (11,12). Table 16.1 shows an inclusive list of reported nonneurological complications. Complications may be underestimated in the setting of very short clinical follow-up and limited life expectancies as well as confounding toxicities related to other treatments like chemotherapy and surgery. These reports highlight the need to limit radiation dose to adjacent organs by contouring them prior to inverse dose planning. Although dose limits for single fractions or hypofractionation schemes are not known, it has been recommended that doses to the gastrointestinal tract be limited to less than 8 or 10 gray (Gy) in order to avoid toxicity (12). Kidney toxicity is uncommon. However, great care should be taken to limit dose to patients with marginal renal function, a transplanted kidney, or a single kidney. To prevent possible injury, Gerszten

TABLE 16.1 Nonneurological Complications Following Spine SRS

Esophageal
Esophagitis
Esophageal ulcer
Esophageal edema
Tracheoesophageal fistula
Pharyngitis
Laryngitis
Tracheitis
Gastrointestinal
Gastritis
Gastrointestinal ulcer
Enteritis
Proctitis
Soft tissue fibrosis
Bone
Vertebral body fracture
Progressive kyphosis
Postsurgical wound complication

et al. (4) limit the dose to each kidney to 2 Gy or less. Often patients who are candidates for spinal SRS have had recent open spinal surgery for tumor debulking and spinal stabilization. Although only reported in limited series, there has not been an increased risk of infection, wound complication, or spinal fluid leak after adjuvant spinal SRS (6,13). Sahgal et al. (13) typically wait until 4 weeks after surgery to begin SRS treatment.

Neurological Toxicity

One of the most dreaded complications following spinal SRS is radiation myelitis, which occurs late and is irreversible, typically occurring 6 or more months after treatment. Acute toxicities are mostly reversible and respond to corticosteroids. Symptoms of radiation-induced spinal cord injury include progressive and permanent motor and sensory deficits with associated myelopathy and pain. On magnetic resonance imaging, radiation myelitis appears as an area of abnormal T2 signal hyperintensity with associated contrast enhancement (Figure 16.1). The precise mechanism is unknown but likely involves a combination of vascular injury, inflammation, and demyelination. The radiation tolerance of the spinal cord to high-dose single-fraction or hypofractionated treatments is not known. For conventional fractionated radiation therapy, it has been predicted that 50 Gy or less to a 5-cm length of full thickness spinal cord limits the 5-year risk of radiation myelitis to 5% (14). However, this prediction cannot be extrapolated to SRS. For single-fraction and hypofractionated approaches there is likely a partial-volume tolerance effect for the spinal cord whereby higher doses can be tolerated if only applied to a very small volume (3,15). Early spine SRS practice was guided by the radiation tolerance of the optic apparatus during intracranial SRS (less than 8–10 Gy). On this

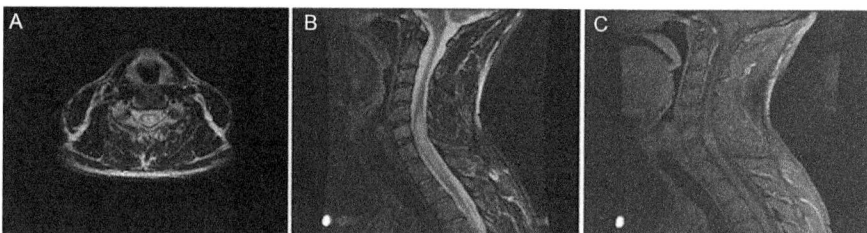

FIGURE 16.1 Magnetic resonance imaging of a patient with radiation myelitis presenting with Brown-Séquard syndrome and back pain. (A, B) Axial and sagittal T2-weighted images showing an area of hyperintensity within the spinal cord. (C) Sagittal T1-weighted image after gadolinium administration showing an area of contrast enhancement in the lower cervical spinal cord.

basis, our best information regarding spinal cord tolerance derives from clinical series.

Ryu et al. evaluated the partial-volume tolerance of the spinal cord following single-dose radiosurgery for 230 lesions in 177 patients not previously irradiated for metastatic spine lesions (3). One patient developed radiation myelitis, and from analysis of the dose/volume histograms from this series Ryu et al. concluded that the partial volume tolerance of the human spinal cord is at least 10 Gy to 10% of the cord volume 6 mm above and below the radiosurgical target. Gibbs et al. retrospectively reviewed the SRS treatments of 1075 patients for various spinal lesions to identify patients who suffered radiation myelitis and determine dosimetric factors associated with its incidence (16). Hypofractionated and single-fraction protocols were used in previously irradiated and radiation-naïve patients. Six of 1075 patients developed radiation myelitis (0.6%), with symptoms that started approximately 6 months following SRS. This group concluded that caution be used when considering radiosurgery plans that expose more than approximately 1 cm^3 of the spinal cord to an 8 Gy or higher dose equivalent.

Sahgal et al. (17) compared five patients who suffered radiation myelitis with 19 who did not, all radiation naïve, following spine SRS using hypofractionation and single-fraction dosing. Due to dosing differences, a biologically effective dose (BED) was calculated to compare regimens. Radiation-induced cord injury was associated with single-fraction point doses to the spinal cord of 10.6, 13.1, and 14.8 Gy. Maximum point doses of 25.6 Gy in two fractions and 30.9 Gy in three fractions also caused cord toxicity. Thus, it was concluded that point doses for SRS should be respected with a maximum point dose for single-fraction treatment limited to 10 Gy. For fractionated treatments a 2-Gy equivalent normalized BED of 30 to 35 Gy to the thecal sac minimizes the risk of cord injury. Although it has been hypothesized that the thoracic cord may be more sensitive to radiation due to its watershed vascular supply, no segment of the cord seemed to be at higher risk.

Many patients who are candidates for spine SRS have previously undergone conventional radiation therapy. The optimum parameters for reirradiation with SRS to prevent radiation myelitis were sought by Sahgal et al. (18). Five radiation myelitis sufferers were compared with 14 patients without radiation myelitis, all of whom had prior conventional fractionated radiation. The 2 Gy equivalent normalized BED for the conventional radiation therapy was between 30 and 50 Gy. After comparing the cohorts, Sahgal et al. concluded that the max point normalized 2 Gy equivalent BED to the thecal sac should not exceed 70 Gy (the total of conventional radiation and SRS). The point maximum 2 Gy equivalent normalized BED for subsequent SRS should not exceed 25 Gy. The BED ratio of SRS to total dose should not exceed 0.5. Finally, no radiation myelitis occurred when conventional radiation and SRS were separated by 5 months or more. Thus, the interval for reirradiation by SRS should be at least 5 months. Table 16.2 summarizes the dose limitations based on current clinical experience.

The cauda equina and nerve roots are felt to have a higher radiation tolerance than the spinal cord, as they are considered part of the peripheral nervous

TABLE 16.2 Select Spinal Cord Dose-Limitation Recommendations

	Dose Tolerance
Ryu et al. (3)	10 Gy to 10% of the cord for single fractions
Gibbs et al. (16)	8 Gy (or dose equivalent) to 1 cm^3
Sahgal et al. (17)	10 Gy maximum point dose for single fractions 30–35 Gy in 2 Gy normalized BED for hypofractionation
Sahgal et al. (18)	70 Gy maximum point dose in 2 Gy normalized BED total 25 Gy maximum point dose in 2 Gy normalized BED for SRS
Gerszten et al. (19)	10 Gy
Kirkpatrick et al. (20)	13 Gy maximum for single fraction, 20 Gy in 3 fractions

system. No clear guidelines for dose limitation to the cauda equina have been delineated. In a large series by Gerszten et al. (21), the maximum dose to the cauda equina was 14 Gy for single-fraction treatments (mean and median doses were 10 Gy). There were no reported cases of radiation toxicity reported in this series. In a subsequent prospective evaluation of spinal cord and cauda equina doses, Gerszten et al. (19) observed no neurological toxicity and concluded that limiting the cauda equina dose to 11 Gy is safe and effective. Thus, limiting doses to the cauda equina is advisable, with 14 Gy being a reasonable dose for single-fraction treatments. In 31 patients, Benzil et al. (11) noted two cases of transient radiculitis following SRS. In 59 reirradiated patients treated by SRS, Garg et al. (22) observed two cases of grade three neurological toxicity as a result of radiation-induced lumbar plexopathy. These patients had persistent neuropathy and foot drop.

Overall, neurological toxicity in the current published experience has proven rare at reported doses. However, many factors, including medical comorbidities and previous treatments, are likely to contribute to continued variability in observed spinal cord tolerance. It is important to keep in mind that many of the patients included in published studies have limited life expectancies, and these patients may not have lived long enough to experience side effects that may take months to manifest. Treatment of benign spinal tumors with SRS may yield further long-term observations about toxicity.

DOSE SELECTION

Several factors must be considered when choosing an SRS dose for spinal lesions, including indication, tumor/lesion histology, treatment volume, normal tissue tolerance, and previous treatments. Single-fraction dosing for various lesions is based in part on experience with intracranial radiosurgery. The current published experience has proven variable and appears to be based on institutional preferences. At present, spinal metastases are the most commonly treated lesions via

SRS, with benign extramedullary tumors, primary spine tumors, arteriovenous malformations (AVMs), and intramedullary cord tumors making up the remainder of the experience (23).

Spine Metastases

The goals of SRS for metastatic spine disease are tumor control and pain relief. There is no consensus regarding prescription dosing for metastases. At the University of Pittsburgh a single-fraction approach has been employed on the basis of the institutional experience with Gamma Knife. For metastatic lung cancer, a mean single-fraction dose of 20 Gy was used (range 15–25 Gy) to the 80% isodose line in 77 patients with 87 spine tumors (21). No radiation toxicity was observed during a median follow-up period of 16 months. As a primary modality, SRS achieved 100% tumor control and 89% of patients who presented with pain reported long-term improvement. A mean dose of 19 Gy contoured to the 80% isodose line (range 15–22 Gy) was used in a series of 50 patients harboring 68 metastatic breast tumors to the spine (24). Again, tumor control during a median follow-up of 16 months was 100% and there was no radiation toxicity. Of the patients presenting with pain as their primary complaint, 96% reported long-term improvement. Similar dosing was used to treat spinal metastases from renal cell carcinoma (mean maximum dose of 20 Gy, range 17.5–25 Gy; 25). Single-fraction therapy as a boost after conventional fractionated radiation therapy has also been reported (26). Ryu et al. delivered single-fraction doses of 6 to 8 Gy following 25 Gy in 10 fractions of conventional fractionated therapy to metastatic tumors.

When fractionation is used, a wide variety of dosing has been reported. At Memorial Sloan-Kettering a maximum dose of 20 Gy is administered in five fractions (27,28). The group at Georgetown reported a mean dose of 21 Gy delivered in three fractions (29). The MD Anderson group gave a maximum dose of 27–30 Gy over three to five fractions (30,31). Regardless of the scheme, fractionation has proven valuable in reducing pain and controlling tumors. Wang et al. (31) reported a twofold increase in the proportion of patients reporting no pain (26% to 54% over 6 months) following SRS for spinal metastases. Bilsky et al. (27) observed 87% tumor control during a median of 12 months follow-up after hypofractionated SRS for multiple histologies. Overall, these data suggest that most current dosing regimens are effective in achieving tumor control and pain relief. It is noteworthy that in reported failures, maximum prescribed doses were lower than the mean maximum tumor doses for the overall cohort (failed renal cell patients: maximum doses in failures 17.5 Gy, mean maximum dose in cohort 20 Gy; 25). Table 16.3 summarizes dose prescriptions for metastatic spine disease. Finally, many radiosurgical patients have undergone previous conventional fractionated radiation. For some groups, depending on the interval between treat-

TABLE 16.3 Select Dose Prescriptions for Metastatic Spine Disease

	Histology and Dose
Gerszten et al. (21)	Lung, 15–25 Gy, single fraction
Gerszten et al. (24)	Breast, 15–22 Gy, single fraction
Gerszten et al. (25)	Renal cell, 17.5–25 Gy, single fraction
Memorial Sloan-Kettering (5,27,28)	Multiple, 18–24 Gy, single fraction Multiple, 20 Gy in 5 fractions
Georgetown (29)	Multiple, 21 Gy in 3 fractions
MD Anderson (30,31)	Multiple, 27–30 Gy in 3–5 fractions
Ryu et al. (26)	Multiple, 6–8 Gy, single-fraction boost therapy

ments, the typical dose will be reduced (e.g., if 6 months or less between radiation therapies, dose will be reduced by 2 Gy; 3).

Benign Extramedullary Spine Tumors

Although surgery is the primary treatment modality for benign extramedullary tumors like schwannomas and meningiomas, several series have reported on the utility of spine SRS as adjuvant or primary therapy. Dosing is again based on the intracranial experience. Both single-fraction therapy and hypofractionation have been employed. Gerszten et al. (32) treated a mixture of 72 patients harboring schwannomas, meningiomas, and neurofibromas with a single fraction. Using maximum tumor doses of 15 to 25 Gy (mean 21.6 Gy) pain control was achieved in 73% of patients. No tumors progressed on imaging during follow-up, although one patient went on to have surgery for worsening symptoms. Three patients (4.2%) in this series developed radiation myelitis 5 to 13 months after treatment, a rate several fold higher than that experienced with metastatic lesions. The etiology for this remains unclear. In a subsequent series by Gerszten et al. (33), the mean prescribed dose to a second cohort of 40 patients was 14 Gy (range 11 to 17 Gy) in a single fraction. For tumors distorting the spinal cord, 18 to 21 Gy was delivered to the GTV in three fractions. 100% tumor control was achieved without spinal cord toxicity during follow-up. Dodd et al. (34) treated 51 patients with a mixture of 55 benign extramedullary tumors with 16 to 30 Gy in one to five fractions. More than half of these patients had at least 2-year follow-up with only one radiographic failure and three patients going on to surgery. Radiation myelitis occurred in one patient (2%) 8 months after treatment. A follow-up report from Stanford in 87 patients with 103 benign extramedullary tumors indicated that a mean prescription dose of 19.4 Gy (range 14 to 30 Gy) in one to five fractions was employed (35). Similar clinical results were achieved with only one case of transient radiation myelitis observed. Overall, with limited experience as a basis, SRS for benign extramedullary tumors has utility despite an apparently higher risk of radiation injury. More data are necessary to identify the best dosing schemes for these lesions.

Primary Spine Tumors

Primary tumors of the spine make up a very small proportion of SRS candidate lesions and specific dose recommendations are lacking. Most of these tumors are radioresistant and theoretically respond better to high single-fraction doses (greater than 15 Gy). In a case report from Memorial Sloan Kettering, a patient with lumbar chordoma was treated with 24 Gy in a single fraction with near complete pathological response of the tumor (36). Henderson et al. (37) treated 11 patients with spinal chordomas by SRS with a median of 35 Gy (range 24–40 Gy) in five fractions. The actuarial control rate in this series at 5 years was 59.1%. Levine et al. (38) performed fractionated SRS to 14 patients with primary spinal sarcomas with a treatment dose that ranged from 20 to 36 Gy (median, 30 Gy to the 70%–85% isodose line), administered in one to five fractions. In this series, 10 of 14 patients had either a complete or a partial response to treatment and were still alive at the time of the publication. In total, the experience with primary spine tumors remains limited. Despite this, a consensus exists that these tumors require a substantially higher dose than other spine SRS lesions for adequate tumor control.

Spinal Arteriovenous Malformations

Cerebral AVMs have been treated for over 20 years by SRS. SRS to AVMs of the spinal cord thus represents a reasonable extension of the technology. Like the experience with primary spine tumors, AVM treatment is in its infancy; so only a few conclusions can be drawn about specific dose guidelines. Treatment of spinal AVMs is particularly challenging because of the anatomic proximity or incorporation of the target within the spinal cord itself. The largest series to date comes from the group at Stanford (39,40). Chang et al. suggest that spine SRS is only of utility in patients harboring type II or, rarely, type III AVMs who are not candidates for microsurgery or embolization. In their reported series of 23 patients, they used mean marginal doses of 16 to 21 Gy and treated patients in two to four fractions. Two patients with conus region AVMs were treated with a single-fraction approach. No patient had a subsequent hemorrhage following SRS and although follow-up imaging showed reduction in nidus volume for all AVMs, only three were documented to have been obliterated. Two patients suffered radiation-induced spinal cord injury.

Intramedullary Spinal Cord Tumors

Experience with intramedullary tumors is sparse. In a small radiosurgical series by Shin et al. (41) that included seven patients with intramedullary spinal cord metastases, tumors were treated in a single session with 10 to 16 Gy at the margin (mean, 14 Gy) to the 90% isodose line. In the six patients with follow-up, all but one had symptomatic improvement and none had radiographic progression. No toxicity was noted during follow-up that was limited due to an average survival of 8.5 months. In a series of 16 patients with spinal hemangioblastomas, a median dose of 21 Gy (range 21–25 Gy) was used over one to three sessions (42). Fifteen of these tumors shrank or remained stable without any evidence of radiation myelitis. No meaningful consensus regarding dose to intramedullary tumors is available from the published literature.

CONCLUSIONS

Spine SRS has evolved from the footprint of intracranial SRS as a useful adjuvant or primary treatment for a variety of spinal lesions. Although it offers the advantage of high conformality and sharp dose falloff, the risk of radiation toxicity remains, albeit extremely low. There are no prospective randomized data regarding the risk of radiation toxicity, the appropriate dose limitations to the spinal cord and surrounding tissues, or best dosing regimens. The current data are experiential and suggest that with careful dose limitations to normal tissues the current dosing regimen for spine SRS is both safe and effective.

REFERENCES

1. Leksell L. The stereotaxic method and radiosurgery of the brain. *Acta Chir Scand.* 1951;102(4):316–319.
2. Hamilton AJ, Lulu BA, Fosmire H, Stea B, Cassady JR. Preliminary clinical experience with linear accelerator-based spinal stereotactic radiosurgery. *Neurosurgery.* 1995;36(2):311–319.
3. Ryu S, Jin JY, Jin R, et al. Partial volume tolerance of the spinal cord and complications of single-dose radiosurgery. *Cancer.* 2007;109(3):628–636.
4. Gerszten PC, Burton SA, Ozhasoglu C, Welch WC. Radiosurgery for spinal metastases: clinical experience in 500 cases from a single institution. *Spine.* 2007;32(2):193–199.
5. Yamada Y, Bilsky MH, Lovelock DM, et al. High-dose, single-fraction image-guided intensity-modulated radiotherapy for metastatic spinal lesions. *Int J Radiat Oncol Biol Phys.* 2008;71(2):484–490.

6. Moulding HD, Elder JB, Lis E, et al. Local disease control after decompressive surgery and adjuvant high-dose single-fraction radiosurgery for spine metastases. *J Neurosurg Spine*. 2010;13(1):87–93.
7. Sheehan JP, Shaffrey CI, Schlesinger D, Williams BJ, Arlet V, Larner J. Radiosurgery in the treatment of spinal metastases: tumor control, survival, and quality of life after helical tomotherapy. *Neurosurgery*. 2009;65(6):1052–61; discussion 1061.
8. Cox BW, Jackson A, Hunt M, Bilsky M, Yamada Y. Esophageal toxicity from high-dose, single-fraction paraspinal stereotactic radiosurgery. *Int J Radiat Oncol Biol Phys*, 2012, Epub ahead of print.
9. Rose PS, Laufer I, Boland PJ, et al. Risk of fracture after single fraction image-guided intensity-modulated radiation therapy to spinal metastases. *J Clin Oncol*. 2009;27(30):5075–5079.
10. Damast S, Wright J, Bilsky M, et al. Impact of dose on local failure rates after image-guided reirradiation of recurrent paraspinal metastases. *Int J Radiat Oncol Biol Phys*. 2011;81(3):819–826.
11. Benzil DL, Saboori M, Mogilner AY, Rocchio R, Moorthy CR. Safety and efficacy of stereotactic radiosurgery for tumors of the spine. *J Neurosurg*. 2004;101 (suppl 3):413–418.
12. Ryu S and Gerszten PC. Treatment failure and complications. In: Gerszten PC, Ryu S, (eds. *Spine Radiosurgery*. New York: Thieme, 2009:104–111.
13. Sahgal A, Bilsky M, Chang EL, et al. Stereotactic body radiotherapy for spinal metastases: current status, with a focus on its application in the postoperative patient. *J Neurosurg Spine*. 2011;14(2):151–166.
14. Emami B, Lyman J, Brown A, et al. Tolerance of normal tissue to therapeutic irradiation. *Int J Radiat Oncol Biol Phys*. 1991;21(1):109–122.
15. Daly ME, Choi CY, Gibbs IC, et al. Tolerance of the spinal cord to stereotactic radiosurgery: insights from hemangioblastomas. *Int J Radiat Oncol Biol Phys*. 2011;80(1):213–220.
16. Gibbs IC, Patil C, Gerszten PC, Adler JR Jr, Burton SA. Delayed radiation-induced myelopathy after spinal radiosurgery. *Neurosurgery*. 2009;64(2 suppl):A67–A72.
17. Sahgal A, Ma L, Gibbs I, et al. Spinal cord tolerance for stereotactic body radiotherapy. *Int J Radiat Oncol Biol Phys*. 2010;77(2):548–553.
18. Sahgal A, Ma L, Weinberg V, et al. Reirradiation human spinal cord tolerance for stereotactic body radiotherapy. *Int J Radiat Oncol Biol Phys*. 2012;82(1):107–116.
19. Gerszten PC, Quader M, Novotny JJ, Flickinger JC. Prospective evaluation of spinal cord and cauda equina dose constraints using cone beam computed tomography (CBCT) image guidance for spine radiosurgery. *J Radiosurg SBRT*, 2011; 1,197–202.
20. Kirkpatrick JP, van der Kogel AJ, Schultheiss TE. Radiation dose-volume effects in the spinal cord. *Int J Radiat Oncol Biol Phys*. 2010;76(3 suppl):S42–S49.
21. Gerszten PC, Burton SA, Belani CP, et al. Radiosurgery for the treatment of spinal lung metastases. *Cancer*. 2006;107(11):2653–2661.
22. Garg AK, Wang XS, Shiu AS, et al. Prospective evaluation of spinal reirradiation by using stereotactic body radiation therapy: The University of Texas MD Anderson Cancer Center experience. *Cancer*. 2011;117(15):3509–3516.
23. Gerszten PC, Mendel E, Yamada Y. Radiotherapy and radiosurgery for metastatic spine disease: what are the options, indications, and outcomes? *Spine*. 2009;34(22 suppl):S78–S92.
24. Gerszten PC, Burton SA, Welch WC, et al. Single-fraction radiosurgery for the treatment of spinal breast metastases. *Cancer*. 2005;104(10):2244–2254.
25. Gerszten PC, Burton SA, Ozhasoglu C, et al. Stereotactic radiosurgery for spinal metastases from renal cell carcinoma. *J Neurosurg Spine*. 2005;3(4):288–295.

26. Ryu S, Fang Yin F, Rock J, et al. Image-guided and intensity-modulated radiosurgery for patients with spinal metastasis. *Cancer*. 2003;97(8):2013–2018.
27. Bilsky MH, Yamada Y, Yenice KM, et al. Intensity-modulated stereotactic radiotherapy of paraspinal tumors: a preliminary report. *Neurosurgery*. 2004;54(4):823–30; discussion 830.
28. Yamada Y, Lovelock DM, Yenice KM, et al. Multifractionated image-guided and stereotactic intensity-modulated radiotherapy of paraspinal tumors: a preliminary report. *Int J Radiat Oncol Biol Phys*. 2005;62(1):53–61.
29. Degen JW, Gagnon GJ, Voyadzis JM, et al. CyberKnife stereotactic radiosurgical treatment of spinal tumors for pain control and quality of life. *J Neurosurg Spine*. 2005;2(5):540–549.
30. Chang EL, Shiu AS, Lii MF, et al. Phase I clinical evaluation of near-simultaneous computed tomographic image-guided stereotactic body radiotherapy for spinal metastases. *Int J Radiat Oncol Biol Phys*. 2004;59(5):1288–1294.
31. Wang XS, Rhines LD, Shiu AS, Yang JN, Selek U, Gning I, Liu P, Allen PK, Azeem SS, Brown PD, Sharp HJ, Weksberg DC, Cleeland CS, Chang EL. Stereotactic body radiation therapy for management of spinal metastases in patients without spinal cord compression: a phase 1–2 trial. *Lancet Oncol*, 2012, Epub ahead of print.
32. Gerszten PC, Burton SA, Ozhasoglu C, McCue KJ, Quinn AE. Radiosurgery for benign intradural spinal tumors. *Neurosurgery*. 2008;62(4):887–95; discussion 895.
33. Gerszten PC, Quader M, Novotny J Jr, Flickinger JC. Radiosurgery for benign tumors of the spine: clinical experience and current trends. *Technol Cancer Res Treat*. 2012;11(2):133–139.
34. Dodd RL, Ryu MR, Kamnerdsupaphon P, Gibbs IC, Chang SD Jr, Adler JR Jr. CyberKnife radiosurgery for benign intradural extramedullary spinal tumors. *Neurosurgery*. 2006;58(4):674–85; discussion 674.
35. Sachdev S, Dodd RL, Chang SD, et al. Stereotactic radiosurgery yields long-term control for benign intradural, extramedullary spinal tumors. *Neurosurgery*. 2011;69(3):533–9; discussion 539.
36. Wu AJ, Bilsky MH, Edgar MA, Yamada Y. Near-complete pathological response of chordoma to high-dose single-fraction radiotherapy: case report. *Neurosurgery*. 2009;64(2):E389–90; discussion E390.
37. Henderson FC, McCool K, Seigle J, Jean W, Harter W, Gagnon GJ. Treatment of chordomas with CyberKnife: Georgetown University experience and treatment recommendations. *Neurosurgery*. 2009;64(2 suppl):A44–A53.
38. Levine AM, Coleman C, Horasek S. Stereotactic radiosurgery for the treatment of primary sarcomas and sarcoma metastasis of the spine. *Neurosurgery*. 2009;64(2 suppl):A54–A59.
39. Sinclair J, Chang SD, Gibbs IC, Adler JR Jr. Multisession CyberKnife radiosurgery for intramedullary spinal cord arteriovenous malformations. *Neurosurgery*. 2006;58(6):1081–9;discussion 1081.
40. Chang SD, Hancock SL, Gibbs IC, Adler JRJ. Spinal cord arteriovenous malformation radiosurgery. In: Gerszten PC, Ryu S, eds. *Spine Radiosurgery*. New York: Thieme, 2009: 123–127.
41. Shin DA, Huh R, Chung SS, Rock J, Ryu S. Stereotactic spine radiosurgery for intradural and intramedullary metastasis. *Neurosurg Focus*. 2009;27(6):E10.
42. Moss JM, Choi CY, Adler JR Jr, Soltys SG, Gibbs IC, Chang SD. Stereotactic radiosurgical treatment of cranial and spinal hemangioblastomas. *Neurosurgery*. 2009;65(1):79–85; discussion 85.

Index

alpha cradle, 28
anesthesia dolorosa, radiosurgery and, 158
aneurysmal bone cysts, 188
anticonvulsants, 155
arteriovenous malformation (AVMs), 162
   classification of, 124–125
   incidence of, 123
   radiosurgery for, 123–131
      complications, 131
      follow-up, 130–131
      hypofractionated stereotactic, 128–129
      imaging and selection of, 126
      imaging changes following, 114
      indications, 125
      large lesions, 127–128
      multimodal treatment, 129–130
      small lesions, 127
      staged treatment, 129
      stereotactic, 126–127
   salvage therapy for, 128
   spinal, 221–223, 233
astrocytomas, radiosurgery for, 36
   intramedullary spinal cord, 204–205
   low-grade, 36
AVMs. *See* arteriovenous malformation
axial computed tomography, 15

baclofen, for trigeminal neuralgia, 155
balloon compression (BC)
   for trigeminal neuralgia, 155, 157
BC. *See* balloon compression
BED. *See* biologically effective dose
benign extramedullary spine tumors
   dose selection, for radiosurgery, 232
biologically effective dose (BED), 229
BodyFix vacuum body-fixing device, 28

borden classification, of dural arteriovenous fistulae, 138
bothersome dysesthesia, radiosurgery and, 158
brain metastases
   surgery for, 51
   whole-brain radiotherapy for, 46–54
      dose selection, 52–54
      historical standard of, 46–47
      intensified local treatment with, 47–48
      radiosurgery without, 51–52
      toxicity of, 48–50
      tumor bed radiosurgery after resection, 50–51
brain tumors, primary, 35–40
   ependymoma, 36–37
   glioblastoma multiforme, 35–36
   hemangioblastoma, 38–40
   low-grade astrocytoma, 36
   neurocytoma, 37–38
   oligodendroglioma, 37

carbamazepine, for trigeminal neuralgia, 155
carbon ion radiotherapy, for chordomas, 215
C-arm conebeam computerized tomography angiography, for arteriovenous malformations, 126
carotid-cavernous fistulae (CCF), 139–141
cavernous hemangioma, 223
CCF. *See* carotid-cavernous fistulae
central neurocytoma (CN)
   radiosurgery for, 37–38
cerebral angiography, for dural arteriovenous fistulae, 138

cerebral cavernous malformations (CMs), 147–152
  epidemiology of, 147
  management of, 148
  microsurgical resection of, 148–149
  natural history of, 148
  presentation of, 148
  radiosurgery for, 149
    complications of, 150–151
    effect on bleeding/rebleeding, 150
    epilepsy associated with, 151
    histopathological effects of, 149–150
    radiographic changes following, 151
chemotherapy
  for Ewing's sarcoma, 187
  for multiple myeloma, 187
  for osteoblastomas, 189
  for osteoid osteomas, 189
  for osteosarcomas, 186
  for skull base meningioma, 60
chondromas, radiotherapy for, 185
chondrosarcomas, radiotherapy for, 185
chordomas, radiotherapy for, 184–185
  complications of, 214
  sacral, 214–216
cisplatin
  for Ewing's sarcoma, 187
  for osteoblastomas, 189
  for osteoid osteomas, 189
  for osteosarcomas, 186
clinical differential effect, 162–164
clinical target volume (CTV), 226
CMs. See cerebral cavernous malformations
CN. See central neurocytoma
cobalt-60 (^{60}Co), 4
compensator based intensity-modulated radiation therapy, 16
complications, of radiotherapy, 22, 30–31, 63–64, 109, 131, 142, 150–151, 207–208, 214, 218, 225–230
computed tomography (CT) scan
  for arteriovenous malformations, 126
  axial, 15
  -based intensity-modulated radiation therapy, 28–29
  for optic nerve sheath meningiomas, 94–96
  of sellar lesions, 104
  single photon emission, 15
  for spinal arteriovenous malformation, 222
  for spinal tumors, 27, 29
conventional radiotherapy, radiobiology of, 6–8
cranial radiosurgery, 13–24
  fractionated radiation therapy, 13–15
  for intracranial lesions, 14
  stereotactic radiosurgery. See stereotactic radiosurgery
craniopharyngiomas, sellar region affected by, 104
  radiation dosing for, 107
  sellar region affected by, 104
CT. See computed tomography scan
CTV. See clinical target volume
CyberKnife radiosurgery, 16, 21–22, 28, 183
  for craniopharyngiomas, 107
  for glomus jugulare tumors, 78, 80
  for hemangiopericytomas, 72–73
  for optic nerve sheath meningiomas, 97
  for sellar lesions management, 106
  for skull base meningioma, 61–63
    complications of, 63
  for vestibular schwannomas, 85
cyclophosphamide, for osteosarcomas, 186

dAVF. See dural arteriovenous fistulae
dexamethasone, for spinal arteriovenous malformation, 223
DNA, radiation injuries to, 6
dose selection, for radiosurgery, 230–234
  benign extramedullary spine tumors, 232
  brain metastases, 52–54
  intramedullary spinal cord tumors, 233–234
  primary spine tumors, 233
  spinal arteriovenous malformations, 233
  spine metastases, 231–232
doxorubicin
  for Ewing's sarcoma, 187
  for osteoblastomas, 189
  for osteoid osteomas, 189
  for osteosarcomas, 186
drug-resistant epilepsies
  hypothalamic hamartomas, 164–168
  mesial temporal lobe epilepsy, 168–172
  radiosurgery for, 161–174
  rationale for, 162–164
dural arteriovenous fistulae (dAVF), 137–143
  background of, 137
  Borden classification of, 138

clinical presentation of, 137–138
natural history of, 137–138
radiotherapy for
 algorithm of, 141
 complications of, 142
 dose calculation, 140
 historical evidence and current
  data, 139–140
 in combination with embolization, 141
 pathophysiology, 140
 planning, 140
 salvage therapy, 141
 sole upfront therapy, 140
 treatment modalities for, 138–139
  conservative, 139
  endovascular embolization, 139
  microsurgery, 139

EBRT. *See* external-beam radiotherapy
EC. *See* entorhinal cortex
electromagnetic radiation, 3–4
en bloc resection
 for chordomas, 184
 for giant cell tumors, 188
 for osteosarcomas, 186
endovascular embolization
 for dural arteriovenous fistulae, 139
 in combination with
  embolization, 141
 for spinal arteriovenous
  malformation, 222
entorhinal cortex (EC)
 role in epilepsy, 171–172
EORTC. *See* European Organisation for
 Research and Treatment of Cancer
 clinical trials
ependymomas
 intramedullary spinal cord,
  radiotherapy for, 206–207
 radiosurgery for, 36–37
 supratentorial, 36
epilepsy
 associated with cerebral cavernous
  malformations, radiosurgery
  for, 151
 drug-resistant. *See* drug-resistant
  epilepsies
European Organisation for Research and
 Treatment of Cancer (EORTC)
 clinical trials
 brain metastases, whole-brain
  radiotherapy for, 50

Ewing's sarcoma, 186–187
ExacTrac alignment system, 28
external-beam radiotherapy (EBRT)
 for chordomas, 215
 for ependymoma, 36, 37
 for sacral metastases, 217

facial numbness, radiosurgery and, 158
FDG-PET. *See* 18F-fluorodeoxyglucose
 positron emission tomography
FLAIR. *See* fluid-attenuated inversion
 recovery MRI
fluid-attenuated inversion recovery
 (FLAIR) MRI
 for arteriovenous malformations, 126
18F-fluorodeoxyglucose positron emission
 tomography (FDG-PET)
 of metastatic intracranial tumors, 113
fractionated stereotactic radiation
 therapy, 13–15
 for optic nerve sheath
  meningiomas, 93–101
free radicals, 5–6

gabapentin, for trigeminal neuralgia, 155
Gamma Knife (GK) radiosurgery, 17–18,
 28, 156, 183
 for arteriovenous malformations, 126
 for cerebral cavernous malformations,
  150, 151
 dose characteristics of, 17
 for glomus jugulare tumors, 78
 for hemangioblastoma, 39
 for hemangiopericytomas, 70–72
 for hypothalamic hamartoma, 165–168
 for mesial temporal lobe epilepsy, 162,
  164, 168–172
 for metastatic intracranial tumors,
  imaging changes following, 113
 for pituitary adenomas, 107
 for sellar lesions management, 106
 for skull base meningioma, 61
  complications of, 63
 for vestibular schwannomas, 85, 87
GBM. *See* glioblastoma multiforme
giant cell tumors, radiotherapy
 for, 188–189
 complications of, 214
 sacral, 214, 215
GK. *See* Gamma Knife radiosurgery
glioblastoma multiforme (GBM)
 radiosurgery for, 35–36

glomus jugulare tumors, stereotactic radiosurgery for, 77–80
   methods of, 78
   outcomes of, 79–80
glycerol injection, for trigeminal neuralgia, 155
gross tumor volume (GTV), 226
GTV. *See* gross tumor volume

hemangioblastoma, radiosurgery for, 38–40
hemangiomas, 189–190
hemangiopericytomas (HPCs)
   radiosurgery for, 67–74
      CyberKnife, 72–73
      dose, 68–70
      external beam radiotherapy for, 70
      Gamma Knife, 70–72
      long-term prognosis of, 73
      outcomes, 70
      planning and techniques, 68
      rationale, 67–68
hexamethylpropyleneamine oxime (HMPAO) SPECT imaging for metastatic intracranial tumors, 113
HFSR. *See* hypofractionated stereotactic radiosurgery
HH. *See* hypothalamic hamartomas
HMPAO. *See* hexamethylpropyleneamine oxime SPECT imaging
HPCs. *See* hemangiopericytomas
hypofractionated stereotactic radiosurgery (HFSR), 183
   for arteriovenous malformations, 128–129
hypothalamic hamartomas (HH) radiosurgery for, 164–168

imaging changes following radiosurgery, 111–118
   for arteriovenous malformations, 114
   biology of, 115
   case study, 116
   for metastatic intracranial tumors, 112–114
   recommendations for, 116–118
immobilization, for spinal tumors, 28–29
IMRT. *See* intensity-modulated radiation therapy
IMSCT. *See* intramedullary spinal cord tumors

intensity-modulated radiation therapy (IMRT), 15–16
   CT-based, for spinal tumors, 28–29
   for optic nerve sheath meningiomas, 98–101
   for sacral metastases, 218
intracranial lesions, radiosurgery for, 14
intralesional excision, for giant cell tumors, 214
intramedullary spinal cord tumors (IMSCT), 203–208
   astrocytomas, 204–205
   dose selection, for radiosurgery, 233–234
   ependymomas, 206–207
   in pediatric population, 207
   stereotactic radiotherapy for, 207
      complications of, 207–208
intraparenchymal tumors
   brain metastases, 45–54
   primary brain tumors, 35–40
ionizing radiation
   defined, 3
   types of, 3–5

Kaplan–Meier analysis, 113
Karnofsky Performance Status (KPS), 35, 36, 217
Koos criteria, for grading vestibular schwannomas, 83–84
KPS. *See* Karnofsky Performance Status

lamotrigine, for trigeminal neuralgia, 155
Leksell Gamma Unit (Gamma Knife), 17–18
   dose characteristics of, 17
L'Hermitte's sign, 31
LINAC. *See* linear accelerator radiosurgery
linear accelerator (LINAC) radiosurgery, 20–21, 156, 225
   for arteriovenous malformations, 126–127
   dose characteristics of, 17
   for drug-resistant epilepsy, 164
   fixed, 28
   for glomus jugulare tumors, 78
   for hemangiopericytomas, 72
   for optic nerve sheath meningiomas, 97
   portable, 28
   for skull base meningioma, 61
   for vestibular schwannomas, 85, 87

logistic regression analysis, 159
low-grade astrocytoma, radiosurgery for, 36

magnetic resonance angiography (MRA)
  for arteriovenous malformations, 126
magnetic resonance imaging (MRI)
  for arteriovenous malformations, 126
  for cerebral cavernous malformations, 147, 151
  of dural arteriovenous fistulae, 139
  fluid-attenuated inversion recovery, 126
  for hypothalamic hamartoma, 166
  for neurocytoma, 38, 39
  for optic nerve sheath meningiomas, 96
  of sellar lesions, 104
  serial, 112
  for skull base meningioma, 60
  for spinal arteriovenous malformation, 222
  for spinal tumors, 27, 29
  for trigeminal neuralgia, 157, 159
  for vestibular schwannomas, 84, 85
meningiomas
  optic nerve sheath, 93–101
  radiation dosing for, 108
  sellar region affected by, 104
  skull base, 59–64
    diagnosis of, 60
    evaluation of, 60
    overview of, 59–60
    stereotactic radiosurgery for, 60–64
    treatment for, overview of, 60–61
mesial temporal lobe epilepsy (MTLE)
  radiosurgery for, 168–172
    dose selection, 170–171
    indications of, 173–174
    patient selection, 172–173
    potential concerns, 173
    target definition, 171–172
metastases, sacral
  radiosensitivity of, 217
  radiotherapy for, 216–218
    complications of, 218
    recommendations for, 218
metastasis, sellar region affected by, 104
metastatic intracranial tumors, imaging changes following radiosurgery for, 112–114

metastatic spinal tumors, stereotactic radiosurgery for, 195–201
  combination with surgery, 200
  dose selection, 231–232
  efficacy of, 198–199
  impact on neurologic outcomes, 199
  side effects of, 200–201
methotrexate
  for Ewing's sarcoma, 187
  for osteosarcomas, 186
microsurgery
  for cerebral cavernous malformations, 148–149
  for dural arteriovenous fistulae, 139
  for spinal arteriovenous malformation, 222
  for vestibular schwannomas
    following radiosurgery, 87–88
    radiosurgery following, 87
microvascular decompression (MVD)
  for trigeminal neuralgia, 155, 157
Mini-Mental State Examination, 47
motor neuron disease, 31
MRA. *See* magnetic resonance angiography
MRI. *See* magnetic resonance imaging
MTLE. *See* mesial temporal lobe epilepsy
multiple myeloma, 187
MVD. *See* microvascular decompression
myelography, for spinal arteriovenous malformation, 222

neurocytoma, radiosurgery for, 37–38
neurofibromatosis type 2 (NF2), 84–85
neurological toxicity, following spinal stereotactic radiosurgery, 228–230
Neuro-Oncology Working Group, 112
NF2. *See* neurofibromatosis type 2
nonneurological toxicity, following spinal stereotactic radiosurgery, 226–228
Novalis TX, 28, 183
numbness, facial, 158

oligodendroglioma, radiosurgery for, 37
ONSMs. *See* optic nerve sheath meningiomas
optic nerve sheath meningiomas (ONSMs)
  clinical manifestations of, 94
  imaging of, 94–96
  management of, 96–101
  stereotactic fractionated radiation therapy for, 93–101

osseous spinal tumors, stereotactic radiosurgery for
  metastatic spinal tumors, 195–201
  primary, 183–190
osteoblastomas, 189
osteoidosteomas, 189
osteosarcomas, 186
oxcarbazepine, for trigeminal neuralgia, 155

particle radiation, 5
PBRT. *See* proton beam radiotherapy
pediatric population
  intramedullary spinal cord tumors, radiotherapy for, 207
PET. *See* positron emission tomography
phenytoin, for trigeminal neuralgia, 155
pituitary adenomas
  radiation dosing for
    nonsecretory, 107
    secretory, 107
  sellar region affected by, 103–104
planning target volume (PTV), 226
plasmacytomas, 187
positron emission tomography (PET), 15
  for metastatic intracranial tumors, 113
  for spinal tumors, 29
primary brain tumors, radiosurgery for, 35–40
  ependymoma, 36–37
  glioblastoma multiforme, 35–36
  hemangioblastoma, 38–40
  low-grade astrocytoma, 36
  neurocytoma, 37–38
  oligodendroglioma, 37
primary osseous spinal tumors, stereotactic radiosurgery for, 183–190
  aneurysmal bone cysts, 188
  chondromas, 185
  chondrosarcomas, 185
  chordomas, 184–185
  Ewing's sarcoma, 186–187
  giant cell tumors, 188–189
  hemangiomas, 189–190
  multiple myeloma, 187
  osteoblastomas, 189
  osteoidosteomas, 189
  osteosarcomas, 186
primary spine tumors, radiosurgery for
  dose selection, 233
  osseous. *See* primary osseous spinal tumors, stereotactic radiosurgery for

proton beam radiotherapy (PBRT), 18–20
  for arteriovenous malformations, 127
  for chondrosarcomas, 185
  for chordomas, 215
  dose characteristics of, 17
  for vestibular schwannomas, 85
pseudoprogression, 111–112, 113, 115, 118
  diagnosing, 115–116
  distinguished from radiation necrosis, 115–116
  managing, 115–116
PTV. *See* planning target volume

radiation
  critical structures, strategies to prevent, 23
  injuries to DNA, 6
  Radiation Therapy Oncology Group (RTOG), 46
    Acute and Long-term Morbidity Scoring Criteria, 23
    brain metastases, whole-brain radiotherapy for (clinical trial), 46, 47, 54
radiobiology
  of conventional radiotherapy, 6–8
  of radiosurgery, 8–9
radiochemistry
  free radicals, 5–6
  radiation injuries to DNA, 6
radiofrequency rhizotomy (RFR)
  for trigeminal neuralgia, 155, 157
recursive partitioning analysis (RPA), 46
RFR. *See* radiofrequency rhizotomy
Robotic LINAC IMRT (CyberKnife), 16, 21–22
RPA. *See* recursive partitioning analysis
RTOG. *See* Radiation Therapy Oncology Group

sacral tumors, 213–218
  chordomas, 214–216
  giant cell tumors, 214
  metastases, 216–218
salvage therapy
  for arteriovenous malformations, 128
  for dural arteriovenous fistulae, 141
  for hypothalamic hamartoma, 166
SEEG. *See* stereoelectroencephalographic radiosurgery
sellar lesions, 103–109
  craniopharyngiomas, 104

INDEX **243**

evaluation and diagnosis of
    endocrine, 105
    imaging, 104
    ophthalmological evaluation, 105
  meningiomas, 104
  metastasis, 104
  overview of, 103
  pituitary adenomas, 103–104
  radiosurgery for
    complications of, 109
    dosing, 106–108
    management strategies, 105
    outcomes of, 108
    planning and technique, 106
    prognosis of, 108
    sample plan, 108
    treatment goals and
      indications, 105–106
serial magnetic resonance imaging, 112
single photon emission computed
    tomography (SPECT), 15
  hexamethylpropyleneamine oxime, 113
  of metastatic intracranial tumors, 113
"skin-sparing" effect, 4
skull base tumors
  glomus jugulare tumors, 77–80
  hemangiopericytomas, 67–74
  meningioma, 59–64
  optic nerve sheath meningiomas, 93–101
  sellar lesions, 103–109
  vestibular schwannomas, 83–90
sole upfront therapy, for dural
    arteriovenous fistulae, 140
SPECT. *See* single photon emission
    computed tomography
spinal arteriovenous malformation, 221–223
  clinical presentation of, 221
  dose selection, for radiosurgery, 233
  evaluation of, 222
  treatment for, 222–223
spinal lesions, radiosurgery for
  complications of
    neurological toxicity, 228–230
    nonneurological toxicity, 226–228
    treatment planning, 225–226
  dose selection, 230–234
    benign extramedullary spine
      tumors, 232
    intramedullary spinal cord
      tumors, 233–234
    primary spine tumors, 233
    spinal arteriovenous malformations, 233

    spine metastases, 231–232
spinal radiosurgery, 27–31
  avoidance of, 30–31
  complications of, 30–31
  current technologies of, 28–29
  dose considerations of, 29–30
  immobilization, 28–29
  targeting, 29
SRS. *See* stereotactic radiosurgery
stereoelectroencephalographic (SEEG)
    radiosurgery, 172
stereotactic radiosurgery (SRS), 8, 14,
    16–22, 29, 111
  for aneurysmal bone cysts, 188
  for arteriovenous malformations,
    125, 126–127
  for cerebral cavernous malformations,
    150, 151
  for chondromas, 185
  for chondrosarcomas, 185
  for chordomas, 184–185, 215
  complications following, 22
  CyberKnife. *See* CyberKnife radiosurgery
  dose characteristics of, 17
  dose tolerances of, 23
  for ependymoma, 36–37
  for Ewing's sarcoma, 186–187
  fractionated. *See* fractionated radiation
    therapy
  Gamma Knife. *See* Gamma Knife
    radiosurgery
  for giant cell tumors, 188–189
  for glioblastomamultiforme, 35–36
  for glomus jugulare tumors, 77–80
  for hemangioblastoma, 40
  for hemangiomas, 189–190
  for hemangiopericytomas, 70–73
  hypofractionated, 128–129, 183
  for intramedullary spinal cord
    tumors, 207
    complications of, 207–208
  linear accelerator, 20–21
  for low-grade astrocytoma, 36
  for metastatic spinal tumors, 195–201
  for multiple myeloma, 187
  for neurocytoma, 38
  for oligodendroglioma, 37
  for osteoblastomas, 189
  for osteoid osteomas, 189
  for osteosarcomas, 186
  for primary osseous spinal
    tumors, 183–190

stereotactic radiosurgery (SRS) (*Cont.*)
  proton beam, 18–20
  for sacral metastases, 217
  for sellar lesions management, 106
  for skull base meningioma, 60–64
    complications of, 63–64
  for spinal lesions
    dose-limitations recommendations for, 230
    neurological toxicity following, 228–230
    nonneurological toxicity following, 226–228
    treatment planning, complications associated with, 225–226
  for spinal tumors, 27
    avoidance of, 30–31
    complications of, 30–31
    current technologies of, 28–29
    dose considerations, 29–30
    targeting, 29
  for trigeminal neuralgia, 157
  for vestibular schwannomas, 85
sudden unexplained death in epileptic patients (SUDEP), 173
SUDEP. *See* sudden unexplained death in epileptic patients
supratentorial ependymomas, 36
synergy, 183

target volume
  clinical, 226
  gross, 226
  planning, 226
3DCRT. *See* three-dimensional conformal radiotherapy
three-dimensional conformal radiotherapy (3DCRT), 15
TN. *See* trigeminal neuralgia
"tram-track" sign, 94–96
trigeminal neuralgia (TN), 155–159
  management of, therapeutic options for, 155–156
  radiosurgery for, 157–159
  treatment algorithm for, 156–157
tumor necrosis-associated neurological damage, 31
tumors. *See specific tumor types*

ultrasound image-guided radiosurgery, for spinal tumors, 28

valproate, for trigeminal neuralgia, 155
vascular disorders
  cavernous hemangioma, 223
  spinal arteriovenous malformation, 221–223
vascular injury, 109
vertebral compression fracture, 201
vestibular schwannomas (VSs)
  radiosurgery for, 83–90
    clinical results of, 85–87
    complications, 89
    diagnostic imaging, 84
    following microsurgery, 87
    follow-up, 88
    indications, 83–84
    Koos criteria, 83–84
    microsurgery following, 87–88
    neurofibromatosis type 2 patients, considerations for, 84–85
    pre-treatment work-up, 84
    stereotactic, 85
    success assessment, 88
VHL. *See* Von Hippel–Lindau-associated hemangioblastomas
vincristine
  for Ewing's sarcoma, 187
  for osteosarcomas, 186
Von Hippel–Lindau (VHL)-associated hemangioblastomas, 38, 40
VSs. *See* vestibular schwannomas

WBRT. *See* whole-brain radiotherapy
whole-brain radiotherapy (WBRT), 22
  for brain metastases, 46–47
  dose selection, 52–54
  historical standard of, 46–47
  intensified local treatment with, 47–48
  radiosurgery without, 51–52
  toxicity of, 48–50
  tumor bed radiosurgery after resection, 50–51

x-rays
  bremsstrahlung, 4
  characteristic, 4
Xsight Spine tracking system, 28